Medicinal Plants :
Hypolipidemic, Hypocholesterolemic and Anti-atherosclerotic Properties

J. P. N. Chansouria
Senior Research Officer (Retd.)
Centre of Experimental Medicine and Surgery
Institute of Medical Sciences
Banaras Hindu University
Varanasi 221 005, U. P., INDIA

A. B. Ray
Professor of Medicinal Chemistry (Retd.)
(Banaras Hindu University)
C-38, Ashokpuram Colony
Dafi, Varanasi 221005, U.P., INDIA

S. Hemalatha
Reader
Department of Pharmaceutics
Institute of Technology
Banaras Hindu University
Varanasi 221 005, U. P., INDIA

IBDC

International Book Distributing Co.
(Publishing Division)

Published by

INTERNATIONAL BOOK DISTRIBUTING CO.
(Publishing Division)
Chaman Studio Building, 2nd Floor,
Charbagh, Lucknow 226 004 U.P. (INDIA)
Tel. : Off. : 2450004, 2450007, 2459058 Fax : 0522-2458629
E-Mail : ibdco@sancharnet.in

First Edition 2006

Price: Rs. 995/-

ISBN 81-8189-128-7

Composed & Designed at :

Panacea Computers
2nd Floor, Agarwal Sabha Bhawan, Subhash Mohal
Sadar Cantt. Lucknow-226 002
Phone : 9335927082, 2480875
E-mail : prasgupt@rediffmail.com

Printed at:

Salasar Imaging Systems
C-7/5, Lawrence Road Industrial Area
Delhi - 110 035
Tel. : 011-27185653, 9810064311

FOREWORD

Plants have been the eternal source of food and medicine since antiquity in all traditions and cultures. The exponents of Ayurvedic Medicine in India and Traditional Chinese Medicine in China develoepd great theoretical insights into the subject with comprehensive concepts of plant medicine and they codified these medicines in terms of their probable pharmacodynamics. The use of plants as medicine did not remain a folklore rather it was developed into a rational drug science even in the classical age. Ayurved and traditional Chinese Medicine and the use of medicinal plants flourished to great heights till recent past, which was followed by emergence of the chemotherapeutic approach of Western Modern Medicine shrouded by use of chemicals as medicine. This new-system of therapeutics has been flourishing world over because of rapid specific action of many drugs. But because of increasing occurrence of grave side effects of chemical medicines and a number of other therapeutic limitations of their use, observed in recent years, a stage of caution has come. As a result, the green resource of medicine i.e. medicinal plants is re-emerging fast in the field of health care with Green Pharmacy gradually occupying the central place in Pharmaceutical Industry. The increasing craze for use of green pharma products as medicine and food-supplements has now revolutionised the global market which is claimed to have crossed over 100 billion US dollars with sustained further rise likely to reach five trillion US dollars by the middle of this Century.

This global scenario warrants stock-taking at home to be able to profitably share the global demand. Besides, enforcing GMP regulations and establishing good pharmacies, attempts are being made to regulate and to expand raw material resources. Natural sources of green materials from forests and waste lands have to be now registered and regulated to avoid undue exploitation in addition to extended attempts of conservation and cultivation of medicinal plants with appropriate value addition utilising the good agricultural and collection practices (GACP, defined by WHO.

Besides conservation, cultivation and pharmacy aspects of medicinal plants, it is imperative to put serious efforts on documentation of medicinal plants and their good use on scientific lines establishing their efficacy and safety. Besides conceptual and literary information on these plants in Ayurvedic texts and Nighantus, lot of modern research has been done in recent years on pharmacognostical, pharmaceutical and pharmacological aspects of these medicinal plants including clinical trials. These researches have not been done in an organised way and the available information has not been properly documented. Such a documentation is greatly needed for identifying the leads for further research.

Some efforts have been made in this direction in the form of review publications by CDRI and ICMR. The present effort of Dr. J.P.N. Chansouria and his group is a step in the same direction.

The recent researches on single plant drugs have succeeded in identifying certain areas of therapeutic application where these drugs have shown promising potential. The areas of therapeutic indication which are professionally important and where modern medicine has nothing much to offer and where medicinal plants have shown promises, are - Antistress and Adoptogens, Memory enhancers, Hypolipidemic and Antiatherosclerotic agents and Immunomodulators, Anti-aging drugs.

The authors of this book have rightly chosen to review the scientific leads available on the Hypolipidemic and anti-atherosclerotic efficacy of the medicinal plants. The lipid disorder has been posing a great health hazard in present times world over involving major complications like Coronary Artery disease, Cerebrovascular accidents and a range of associated angiopathic problems. The western modern medicine has not succeeded to search a safe and effective medicinal remedy for such ailments. The problem largely remains preventive and protective than curative. And hence it seems logical to explore the natural green resources to tackle this problem. The medicinal plants like ***Guggulu, Puskarmula, Vacha*** and ***Arjun*** have already been shown to possess significant hypolipidemic effect. A large number of other plants are also claimed for similar efficacy and there is an urgent need to investigate them.

The first author of this monograph has adequate credentials to undertake such a work as he is an expert of both Ayurveda and modern biomedical sciences. He is known for his scientific work on a wide range of topics of current interest. The co-authors, as I know, are also experts in their respective fields. I congratulate the authors for compiling the present book which is likely to be of immense value for students and researchers in this fast emerging field of investigation.

Aug. 31, 2005

Prof. Ram Harsh Singh
Vice Chancellor
Rajasthan Ayurved University,
Jodhpur
Formerly Professor - Head,
Kayachikitsa,
and Dean, Faculty of
Ayurveda,
Banaras Hindu University,
Varanasi

Preface

Medicinal properties of plants are well known. In traditional systems of medicine, remedies for virtually all types of diseases are found in plants and cardiovascular disorders, responsible for untimely deaths, are no exception. However, a perfect blend of traditional concepts with modern ideas and methodologies are essential for exploring the full potential of the herbal drugs. It is because of this reason that considerable research work has been done on a variety of plants and their hypolipidemic potential has been assessed and also the mechanisms of action of effective plant drugs have been studied. It is essential for the researchers in this area to have a thorough knowledge of the work already done in this area so that they can extend the work to further heights and develop appropriate methods to utilise the plant drugs as safe and effective hypocholesterolemic, hypolipidemic and antiatherosclerotic agents with reproducible results. As there is no systematic compilation of literature of plants showing the above-mentioned activities, it was felt desirable to compile the available information of plants known to correct lipid disorders in the form of a glossary. Based primarily on Biological Abstracts, Medicinal and Aromatic Plant Abstracts and online data bases from Pub Med, the glossary presents brief abstracts of papers in this area on different plants published during the last 35 years with complete references in a chronological order. Hindi (H.) and Sanskrit (S.) synonyms of the plants have been provided wherever possible and a content has been added at the end. The authors are grateful to Professor R.H. Singh, Vice-Chancellor, Rajasthan Ayurveda University, Jodhpur, for writing the 'Foreword' for the volume. The facilities provided by Professor G. Singh, Director, Institute of Medical Sciences, Banaras Hindu University and Dr. A.N. Gangopadhyay, Professor-in-Charge of the Centre for Experimental Medicine and Surgery of the Institute in the compilation of this volume are gratefully acknowledged. Thanks are also due to Shri Lalit Kumar, Research Scholar of the above Centre, for his kind help in some typing work.

JPN Chansouria

AB Ray

S Hemalatha

Introduction

Recent years have witnessed a steady increase in the incidence of cardiovascular diseases, which, according to an estimate, are responsible for about 30% of total untimely deaths. Coronary heart diseases, reported to be the fifth leading cause of death in the year 1990 by the World Health Organization, are estimated to top the list of causes of untimely deaths by the year 2020. It is now well established that elevated levels of cholesterol, triglycerides, low-density lipoprotein cholesterol (LDL-c), very low-density lipoprotein cholesterol (VLDL-c) and decreased level of high-density lipoprotein cholesterol (HDL-c) are closely associated with coronary heart ailments and also atherosclerosis. While any of these factors may be an independent predictor of coronary heart diseases, a combination of such lipid abnormalities may further enhance the risk of the heart disease.

In view of the observations that the incidence of deaths due to coronary disorders is reduced by treatment with drugs capable of lowering LDL- cholesterol level and that the risk of coronary heart diseases increases with decreasing HDL- cholesterol levels, it is currently believed that a reduction of total and LDL-cholesterol and an increase of HDL-cholesterol decrease the risk of coronary heart diseases. Atherosclerosis is the name of a disease in which deposits of fat, cholesterol and other cellular waste products build up along the walls of the arteries, thickens, hardens and form "atheromas" or plaques. Plaques can grow large enough to reduce the flow of blood through an artery but the maximum damage takes place when the plaque becomes fragile and ruptures.The broken plaques may travel to another part of the body and block the blood vessels; if it blocks the blood vessel that feeds the heart, it causes a heart attack, if it blocks the blood vessel that feeds the brain, it causes a stroke. For the development of atheroma and its progression or regression, the key issue factor is not the cholesterol concentration but its transport pattern.

Cholesterol cannot travel freely through blood because it is insoluble in water. Lipoproteins are responsible for carrying cholesterol and other fats through the bloodstream as little packages. A lipoprotein is a biochemical assembly of both proteins and lipids. Lipoproteins of different size and density are known. Larger and less dense (more fat than protein) low density lipoprotein is known to carry cholesterol from the liver to cells and is popularly known as 'bad cholesterol' because it is responsible for cholesterol build up and blockage in the arteries. On the other hand, smaller and more dense (more protein than fat) high density lipoprotein collects cholesterol from body tissues and brings it back to the liver and thus prevents accumulation of cholesterol in the blood. High density lipoprotein also plays an important role in preventing atherosclerosis by facilitating reverse transport of cholesterol from peripheral tissues to the liver resulting in decreased uptake of cholesterol by macrophages. It also inhibits LDL oxidation and reduces vascular oxidative stress. Majority of clinical studies suggest that lipid-modifying agents , which are capable of decreasing LDL-c levels and enhancing HDL-c levels, are more useful in reducing the risk of coronary heart diseases. The inverse relationship between plasma high density lipoprotein levels and coronary heart disease has been attributed to the role that HDL and its major constituent, apolipoprotein A-I (apoA-I), play in reverse cholesterol transport.

While life-style change (regular exercise, exclusion of certain food items and inclusion of some others in the diet, etc.) is recommended for avoiding hyperlipidemia and the associated risks, there is need for appropriate lipid-modifying agents, once a person is diagnosed as hyperlipidemic. This necessity prompted scientists all over the world to make systematic search for effective and safe antihyperlipidemic and antiatherosclerotic agents and obtain them either from natural resources or by synthesis. The progress made so far in this direction is discussed briefly in the sequel.

It would be pertinent to mention in this connection that cholesterol and other fats (collectively known as lipids) are essential for life. Cholesterol is a component in the membrane of our cells. It is used for making several hormones, important in every day life. Some fatty acids are also essential nutrients and their deficiency can be harmful, yet too much of a good thing can be bad and thus hypercholesterolemia and hyperlipidemia are conditions of concern and require immediate attention. The body can get rid of excess cholesterol in two ways; it can either reduce the synthesis of cholesterol by inhibiting 3-hydroxy-3-methylglutaryl coenzyme A (HMG CoA), the key enzyme for the synthesis of endogenous cholesterol or it can enhance the elimination of cholesterol by use of bile acid sequestrants. Bile acids are produced in the liver from cholesterol and secreted into the small intestine to help the emulsification of dietary fat and cholesterol. Bile acid sequestrants act at the level of small intestine and bind to bile to form an insoluble complex and thus prevent reabsorption of cholestrol into circulation and help being excreted in faeces. Cholestyramine and colestipol are the two common drugs of this group that were developed and found effective. The usual effect of bile acid sequestrants is to lower LDL-cholesterol. This group of drugs also suffer from certain limitations. There are reports that certain bile acid sequestrants may prevent absorption of folic acid, fat soluble vitamins, carotenoids and metals like Calcium and Zinc.

The potent naturally-occurring hypolipidemic agents include fungal metabolites compactin, isolated from the cultures of *Penicillium brevicompactum* and mevinolin from *Aspergillus terreus*. Derivatives of these compounds, simvastatin and pravastatin elicited promising hypolipidemic activity. A number of this group of compounds, known as 'statins' (fluvastatin, atorvastatin, cerivastatin, etc.) have now been synthesised and are being used for treating hypercholesterolemia. Statins, the most effective drugs for lowering LDL-cholesterol, competitively inhibit HMG-CoA reductase. The resultant reduction in hepatocyte cholesterol concentration triggers increased expression of hepatic LDL receptors, which, in turn, clears LDL from the circulation. Statins have become the most prescribed cholesterol-loweing medicine. Though some researchers theorise that blocking cholesterol production, as statins do, interferes with brain's performance and cause, muddled thinking and memory loss, statins, by and large, are well tolerated by most people and serious side effects are claimed to be rare. HMG-CoA reductase inhibitors and bile acid sequestrants are good combination therapy in patients with resistant hypercholestrolemia.

Niacin (nicotinic acid, also known as vitamin B_3), present in a number of legumes and cereals, has earned a reputation as a natural cholesterol-lowering agent. It reduces total cholesterol, LDL-c and triglycerides and increases HDL-c and, therefore, may be regarded as a very good hypolipidemic agent with attractive features. However, the major drawback in its use is the associated side effects (flushing, itching, headache and palpitation) and reported hepatotoxicity.

Plants, an established storehouse of a variety of chemicals, have always been the source of our foods and drugs. Further, a drug of plant origin is often regarded as one with minimum or no side effects. Certain vegetable proteins have been reported to be superior to animal proteins in taking care of excess cholesterol and lipids in the system. Some soluble plant fibres were found to be efficient in the removal of surplus chlesterol from the system. Dietary soluble fibre supplementation has been found to be a very effective natural approch to cholesterol lowering. Besides, a variety of phytochemicals (flavonoids, tocols, steroids, triterpenoids, saponins etc.), isolated from different plant sources, showed a wide range of hypocholestrolemic, hypolipidemic and antiatherosclerotic activity.

While modern approach is to find out a single chemical entity from a plant (active compound), that is responsible for the therapeutic efficacy, it is generally believed by the scholars of Ayurveda and of other traditional systems of medicine that the forms in which the plant parts are used in these systems are useful for the treatment. But whatever may be the outlook in this matter, what is important is the systematic scientific investigation of the plant drugs and a researcher in the field should be familiar with the work that has already been done on different plants and the results obtained. With this objective in mind, the authors present in this volume, brief abstracts of scientific papers on different plants published during the last 35 years. It is expected that the book will be helpful to researchers in this field to plan their investigation on the basis of the work already done in the area. We believe that a perusal of this volume will largely prevent repetition of the work and help the researcher to plan the work in a proper way so that new light can be thrown on the subject and newer and effective plant-derived hypolipidemic and antiatherosclerotic drugs can be developed. We hope that the present volume will be well accepted by the scientists, who are keen to know the contribution of plants in the management of cardiovascular diseases and by the researchers engaged in this area of investigation.

A

Acacia catechu (H. Katha, S. Khadira): Administration of katha *(0.2%)* to cholesterol fed (1%) rats significantly lowered the serum and hepatic tissue cholesterol levels as compared to untreated hypercholesterolemic rats. *Acacia catechu* also prevented the infiltration of fat in the liver of cholesterol-fed animals. [Choudhary PN, Hatwalne VG; Effect of katha (*Acacia catechu*) on serum and liver cholesterol levels in rats, *Indian J Nutr Diet* **10**, 130-33 (1973)].

***Acacia* species:** See Gum Arabic in Appendix:

Acanthopanax gracilistylus* var. *pubescens (Siberian ginseng): The lipid-lowering effects of saponins from the plant (AGVPS) were evaluated in several rat models. Intraperitoneal administration of the saponins (300mg/kg/d) caused a reduction of serum total cholesterol and phospholipid and an elevation of high density lipoprotein cholesterol (HDL-c). Treatment of atherogenic diet (4% cholesterol and 10% lard)-induced hypercholesterolemic rats with the saponins for 10 days showed signs of hypolipidemic activity with reductions of total cholesterol, VLDL-c and LDL-c, and phospholipid in a good dose-dependent relationship. The ratio of HDL-c / total cholesterol also increased by this treatment. The saponins have an excellent therapeutic potential. [Yan-Y, Yang-S, Xiao-H, Huang-Y, Yang-F; Chou-C; Serum lipid-lowering effects of AGVPS in rats, *Bull Hunan Med College* **12**(3), 217-20 (1987) Article in Chinese].

***Acanthopanax senticocus*:** In 31 hyperlipidemic patients, serum lipids were estimated before and after treatment with a mixture of *A. senticocus* and *Elsholtzia splendens.* These herbal drugs reduced the β-lipoprotein along with enhancement of high density lipoprotein cholesterol (HDL-c) levels. Thus the ratios of HDL-c to total cholesterol (HDL-c/TC) and to LDL-c (HDLc/ LDL-c) were significantly increased with a reduction of arteriosclerosis index. These results suggest that the herbal drug might play an important role in preventing arteriosclerosis. [Zhizhen S, Chenglin L, Ruixian L; Effect of the mixture of *Acanthopanax senticocus and Elsholtzia splendens* on serum lipids in hyperlipidemia patients, *Chin J Integ Trad West Med* **10**(3), 155-56 (1990)].

Administration of various doses (100, 200, 400 mg/kg) of mixed extracts of *Acanthopanax senticosus* and *Eucommiae cortex* to streptozotocin induced diabetic rats, significantly lowered the serum total cholesterol and triglyceride levels in a dose dependant manner. These extracts also prevented stress-induced gastric ulcer in mice. [Whang WK, Choi SB, Kim IH; Physiological activities of mixed extract of *Acanthopanacis senticosi* Radicis cortex and *Eucommiae* cortex, *Korean J Pharmacogn* **27**(1), 65-74 (1996)].

Administration of aqueous extract of stem bark of *A. senticosus* (1ml of 30% extract) to lipid rich diet (15% cholesterol, 1% sodium cholate and 84% corn oil)-induced hyperlipidemic rats for three consecutive days caused a significant reduction in plasma cholesterol and triglyceride concentrations. The treated rats also exhibited significantly enhanced HDL- cholesterol levels. [Lee YS, Jung SH, Lim SS, Ji J, Lee SH, Shin KH; Effect of water extract from the stem bark of *Acanthopanax senticosus* on hyperlipedemia in rats, *Korean J Pharmacogn* **32**(2), 103-07 (2001)].

***Acanthopanax* species:** The pharmacological activities of a variety of phytochemicals, isolated from *Acanthopanax* species, have been reviewed. Many of these phytochemicals were found to exhibit hypocholesterolemic and antioxidant activities. [Shin KH, Lee S; The chemistry of secondary products from *Acanthopanax* species and pharmacological activities, *Nat Prod Sci* **8**(4), 111-26 (2002)].

***Achillea wilhelmsii*:** The flavonoids and sesquiterpene lactones, present in *A. wilhelmsii,* are known to be effective in lowering blood lipids and hypertension. The results of a double-blind placebo controlled clinical trial with Achillea drops (15-20 drops twice daily for more than 6 months) showed a significant decrease in triglycerides after 2 months while decreases in triglycerides, total cholesterol and LDL-cholesterol were significant after 4 months. Levels of HDL-cholesterol were significantly increased after treatment for 6 months. [Asgary S, Naderi GH, Sarrafzadegan N, Mohammadifard N, Mostafavi S, Vakili R; Antihypertensive and antihyperlipidemic effects of *Achillea wilhelmsii, Drugs Exp Clin Res* **26**(3), 89-93 (2000)].

Achyranthes aspera (H. Laljira, S. Apamarga)**:** The alcoholic extract of *A. aspera*, at 100 mg/kg dose lowered serum cholesterol, phospholipid, triglyceride and total lipid levels by 60, 51, 33 and 53%, respectively in triton induced hyperlipidemic rats. The chronic administration of this drug at the same dose to normal rats for 30 days showed, in addition, significant reduction in the levels of hepatic lipids. The drug increased the faecal excretion of cholic acid and deoxycholic acid by 24 and 40%, respectively. The possible mechanism of action of cholesterol lowering activity of *A. aspera* may be due to rapid excretion of bile acids causing low absorption of cholesterol. [Khanna AK, Chander R, Singh C, Srivastava AK, Kapoor NK; Hypolipidemic activity of *Achyranthus aspera* Linn in normal and triton induced hyperlipemic rats, *Indian J Exp Biol* **30**(2), 128-30 (1992)].

Acorus calamus (H. Bach, S. Bhadra)**:** Administration of 50% ethanolic extract of rhizomes of the plant (100 and 200 mg/kg) as well as of saponins (10 mg/kg) isolated from the extract to atherogenic diet-fed rats significantly reduced serum cholesterol and triglycerides along with enhancement of high density lipoprotein cholesterol (HDL-c). Aqueous extract was slightly less active. [Parab RS, Mengi SA; Hypolipidemic activity of *Acorus calamus* L. in rats, *Fitoterapia* **73**(6), 451-55 (2002)].

Administration of aqueous and hydroalcoholic extract of *A. calamus* (100 and 200mg/kg) to hyperlipidemic rats, significantly decreased total cholesterol and triglyceride levels alongwith enhancement of HDL cholesterol. Saponins, isolated from hydroalcoholic extract, also significantly lowered the serum total cholesterol and triglyceride levels. However, the saponins were relatively more effective in increasing the HDL cholesterol levels. Hydroalcoholic extract of the drug was more effective than its aqueous extract. [Parab RS, Mengi SA; Evaluation of hypolipidemic activity of *Acorus calamus* Linn. in rats, *Indian Drugs* 40(1), 25-29 (2003)].

***Adenocalymma alliaceum*:** Dried garlic-smelling flower of *A. alliaceum*, fed at 2% level in diet for 6 weeks to experimental hypercholesterolemic rats, exhibited blood cholesterol lowering effect. Animals fed *A. alliaceum* flowers excreted higher amounts of neutral and acidic sterols in faeces similar to onion or asafoetida fed (at 2% dietary level) rats. *A. alliaceum* significantly lowered the absorption of dietary cholesterol from intestine like other sulphur containing spices, *viz.* garlic oil, onion and asafoetida. [Srinivasan MR, Srinivasan K; Hypocholesterolemic efficacy of garlic-smelling flower of *Adenocalymma alliaceum* Miers. in experimental rats, *Indian J Exp Biol* **33**(1), 64-66 (1995)].

Aegle marmelos (H. Bel, S. Bilva)**:** Administration of *A. marmelos* leaf extract to alloxan diabetic rats, significantly decreased liver glycogen, serum cholesterol and blood urea levels. Same changes were also observed in diabetic rats treated with insulin, which suggests the mode of action of *A. marmelos* leaf extract to be similar to that of insulin. [Ponnachan PTC, Paulose CS, Panikkar KR; Effect of leaf extract of *Aegle marmelos* in diabetic rats, *Indian J Exp Biol* **31**(4), 345-47 (1993)].

***Aesculus hippocastenum*:** Administration of *A. hippocastenum*, a homeopathic herbal drug (3 drops/100ml water), to diet-induced hypercholesterolemic Wistar rats for 4 weeks significantly reduced serum total cholesterol and triglycerides levels. It also raised the level of high density lipoprotein (HDL-cholesterol). However, this drug did not affect serum phospholipids, liver cholesterol and body weight of animals. [Sankhala A, Mathur PN, Sankhala AK, Dashora PK; Hypolipidemic action of homeopathic drug *Aesculus hippocastenum*: in cholesterol fed rats, *Indian J Clin Biochem* **7**(2), 155-58 (1992)].

Akebia quinta (Mokutsu): See *Nelumbo nucifera* (Kayo): [Onishi *et al*.; *Chem Pharm Bull* (Tokyo) **32**(2), 646-50 (1984)].

Albizzia anthelmintica: Traditional healers from Kilosa district, Morogoro region (Tanzania) use this plant for its hypocholesterolemic activity. [Moshi MJ, Mbwambo ZH; Experience of Tanzanian traditional healers in the management of non-insulin dependent diabetes mellitus, *Pharm-Biol* **40**(7), 552-60 (2002)].

Aleurites moluccana (H. Jangli akhrot, S. Akshota): The lipid lowering effect of methanolic extract of the leaves of *A. moluccana* was studied in triton and high fat diet-induced hyperlipidemic rats. The serum lipid and body weight of the hyperlipidemic animals were significantly decreased following administration of methanolic extract of the plant. The hypolipidemic action of this drug was attributed to inhibition of cholesterol biosynthesis and reduced absorption of lipids by the intestines. [Pedrosa RC, Meyre-silva C, Cochinel-Filho V, Benassi JC, Oliveira LFS, Zancanaro V, Magro JD, Yunes RA; Hypolipidemic activity of methanolic extract of *Aleurites moluccana, Phytother Res* **16**(8), 765-68 (2002)].

Alisma plantago-aquatica* var. *orientale: The triterpenoids of rhizomes of the plant have been reported to be hypocholesterolemic. [Hikino H, Iwakawa-T, Oshima-Y, Nishikawa-K, Murata-T, Diuretic principles of *Alisma plantago-aquatica* var. *orientale* rhizomes, *Shoyakugaku Zasshi* **36**(2), 150-53 (1982) Article in Japanese].

Allium bakeri: See *Allium sativum* (Garlic): [Okuyama et *al*., *Planta Med* **55**(3), 242-44 (1989)].

Allium cepa (Onion, H. Piyaz, S. Palandu): In normal growing rats, chronic administration of allyl propyl disulphide, isolated from common onions, led to a significant lowering of serum and liver tissue lipid levels. Such a lipid-lowering effect of disulphide was more marked in the liver than in serum. It did not affect serum protein and blood sugar levels. [Augusti KT; Lipid- lowering effect of allyl propyl disulphide isolated from *Allium cepa* Linn. on long-term feeding to normal rats, *Indian J Exp Biol* **11**(Sept), 264-651974)].

In 10 healthy subjects, the effect of onion juice and its essential oil on alimentary hyperlipemia induced by feeding of 100 g butter was evaluated. Onions significantly prevented fat-induced increase of serum cholesterol levels and reduction of coagulation time and fibrinolytivc actvity. It was suggested that the active principle of the onions is present in its essential oil, which is a sulphur containing compound i.e. allyl propyl disulphide. [Bordia A, Bansal HC, Khabiyaa BL, Arora SK, Singh SV; Effect of essential oil from onion on alimentary lipemia, *Indian Heart J* **26**, 29 31 (1974)].

See *Allium sativum* (Garlic): [Jain RC; *Ind J Med Res* **17**(10), 1509 (1976)].

Effect of aqueous extract of onions on lipid parameters was investigated in sucrose-fed hyperlipidemic rabbits. Onion extract significantly decreased serum, liver and aortic triglycerides contents. Hypolipidemic activity of onions was ascribed to its sulphur containing principles, which oxidize thiol compounds required for lipid synthesis. [Sebastian KL, Zacharias NT, Philip B, Augusti KT; The hypolipidemic effect of onions (*Allium cepa* Linn.) in sucrose fed rabbits, *Indian J Physiol Pharmacol* **23**(1), 27-30 (1979)].

Adminstration of fresh aqueous extract of 50 g of onions (*A. cepa*) and 50g of garlic (*A. sativum*) to different groups of normal human volunteers did not affect the levels of fasting blood cholesterol and its fractions. [Sharma KK, Sharma SP; Effect of onion and garlic on serum cholesterol in normal subjects, *Mediscope* **22**(7), 134-36 (1979)].

Diabetic patients receiving a diet containing 68% carbohydrate, 20% fat, 12% protein plus 3 x 20 g fresh onion per day showed potent hypocholesterolemic effect. [Tjokroprawiro A, Pikir BS, Budhiarta AA, Pranawa, Soewondo H, Donosepoetro M, Budhianto FX, Wibowo JA, Tanuwidjaja SJ, Pangemanan M *et al*; Metabolic effects of onion and green beans on diabetic patients, *Tohoku J Exp Med* 141 Suppl, 671-76 (1983)].

Hypocholesterolemic effect of onion extract on cholesterol-enriched erythrocytes was observed. The cellular cholesterol enrichment induced disturbances in the equilibrium of cholesterol between red cells and plasma was restored by the hypocholesterolemic effect of onions. [Singh M, Kanakaraj P; Hypocholesterolemic effect of onion extract on cholesterol-enriched erythrocytes, *Indian J Exp Biol* 23(8), 456-59 (1985)].

Feeding of diet containing onion and garlic at 20% levels to albino rats for 12 weeks, reduced gain in body weight and lowered serum and liver cholesterol. Onion and garlic supplemented diets also increased prothrombin time and faecal sterol excretion in these rats. However, all these changes were relatively more marked in rats consuming the diet containing garlic than those having onions in their diet. [Bakhsh R, Chughtai MID; Comparative study of onion and garlic on serum cholesterol, liver cholesterol, prothrombin time and faecal sterol excretion in male albino rats, *J Chem Soc Pak* **7**(4), 285-88 (1985)].

See Polysaccharides in Appendix: [Khushbaktova *et al.*; *Khim Farm Zh* **21**(11), 1348-52 (1987)].

Onion extract and residue showed hypercholesterolemic effect, while whole onion showed hypocholesterolemic effect in blood. In erythrocyte membranes, all the fractions had hypocholesterolemic and hypolipidemic effect, which was accompanied by changes in the erythrocyte membrane enzymes studied, i.e., alkaline and acid phosphatase, 5'-nucleotidase, total and Mg^{2+} ATPase. The above study indicated that it is safer to take whole onion rather than onion residue or extract; because whole onion can lower the blood cholesterol level even in normal condition and has a less pronounced effect on the microenvironment of the cells. [Ahluwalia P, Mohindroo A; Effect of oral ingestion of different fractions of *Allium cepa* on the blood and erythrocyte membrane lipids and certain membrane-bound enzymes in rats, *J Nutr Sci Vitaminol* (Tokyo) **35**(2), 155-61 (1989)].

See *Brassica nigra* (Mustard): [Sambaiah & Srinivasan; *J Food Sci Technol* **28**(1), 35-38 (1991)].

See Flavonoids in Appendix: [Khushbaktova *et al.*; *Khim Farma Zh* **25**(4), 53-57 (1991)].

S-methyl cysteine sulphoxide, a sulphur containing amino acid isolated from onion, showed antidiabetic and antihyperlipidemic effects. Oral administration of the amino acid to alloxan diabetic rats daily at a dose of 200 mg/kg body weight for a period of 45 days controlled significantly their blood glucose and lipids in serum and tissues and altered the activities of liver hexokinase, glucose 6-phosphatase and HMG CoA reductase towards normal. [Kumari K, Mathew BC, Augusti KT; Antidiabetic and hypolipidemic effects of S-methyl cysteine sulphoxide isolated from *Allium cepa* Linn., *Indian J Biochem Biophys* **32**(1), 49-54 (1995)].

See *Adenocalymma alliaceum* [Srinivasan & Srinivasan, *Indian J Exp Biol* **33**(1), 64-66 (1995)].

Onion and garlic contain many sulphur containing active principles, which decompose into a variety of volatile products by the action of the enzyme allinase during extraction. These decomposed products, present in the oils of onion and garlic, possess hypocholesterolemic, antidiabetic, antibiotic, fibrinolytic and various other biological actions..[Augusti KT; Therapeutic values of onion (*Allium cepa* L.) and garlic (*Allium sativum* L.), *Indian J Exp Biol* **34**(7), 634-40 (1996)].

Effects of feeding 3% freeze dried onion powder containing diet as well as of 15 mg% capsaicin (a constituent of *Capsicum annuum*) were examined in albino rats rendered diabetic with streptozotocin injection. Diabetic rats fed onion diet exhibited lowered lipid peroxides in circulation and in urine when compared to diabetic control group. Blood cholesterol was lowered significantly by dietary onion in diabetic animals. Cholesterol decrease was exclusively from LDL-and VLDL fractions. Significant decrease in blood phospholipids and triglycerides was also brought about by dietary onion. Elevation of hepatic cholesterol, triglycerides and phospholipids under diabetic condition was countered significantly by dietary onion. Dietary capsaicin did not have any significant influence on any of the parameters tested in diabetic rats. [Babu PS, Srinivasan K; Influence of dietary capsaicin and onion on the metabolic abnormalities associated with streptozotocin induced diabetes mellitus, *Mol Cell Biochem* **175**(1-2), 49-57 (1997)].

The effect of alliums (onion and garlic) on plasma free cholesterol, esterified cholesterol, high density lipoprotein cholesterol (HDL-c), low density lipoprotein cholesterol (LDL-c) and very low density lipoprotein cholesterol (VLDL-c) content was studied on Japanese quails of both sexes. Alliums caused a decrease in the plasma cholesterol on feeding for three weeks and six weeks duration while no effect of sex was observed. The plasma esterified cholesterol content also decreased slightly due to onion and garlic. These results indicate that onion and garlic may not be causing increase in easterification of cholesterol. Further, inconsistent variations in the plasma HDL-c was observed due to dietary onion and garlic given for three weeks and six weeks duration in both sexes. The observation of a decrease in plasma LDL-c as compared to control indicates either much of circulating cholesterol is taken up by liver or rapid recirculation of cholesterol in the body thereby safeguarding against, the possible onset of atherosclerosis. [Kumar VG, Surendranathan KP, Narendranath R; Effect of *Allium cepa* Linn and *Allium sativum* Linn. on plasma free, esterified and lipoprotein cholesterol in Japanese quails (*Coturnix coturnix japonica*), *Indian J Poultry Sci* **33**(2), 142-48 (1998)].

The effect of Alliums (onion and garlic) in the Japanese quails of both sexes was studied. The results indicate that onion and garlic are effective as hypocholesterolemic agents only to limited extent. The cholesterol level was found to be more in the female birds as compared to male birds and was also found to increase with age in both sexes except for the level being lower in the laying birds (nine-week-old) probably due to the diversion of plasma cholesterol towards yolk formation. [Kumar VG, Surendranathan KP, Jayaprakash; Effect of alliums, age and sex on the plasma cholesterol level of Japanese quails (*Coturnix coturnix japonica*), *Indian J Poultry Sci* **35**(1), 95-98 (2000)].

Effect of onion and garlic on total cholesterol in liver and muscle of quails of different age and sex was studied. The total cholesterol contents in the liver and muscle of birds of both sexes at three physiological stages of growth (immature, onset of sexual maturity and mature) were determined. Inconsistent results were obtained when observed between different age groups within a sex or between different sexes within an age group. [Kumar VG, Surendranathan KP; Effect of alliums on total cholesterol content of liver and muscle of Japanese quail (*Coturnix coturnix japonica*), *Indian J-Animal Sci* **71**(7), 670-72 (2001)].

See *Allium sativum* (Garlic): [Augusti *et al.*; *Indian J Exp Biol.* **39**(8), 760-66 (2001)].

Effect of onion and garlic (*Allium sativum*) on muscle triglyceride content in Japanese quails was studied. Dietary onion or garlic was found to have no significant effect on the muscle triglyceride content when fed for three or six week duration in both sexes. The triglyceride level was found to be more in the six-week-old female birds when compared to male birds of similar age group. In the female birds, the muscle triglyceride level was found to increase with age. In the male birds, no significant difference in the muscle triglyceride level was observed when compared between three and six-week of age group, whereas there was significant increase in the nine-week-aold when compared to three and six-week-old male birds. [Kumar VG, Surendranathan KP, Jayaprakash, Devi DR, Gayathri B, Sandhya MR; Effect of onion (*Allium cepa* Linn.) and garlic (*Allium sativum* Linn.) on muscle triglyceride content in Japanese quail (*Coturnix coturnix japonicum*), *Indian J Poultry Sci* **37**(3), 275-77 (2002)].

In growing Japanese quails dietary intake of onions and garlic enhanced the levels of plasma triglycerides, which was attributed to their insulin like activity and other factors that promote lipogenesis during developing stages. The triglyceride levels also varied depending on the age and sex of these birds. Accordingly, plasma triglyceride levels were higher in normal female birds and increased with age. It was suggested that the action of onions and garlic might vary in growing and adult birds. [Kumar G, Surendranathan KP, Umesh KG, Gayathri Devi DR, Belwadi MRS; Effects of onions (*Allium cepa* Linn.) and garlic (*Allium sativum*) on plasma triglyceride contents in Japanese quails (*Coturnix Coturnix japonicum*), *Indian J Exp Biol* **44**(1), 88-90 (2003)].

See *Zingibar officinale:* [Singh VK, Singh S, Singh DK; Pharmacological effects of spices: Recent progress in medicinal plants: Phytochemistry and pharmacology, JN Govil, VK Singh (eds.) Studium press, LLC, Houston, Texas, USA, 2, p 321-353(2003)].

Allium sativum (Garlic, H. Lasan, S. Lashuna)**:** In cholesterol induced atherosclerotic rabbits, the effect of onion and garlic on serum and tissue cholesterol levels was investigated. Severity of aortic atherosclerosis was ascertained by the aortic wall cholesterol contents. Administration of onions to cholesterol-fed rabbits did not affect total, free or ester cholesterol or phospholipids or development of aortic atherosclerosis. However, supplementation of garlic to cholesterol-fed animals elicited significant lowering of total, free and ester cholesterol and phospholipids. Aortic and hepatic cholesterol contents were decreased in garlic treated hypercholesterolemic rabbits. Garlic also prevented the development of atherosclerosis in cholesterol-fed rabbits. [Jain RC; Onion and garlic in experimental cholesterol induced atherosclerosis, *Ind J Med Res* **17**(10), 1509 (1976)].

Feeding of aqueous extract of garlic (0.5ml/kg/d) for two months to hypercholesterolemic patients caused a significant lowering of cholesterol levels. Withdrawal of garlic extract was followed by an increase of cholesterol levels. The hypocholesterolemic activity of garlic was attributed to the presence of sulphur containing compounds in it. [Augusti KT; Hypocholesterolemic effect of garlic (*Allium sativum* Linn.), *Indian J Exp Biol* **15**(6), 489-90 (1977)]

Administration of essential oil of garlic (equivalent of 2 g raw garlic /kg bw) to cholesterol-fed hyperlipidemic rabbits sharply decreased serum cholesterol and triglyceride levels alongwith a significant increase in fibrinolytic activity. Cholesterol induced atherosclerosis also regressed markedly as evidenced by a decrease in grading of atheroma (0.5) as compared to control (2.1) following garlic treatment. [Bordia AK, Verma SK; Garlic on the reversibilty of experimental atherosclerosis, *Indian Heart J* **30**(1), 47 –50 (1978)].

Administration of raw garlic (10 g/d) with diet to normal males (age group 18-35 years) for two months caused a significant reduction of serum cholesterol levels in all the subjects. [Bhushan S, Sharma SP, Singh SP, Agrawal S, Indrayan A, Seth P; Effect of garlic on normal blood cholesterol levels, *Indian J Physiol Pharmacol* **23**(3), 211-14 (1979)].

See *Allium cepa*: [Sharma and Sharma; *Mediscope* **22** (7), 134-36 (1979)].

Administration of garlic powder (25 mg/kg bw) was found to be more effective in lowering the serum cholesterol and triglycerides as compared with that of guggulu (*Commiphora mukul*) when screened in dogs and monkeys. A comparative hypolipidemic action of the two drugs has been discussed. [Dixit VP, Joshi S, Sinha R, Bhargava SK, Varma M; Hypolipidemic activity of guggul resin (*Commiphora mukul*) and garlic (*Allium sativum* Linn.) in dogs (*Canis familiaris*) and monkeys (*Presbytis entellus entellus* Dufresne), *Biochem Exp Biol* **16**(4), 421- 24 (1980)].

In sucrose-fed rabbits, aqueous extract of garlic (10ml/kg/d) significantly increased liver glycogen and amino acid contents alongwith significant lowering of fasting blood sugar, serum, liver and aortic triglycerides and serum and liver protein levels. However, the aqueous extract of garlic did not affect the serum liver and aortic phospholipid and cholesterol. [Zacharias NT, Sebastian KK, Philip B, Augusti KT; Hypoglycemic and hypolipidemic effects of garlic in sucrose-fed rabbits, *Indian J Physiol Pharmacol* **24**(2), 151-54 (1980)].

The essential oil of garlic has been shown to have a distinct hypolipidemic action in both healthy individuals and patients of coronary heart disease. [Bordia A; Effect of garlic on blood lipids in patients with coronary heart disease, *Am J Clin Nutr* **34**(10), 2100-03 (1981)].

The cases of hyperlipidemia were treated with garlic pearls, guggulu (*Commiphora mukul*) and clofibrate. Serum cholesterol was reduced in all the three groups of subjects treated with different drugs for 15 days. However, a significant lowering of cholesterol was noted in subjects treated with garlic pearl (1 pearl BD) and *C. mukul* extract (300 mg BD) after 30 days. Guggulu was more effective than garlic. [Baldwa VS, Ranka PC, Rishi JP, Rai RR; *Commiphora mukul* (Guggulu), garlic extract and clofibrate in hyperlipidemic states, *Rajasthan Med J* **20**(2), 73-76 (1981)].

Oral administration of *A. sativum* (4 cloves, approx. 10 g) to three healthy subjects completely inhibited platelet aggregation. Such an inhibitory effect of garlic lasted for 2.5 hours after its ingestion. [Boulen DJ; Garlic as a platelet inhibitor *Lancet* **1**(8223), 776-77 (1981)].

The hypocholesterolemic and fibrinolysis-enhancing properties of garlic were assessed in patients with ischemic heart disease (IHD) and in healthy control subjects. Garlic therapy for 12 weeks did not cause any appreciable changes in serum triglyceride, β-lipoprotein, plasma fibrinogen levels or coagulation time in either IHD or control subjects. The evidence cited above does not appear to substantiate the prevalent popular belief in the efficacy of garlic in the management of IHD either as a hypocholesterolemic or as a fibrinolytic agent. [Arora RC, Arora S, Gupta RK; The long-term use of garlic in ischemic heart disease—an appraisal, *Atherosclerosis* **40**(2), 175-79 (1981)].

Rats fed with cholesterol and lard diets increased plasma cholesterol and triglycerides compared to controls. Lyophilized garlic supplementation decreased plasma cholesterol in cholesterol and lard-fed rats, but decreased plasma triglycerides only in the lard-fed group. Garlic supplementation decreased very low density lipoprotein cholesterol and increased high density lipoprotein cholesterol. The liver weight, total liver lipid and cholesterol were increased in rats fed with cholesterol diet but a supplementation of garlic decreased those parameters by about 30%. [Chi MS, Koh ET, Stewart TJ; Effects of garlic on lipid metabolism in rats fed cholesterol or lard, *J Nutr* **112**(2), 241-48 (1982)].

Incorporation of freeze dried garlic powder at 0.5 and 1% level in the atherogenic diet-fed rats did not lower cholesterol levels but addition of garlic in the diet at 2 and 3% levels showed significant hypocholesterolemic activity. Maximum effect was noted in the rats fed with 2% garlic in diet. Garlic powder increased the high density lipoprotein (HDL) without affecting high density lipoprotein cholesterol (HDL-c) levels. Administration of garlic pearls (equivalent to 0.15% garlic powder in the diet) significantly reduced the serum and liver cholesterol levels in atherogenic diet-fed rats. Asafoetida (*Ferula asafoetida*) at 1.5% level did not reduce cholesterol in cholesterol-fed rats. [Kamaana VS, Chandrashekhar N; Effect of garlic (*Allium sativum* Linn.) on serum lipoprotein and lipoprotein cholesterol level in albino rats rendered hypercholesterolemic by feeding cholesterol, *Lipids* **17**(7), 483-88 (1982)].

Injection of garlic (*Allium sativum*) extract into **insects** decreased the cholesterol contents of their tissues. Crude garlic extract was most effective. However, higher mortality was noted in crude garlic extract treated insects. [Mandal S, Chaudhary GJ; Cholesterol metabolism in *Lohita grandis* Gray (Hemipetra)), Pyrrhocoridae (Insecta): Effect of Corpora allatectomy and garlic extract, *Curr Sci* **51**(7), 367-69 (1982)].

The effect of different garlic preparations (ethanol extracted garlic residue, ethanol extract of garlic, whole garlic and autoclaved garlic) on lipid metabolism was studied in male rats fed with a diet containing 1% cholesterol. The supplementation of garlic products (other than ethanol extracted garlic residue) at 2% of the diet, reduced plasma and liver cholesterol levels. The reduction in the plasma cholesterol by feeding garlic products was in very low density lipoprotein and low density lipoprotein cholesterol fractions. Animals, fed diets supplemented with garlic, showed decreased liver glucose-6-phosphate dehydrogenase and malic enzyme activities. It also reduced the liver weight, inguinal adipose tissue weight, liver total lipids and plasma triglycerides. [Chi MS; Effects of garlic products on lipid metabolism in cholesterol fed rats, *Proc Soc Exp Biol Med* **171**(2), 174-78 (1982)].

Administration of garlic pearls to normal dogs, produced hypocholesterolemia after initial hypercholesterolemia. [Das SN, Mukherjee BN, Pramanik AK, Mitra SK; Effect of garlic pearls (Ranbaxy) on blood cholesterol levels in normal dogs, *Ind Vet J* **59**(12), 937-38 (1982)].

Administration of garlic (2 pearls TDS for 12 weeks) to hyperlipidemic subjects significantly lowered the serum cholesterol levels. In addition, garlic decreased plasma fibrinogen levels, prolonged coagulation time and increased fibrinolytic activity in some cases. [Sainani GB, Bhalode DP, Natu SM, Pise DV, Kayerkar R; Garlic pearls in cases of hyperlipidemia (A report of a clinical trial), *Antiseptic* **79**(4), 201-04 (1982)].

Studies conducted on the hypocholesterolemic and hypoglycemic activity of *A. sativum* along with its effect on enzyme activity, fibrinolytic activity, rheumatoid arthritis, tumors, urinary disorders, uterine contraction and blood pressure etc. have been reviewed. [Kamanna VS, Chandrashekhar N; Biochemical and physiological effects of garlic (*Allium sativum* Linn.), *J Sci Ind Res* **42**(6), 353-57 (1983)].

Significant decreases in the activities of hepatic 3-hydroxy-3-methylglutaryl-CoA reductase, cholesterol-7α-hydroxylase, fatty acid synthetase and representative pentose-phosphate pathway accompanied the feeding of the petroleum ether, methanol and water-soluble fractions of garlic to white leghorn pullets. Garlic paste and oil also suppressed these activities. Significant decrease in serum lipids occurred in response to the feeding of these garlic fractions; serum total cholesterol by 20-25%, low density lipoprotein cholesterol by 28-41% and triglycerides by 10-26%; but high density lipoprotein cholesterol failed to respond to these treatments. The results confirm that garlic oil and odorous components of garlic lower cholesterol levels. An odorless water-soluble component of garlic also has this effect. The mechanism of the hypocholesterolemic action is at the level of the suppression of cholesterol biosynthesis. [Qureshi AA, Din ZZ, Abuirmeileh N, Burger WC, Ahmad Y, Elson CE; Suppression of avian hepatic lipid metabolism by solvent extracts of garlic: Impact on serum lipids, *J Nutr* **113**(9), 1746-55 (1983)].

Administration of garlic (1g/kg/d) to atherogenic diet (cholesterol 200mg/kg/ d)-fed rabbits decreased the biosynthesis of fatty acids from 2-^{14}C-acetate and glycolipids from 1-^{14}C- palmitate. [Mihadi SA, Ahuja SP, Gupta PP; Effect of garlic (*Allium sativum*) on the lipid composition and lipid biosynthesis in tissues of rabbits during experimental atherosclerosis, *J Nucl Agri Biol* **12**(2), 33-37 (1983)].

The work done on antilipemic, antithrombotic and fibrinolytic activity of *Allium sativum* has been reviewed. [Ernest E; Antiatherosclerotic effects of *Allium sativum*, *Dtsch Apoth Ztg* **123**(13), 625-26 (1983)].

Cholesterol induced hyperlipidemia was controlled by garlic feeding. Garlic treatment did not alter the concentrations of circulating thyroid hormones and thyroidal uptake of radio iodine. The results indicate that the hypolipidemic effect of garlic is probably not mediated through the thyroid. [Chaudhuri BN, Mukherjee SK, Mongia SS, Chakravarty SK; Hypolipidemic effect of garlic and thyroid function, *Biomed Biochim Acta* **43**(7), 1045-47 (1984)].

Feeding of ethanol and a high cholesterol and fat diet to rats markedly increased the total lipids in the liver, cholesterol and triglyceride levels in the serum, liver and kidneys. However, when ethanol mixed with 0.5% garlic oil was fed to animals maintained on the above diet, these lipid levels were significantly reduced to levels near to those seen in untreated control rats. Garlic oil is considered to enhance the catabolism of dietary cholesterol and fatty acids. [Shoetan A, Augusti KT, Joseph PK; Hypolipidemic effects of garlic oil in rats fed with ethanol and a high lipid diet, *Experientia* **40**(3), 261-63 (1984)].

Administration of (*E*, *Z*)–ajoene (20mg/kg bw), a constituent of *A. sativum,* to rabbits, produced 100% inhibition of collagen induced platelet aggregation. Antithrombotic activity of this compound was also investigated. [Block E, Ahmad S, Jain MK, Crecely RW, Apitz-castro R, Cruz MR; (*E*, *Z*)–ajoene, a potent antithrombotic agent from garlic, *J Am Chem Soc* **106**(26), 8275-296 (1984)].

The essential oil and defatted garlic powder caused a lowering in serum and liver cholesterol levels in rats. [Kamanna VS, Chandrasekhara N; Hypocholesterolemic activity of different fractions of garlic (*Allium sativum*), *Indian J Med Res* **79**(Apr.), 580-83 (1984)].

In normal and cholesterol-fed rabbits, the effect of garlic oil and guggulipid on tissue catecholamines and dopamine β-hydroxylase activity was studied. The cholesterol (500mg/kg) -fed hypercholesterolemic rabbits showed decreased catecholamine levels and enzyme activity. Feeding of garlic oil and guggulipid to hypercholesterolemic rabbits led to the recovery of decreased catecholamines biosynthesis. On the other hand, garlic oil (5ml/kg) and guggulipid (100mg/kg)-treated normal rabbits exhibited significantly enhanced activity of dopamine β-hydroxylase activity and catecholamine levels. [Srivastava AM, Nityanand S, Kapoor NK; Effect of hypocholesterolemic agents of plant origin on catecholamine biosynthesis in normal and cholesterol-fed rabbits, *J Biosci* (Bangalore) **6**(3), 277-82 (1984)].

Chemical composition, flavour, and physiological properties of onion and garlic, their extracts, and processed products and particularly their biologically active components have been reviewed. [Fenwick GR, Hanley AB; The genus *Allium* Part 1, *Crit Rev Food Sci Nutr* **22**(3), 199-271 (1985)].

Feeding of a fraction, isolated from garlic, significantly lowered cholesterol, triglyceride, phospholipids and non-esterified fatty acids levels in rats. It also reduced blood sugar levels, which was attributed to enhanced insulin response. [Dixit VP, Sinha R; Hypolipidemic effect of a fraction derived from garlic (*Allium sativum*) in albino rats, house rats and gerbils, *Indian Zoologist* **9**(182), 147-49 (1985)].

The available information on *Allium sativum* with regard to its hypolipidemic, hypotensive, fibrinolytic and antiplatelet aggregatory activity has been reviewed. [Becker H; Garlic-only spice or phytodrug, *Deutsch Apoth Ztg* **125**(34), 1677-80 (1985)].

In streptozotocin induced diabetic rats, administration of garlic oil for 2 months significantly reduced the serum and hepatic cholesterol, triglyceride and total lipid contents. Blood sugar levels were also significantly reduced in these rats. Administration of garlic oil significantly decreased the high fat-induced increases in the level of serum and liver lipids in normal and diabetic rats. In diabetic rats, weight loss was prevented by high fat diet. However, garlic oil did not affect the body weight. [Farva D, Goji IA, Joseph PK, Augusti KT; Effect of garlic oil on streptozotocin–induced diabetic rats maintained on normal and high fat diets, *Indian J Biochem Biophys* **23**(1), 24-27 (1986)].

Serum, hepatic and renal cholesterol and triglyceride levels were enhanced in rats fed with sucrose and high fat containing diet. Feeding of 3% ethanol in place of water to these rats significantly increased liver and kidney cholesterol and triglyceride levels without much change in serum and hepatic lipid levels. However, administration of *A. satium* extract significantly lowered lipid levels in these high fat diet and ethanol fed rats. [Ikpeazu OV, Augusti KT, Joseph PK; Hypolipidemic effect of garlic extract mixed with 3% ethanol in rats fed sucrose-high fat diet, *Indian J Biochem Biophys* **24**(4), 252-53 (1987)].

The hypolipidemic action of garlic was ascribed to its active principle di-allyl-disulphide. It is involved in an exchange reaction between active enzymes and substrates containing thiol group. Garlic oil also enhanced lipase activity, which resulted into enhanced hydrolysis of triacylglycerols. [Adoga GI; The mechanism of the hypolipidemic effect of garlic oil extract in rats fed on high sucrose and alcohol diets, *Biochem Biophys Res Cummun* **142**(3), 1046-52 (1987)].

The hypolipidemic effect of a polyherbal combination containing *Allium sativum, Nepeta hindostana* and *Curcuma longa* was examined in 86 hyperlipidemic and hypercholesterolemic patients. Administration of the formulation (2-3g daily) lowered the serum cholesterol (26%) and triglyceride levels (21%) in these patients. The treated patients also noticed symptomatic improvement. [Arora RB, Kesar DK, Saigal SK, Jameel Ahmad, Quadri IZ; Development of 'Lipotab',; a polypharmaceutical herbal drug for hyperlipidemia and hypercholesterolemia - a double blind clinical study on 86 patients, *Hamdard Medicus* **30**(1-2), 163-74 (1987)].

The efficacy of a herbal formulation containing *Allium sativum, Nepeta hindostana* and *Curcuma longa* was evaluated in 40 hyperlipidemic and hypercholesterolemic patients. This formulation (2-3 g daily) significantly decreased the serum cholesterol and triglyceride levels. Symptomatic relief especially in giddiness, insomnia and constipation etc. became evident in these patients within 2 weeks of treatment. [Arora RB, Roy S, Quadri IZ, Kesar DK; Long-term follow-up of patients of hypercholesterolemia and hyperlipidemia with a herbal polypharmaceutical Lipotab, *Hamdard Medicus* **30**(1-2), 175-84 (1987)].

Administration of a garlic preparation (Wang 1000 kombi –7-fach-kapseln) at a dose of 4/day for 12 weeks to patients of atherosclerosis reduced cholesterol and triglycerides. It also decreased blood pressure, joint pain and improved sleep. [Lutomski J, Mrozikiewicz A; Effect of garlic preparation (Wang 1000 kombi-7-Fach. Kapseln) in early atherosclerosis, *Herba Pol* **34**(4), 231-41 (1988)].

Adenosin, isolated from *n*-butanol soluble fraction of tubers of *Allium bakeri* and *A. sativum*, exihibited significant inhibitory activity against both primary and secondary wave aggregation of human platelets induced by 2 μM ADP. Other compounds isolated from these tubers did not show inhibitory effects. [Okuyama T, Fujita S, Shibata S, Hosor M, Kawsada T, Masoki M Yamate N; Effects of Chinese drug "Xiebari" and "Dasuan" on human platelet aggregation (*A.bakeri, A. sativum*), *Planta Med* **55**(3), 242-44 (1989)].

The effects of feeding fresh garlic cloves and intraperitoneal injection of its total ethanolic extract were studied in adult female Japanese quails. Administration of fresh garlic cloves or its total ethanolic extract significantly reduced serum, egg yolk and liver cholesterol. Alkaline phosphatase was decreased while no definite effect was observed with respect to SGOT and SGPT. Garlic administration was found to increase antibody titre. No significant changes could be obtained in hematological counts. Effects observed were found to be time dependent. In all cases fresh garlic cloves were more effective than its total ethanolic extract. [El Habbak MME, Saleh K, Arbid MS, Hegazi AG, Sofy H, Influence of garlic (*Allium sativum* L.) on some biological and biochemical changes in Japanese quail with special reference to its hypocholesterolemic activity, *Archiv Gefluegelkunde* **53**(2), 73-79 (1989)].

Garlic reduced the serum lipid and cholesterol levels in cholesterol-fed goat kids. Deposition of fatty streaks and spots in aortic intima was also prevented by garlic in these animals. [Kaul PL, Prasad MC; Hypocholesterolemic and anti-atherosclerotic effects of garlic (*Allium sativum* L.) in goats, *Indian Vet J* **67**(12), 1112-15 (1990)].

Addition of garlic to cholesterol-rich diet fed to male rabbits, decreased cholesterol in plasma, aorta and liver. Total lipids, phospholipids and free fatty acids in aorta and liver were also reduced in these animals. Garlic enhanced fibrinolytic activity. The phospolipase activity in the cell-free supernatant of the aorta and liver increased along with a decrease in the cell-free supernatant NADH dehydrogenase of aorta in garlic treated hypercholesterolemic rabbits. Histological studies revealed protective effect of garlic on development of atherosclerosis. [Mirhadi SA, Singh S, Gupta PP; Effect of garlic supplementation of cholesterol rich diet on development of atherosclerosis in rabbits, *Indian J Exp Biol* **29**(2), 162-68 (1991)].

Twenty-six-week-old Single Comb White Leghorn pullets were fed a corn and soybean meal diet with or without .0.2% garlic oil for two 28-day periods. Dietary garlic oil did not affect egg production, egg weight, and feed efficiency. Total plasma lipids, plasma cholesterol and yolk cholesterol were not affected by the dietary treatment. [Reddy RV, Lightsey SF, Maurice-DV; Effect of feeding garlic oil on performance and egg yolk cholesterol concentration, *Poultry Sci* **70**(9), 2006-09 (1991)].

Methanol extract of garlic was found to behave as hypolipidemic drug, increasing the activity of peroxisomal fatty acyl-coenzyme A oxidase and of total carnitine acetyl-coenzyme A transferase in primary cultures of rat hepatocytes. [Orellana A, Kawada ME, Morales MN, Vargas L, Bronfman M; Induction of peroxisomal fatty acyl-coenzyme A oxidase and total carnitine acetyl-coenzyme A transferase in primary cultures of rat hepatocytes by garlic extracts, *Toxicol Lett* **60**(1), 11-17 (1992)].

Administration of the garlic constituent, S-allyl cystein sulphoxide (200mg/kg) to alloxan diabetic rats significantly decreased serum lipids, blood sugar and activity of certain enzymes. This compound also significantly enhanced the hepatic and intestinal HMG Co A reductase and liver hexokinase activity in diabetic rats. [Sheela CG, Augusti KT; Antidiabetic effect of S-allyl cystein sulphoxide isolated from garlic (*Allium sativum* Linn.), *Indian J Exp Biol* **30**(6), 523-26 (1992)].

Chickens were fed 2% lyophilised onion or garlic with different concentrations of disulfides in diets containing 18% soybean oil for 14 days. Hepatic sulphur levels increased almost two-fold in chicks fed garlic. Hepatic cholesterol concentrations were reduced by garlic but not by onions. Garlic decreased total superoxide dismutase (SOD) activity and this was due to reduced activity of the Cu-Zn SOD. However, in contrast, both onions and garlic increased Mn-SOD activity and hepatic glutathione concentrations. Garlic decreased glutathione peroxidase activity. These findings indicate that dietary garlic is more effective as a hypocholesterolemic agent than onion. [Sklan D, Berner YN, Rabinowitch HD; The effect of dietary onion and garlic on hepatic lipid concentration and activity of antioxidative enzymes in chicks, *J Nutr Biochem* **3**(7), 322-25 (1992)].

Administration of garlic powder (equivalent to 8-10 mg of allicin) to patients of cardiovascular disorders for 4 months significantly lowered blood cholesterol and triglycerides contents compared to placebo. Garlic also exhibited antiplatelet aggregatory activity. [Grunwald J; Garlic the best documented medicinal plants in prevention of cardiovascular diseases, *Acta Horticulturae* (332), 115-19 (1993)].

In view of the antioxidant properties of garlic demonstrated *in vitro,* the effects of garlic supplements on lipoprotein oxidation susceptibility in humans were investigated. Administration of garlic powder (600 mg/d) to ten healthy volunteers for two weeks in a placebo-controlled, randomized, double-blind crossover trial, revealed that the *ex vivo* susceptibility of apolipoprotein B-containing lipoproteins to oxidation was significantly decreased (-34%) despite the fact that serum lipid and lipoprotein levels were not lowered in this short time period. The beneficial effects of garlic on serum lipid levels, platelet function, fibrinolysis and blood pressure in conjunction to this effect of retarding lipoprotein oxidation are considered to contribute to the potential antiatherosclerotic effect of garlic. [Phelps S, Harris WS; Garlic supplementation and lipoprotein oxidation susceptibility, *Lipids* **28**(5), 475- 77 (1993)].

Simultaneous feeding of garlic with cholesterol to chickens for 12 weeks significantly reduced levels of blood total cholesterol, triglycerides, LDL and VLDL-cholesterol.

Cholesterol enriched diet-induced aortic damage was also comparatively much less in garlic-fed animals compared to placebo. [Khalid Q, Sultana L, Sarwar M, Ahmed Y; Beneficial effects of *Allium sativum* Linn. in experimental cholesterol atherosclerosis in chickens. Part 1- protective effects, *Pak J Sci Ind Res* **37**(12), 524-27 (1994)].

The mechanism of the cholesterol-lowering effects of garlic was studied using primary hepatocyte cultures. The results of the investigation suggested that the hypocholesterolemic effect of garlic stems, in part, from decreased hepatic cholesterogenesis, whereas the triacylglycerol-lowering effect is due to inhibition of fatty acid synthesis. [Yeh YY, Yeh SM; Garlic reduces plasma lipids by inhibiting hepatic cholesterol and triacylglycerol synthesis, *Lipids* **29**(3), 189-93 (1994)].

In cholesterol-enriched diet-fed rats, S-allyl cysteine sulphoxide isolated from garlic controlled hypercholesterolemia and derangement of enzyme activities. The efficacy of this compound was comparable to gugulipid. The hypolipidemic effect of the compound has been attributed to its inhibitory activity on lipogenic enzymes HMG Co A reductase and stimulatory action on lecithin cholesterol acyl transferase enzyme and faecal excretion of sterols and bile acids. [Sheela CG, Augusti KT; Effects of S-allyl cysteine sulphoxide isolated from *Allium sativum* Linn. and gugulipid on some enzymes and faecal excretion of bile acids and sterols in cholesterol fed rats, *Indian J Exp Biol* **33**(10), 749-51 (1995)].

Administration of fibres from the outer skin of garlic and onion reduced plasma and tissue total lipids, total cholesterol and glyceride levels in albino rats. Garlic skin fibres were more effective as hypolipidemic agent. However, potent antiatherogenic activity was noted in rats, fed fibres of onion skin and this was evidenced by increased HDL-c / LDL-c ratio. Hypocholesterolemic activity of these fibres could not be ascribed to bile acid excretion or cholesterol breakdown. [Vadhera S, Punia AK, Soni GL, Hypocholesterolemic/hypolipidemic effect of dietary fibres from outer dry skin of garlic and onion, *J Food Sci Technol* **32**(1), 62-64 (1995)].

In cholesterol enriched diet-fed (12 weeks) atherosclerotic chickens, administration of garlic led to significant reduction of plasma triglyceride, total cholesterol and LDL +VLDL– cholesterol levels. Aortic damage was also relatively much less in garlic treated chickens. Aqueous extract of garlic also exhibited marked antiplatelet aggregatory activity *in vitro*. [Khalid Q, Sultana L, Sarwar S, Ahmad Y; Beneficial effects of *Allium sativum* Linn. in experimental cholesterol atherosclerosis in chicken. Part II Curative effects, *Pak J Sci Ind Res* 38(1), 11-16 (1995)].

It has been proposed that organic tellurium compounds, found in high concentration in fresh garlic buds, are responsible for the lipid lowering activity of garlic. These compounds may contribute to this action by inhibiting squalene epoxidase, the penultimate enzyme in the synthetic pathway of cholesterol. Weanling rats, fed a diet rich in tellurium, develop a demyelinating polyneuropathy due to inhibition of this enzyme in peripheral nerves. Chronic exposure to small amounts of tellurium found in garlic might reduce endogenous cholesterol production through inhibition of hepatic squalene epoxidase and so reduce cholesterol levels. Tellurium may also contribute to the characteristic odour of garlic since the most obvious clinical sign of tellurium poisoning is a garlic-like odour. [Larner AJ; How does garlic exert its hypocholesterolaemic action? The tellurium hypothesis, *Medical Hypotheses* **44**(4), 295-97 (1995)].

The hypolipidemic effect of *A. sativum* was studied in rabbits and was compared with Gemfibrozil (120 mg/kg), which served as a positive control drug. Aqueous extract of *A. sativum* acted as an effective hypolipidemic agent and this finding was substantiated by the simultaneous histopathological studies carried out. The indigenous drug was capable of correcting the fatty changes produced by the fat containing diet to a considerable extent. The efficacy in lowering plasma cholesterol and triglyceride was comparable to that of Gemfibrozil. [Mini KP, Kumar NG; Hypolipidaemic effect of *Allium sativum* in rabbits, *J Vet Animal Sci* **26**(1), 40-43 (1995)].

See *Adenocalymma alliaceum:* [Srinivasan and Srinivasan; *Indian J Exp Biol* **33**(1), 64-66 (1995)].

Both garlic protein (16% of diet) and garlic oil (100 mg/kg bw/d) exhibited significant lipid lowering effects. The hypolipidemic action was primarily due to a decrease in hepatic cholesterogenesis in the treated rats. Garlic protein, though less effective than garlic oil, is more palatable. [Mathew BC, Daniel RS, Augusti KT; Hypolipidemic effect of garlic protein substituted for casein in diet of rats compared to those of garlic oil, *Indian J Exp Biol* **34**(4), 337-40 (1996)].

Feeding of garlic oil to radio active calcium (74KBq/g/bw)-administered mice prevented radiation induced increase in hepatic total lipids, triglycerides, phospholipids and free fatty acids. These observations suggested the presence of radioprotective activity in garlic. [Gupta NK; Modification of radiation induced changes in murine hepatic lipid profiles by garlic (*Allium sativum* Linn.) unsaturated oils, *Indian J Exp Biol* **34**(9), 851-53 (1996)].

Allicin has been described as a hypolipidemic drug of the future. [Eilat S, Avramovitch D, Rabinkov A, Mirelman D, Battler A, Eldar M, Vered Z; Allicin: Hypolipidemic, *Drugs of the Future* **21**(11), 1101-04 (1996)].

Administration of diallyl disulphide and allyl propyl disulphide extracted from garlic to mice prior to irradiation showed less significant increase in total lipid, phospholipid and triglyceride levels suggestive of radioprotective activity of *Allium sativum.* Such a lipid lowering activity of garlic in irradiated mice could be ascribed to inactivation of SH compounds by organic disulphides of garlic. [Gupta NK; Possible mechanism underlying the hypolipidemic activity of garlic in irradiated mice, *International Seminar on Free Radical Mediated Diseases and Ayurveda,* Faculty of Ayurveda, IMS, BHU, Varanasi, India, (A-25) September 2-4, 1996].

Plants with hypolipidemic, antiplatelet, cardioprotective, hypoglycemic and hypotensive activities were enlisted. Cardiovascular activity of *Allium satium, Cicer arietinum, Commiphora mukul, Coleus froskohlii, Curcuma longa, Embellica officinale, Inula racemosa, Ocimum sanctum, Pterocarpus marsupium, Terminalia arjuna* and *Trigonella foenum – graecum* was discussed. [Dwivedi S; Putative uses of Indian cardiovascular friendly plants in preventive cardiology, *Ann Natl Acad Med Sci* (India) **32**(3&4), 159-75 (1996)].

See *Allium cepa*: [Augusti KT; *Indian J Exp Biol* **34**(7),: 634-40 (1996)].

Fish consumption has been shown to influence epidemiology of heart disease and garlic has been shown to influence triglyceride levels. The effect of fish oil and garlic combination as a dietary supplement on the lipid subfractions was evaluated. In addition to the known anticoagulant and antioxidant properties of both fish oil and garlic, the combination caused favourable shifts in the lipid subfractions within one month. Triglycerides were affected to the largest extent. The cholesterol lowering and improvement in lipid / HDL risk ratios suggested that these combination might have antiatherosclerotic properties and protect against the development of coronary artery disease. [Morcos NC; Modulation of lipid profile by fish oil and garlic combination, *J Natl Med Assoc* **89**(10), 673-78 (1997)].

The use of garlic and garlic preparations as agents for prevention and treatment of atherosclerosis and atherosclerosis-related diseases has been reviewed. The effect of garlic on atherosclerosis is considered to be indirect; it acts by reduction of hyperlipidemia and hypertension, and by prevention of thrombus formation. In animal models, garlic causes direct antiatherogenic (preventive) and antiatherosclerotic (causing regression) effects at the level of artery wall. Garlic's direct effect on atherosclerosis may be explained by its capacity to reduce lipid content in arterial cells and to prevent intracellular lipid accumulation. This effect, in turn, is accompanied by other atherosclerotic manifestations, i.e., stimulation of cell proliferation and extracellular matrix synthesis. The possible positive results of garlic therapy on human atherosclerosis may open a new era in the use of garlic for prevention and treatment of many atherosclerosis-related diseases. [Orekhov AN, Grunwald J; Effects of garlic on atherosclerosis, *Nutrition* **13**(7-8), 656-63 (1997)].

Hypolipidemic activity of allicin in combination with essential phospholipids was examined in 25 patients of atherosclerosis. The hypolipidemic effect of allicin was potentiated by essential phospholipids. These essential phospholipids directly lowered the lipids and also acted as carrier for allicin. [Samochowiec J, Czerny B; The influence of essential phospholipids (EPL) and allicin on lipid metabolism in man, *Herba Pol* **43**(1), 53-57 (1997)].

Pharmacological and clinical investigations, done on medicinal plants with hypolipidemic activity, have been reviewed. Of the plants investigated, *Allium sativum, Commiphora mukul, Inula racemosa, Terminalia arjuna, Cicer arietinum, Curcuma longa, Emblica officinalis* and *Trigonella foenum graecum* were found to possess potent hypolipidemic activity. These drugs also exhibited antiplatelet and antioxidant effects. [Sharma SB, Dwivedi S; Medicinal plants with hypolipidemic activity, *Indian*

Drugs **34**(5), 242-51 (1997)].

The commercial garlic oil preparation, showed no influence on serum lipoproteins, cholesterol absorption, or cholesterol synthesis. Garlic therapy for treatment of hypercholesterolemia cannot be recommended on the basis of the study undertaken by the authors. [Berthold HK, Sudhop T, von Bergmann K; Effect of a garlic oil preparation on serum lipoproteins and cholesterol metabolism: A randomized controlled trial, *J Am Med Assoc* **279**(23), 1900-02 (1998)].

The water-soluble protein fraction of garlic was tested for its hypolipidemic action on alcohol (3.76 g/kg.bw/day)-induced hyperlipidemic rats. Garlic protein (500 mg/kg.bw/d) showed significant hypolipidemic action, comparable to a standard dose of guggulipid (50 mg/kg.bw/d). The hypolipidemic action was mainly due to an increase in cholesterol degradation to bile acids and neutral sterols and mobilization of triacyl glycerols. [Rajasree CR, Rajamohan T, Augusti KT; Biochemical effects of garlic protein on lipid metabolism in alcohol-fed rats, *Indian J Exp Biol* **37**(3), 243-47 (1999)].

Experimental hypercholesterolemia and its modulation by some natural dietary supplements (pectin, garlic and ginseng) and by the drug gemfibrozil were studied in rabbits. Garlic and pectin were successful in reduction of hypercholesterolemia in a significant way, comparable to gemfibrozil. Garlic was also shown to have antilipid peroxidative property. Ginseng administration failed to exert any significant protection from the hypercholesterolemia or atherosclerosis associated with the cholesterol-enriched diet. [Ismail MF, Gad MZ, Hamdy MA; Study of the hypolipidemic properties of pectin, garlic and ginseng in hypercholesterolemic rabbits, *Pharmacol Res* **39**(2), 157-66 (1999)].

Continuous intake of high-dose of garlic powder significantly reduced the increase in arteriosclerotic plaque volume by 5-18% or even effected a slight regression within the observational period of 48 months. The results of the investigation substantiated that not only a preventive but also possibly a curative role in arteriosclerosis therapy (plaque regression) may be ascribed to garlic remedies. [Koscielny J, Klussendorf D, Latza R, Schmitt R, Radtke H, Siegel G, Kiesewetter H; The antiatherosclerotic effect of *Allium sativum*, *Atherosclerosis* **144**(1), 237-49 (1999)].

Oral feeding of garlic extract (100 mg/kg bw) to streptozotocin-induced diabetic rats was found to increase the cardiovascular functions, prevent the abnormality of lipid profile and increase fibrinolytic activities with the decrease of platelet aggregation. However, due to the high incidence of atherosclerosis in diabetes, the effect of garlic extract on the coronary vascular ultrastructural changes was studied. From the results of the investigation, the authors are of the opinion that garlic extract may open a new era in the medicinal use of garlic to prevent diabetic cardiovascular complications. [Patumraj S, Tewit S, Amatyakul S, Jariyapongskul A, Maneesri S, Kasantikul V, Shepro D; Comparative effects of garlic and aspirin on diabetic cardiovascular complications, *Drug Deliv* 7(2), 91-96 (2000)].

Garlic treatment has been shown to ameliorate hyperlipidemia and renal damage in chronic nephrotic syndrome, which is unrelated to proteinuria or antioxidant enzymes. [Pedraza Chaverri J, Medina Campos ON, Granados Silvestre MA, Maldonado PD, Olivares Corichi IM, Hernandez Pando R; Garlic ameliorates hyperlipidemia in chronic aminonucleoside nephrosis, *Mol Cell Biochem* **211**(1-2), 69-77 (2000)].

Cholesterol-lowering effect of steroid saponin from the active fraction of garlic in the cholesterol-enriched diet (16 weeks)-induced hyperlipidemic model was studied. Feeding of crude saponin fraction, prepared from methanolic extract of garlic, produced significant lowering of total cholesterol. It was suggested that the steroid saponins should be one of the active compounds responsible for hypocholesterolemic action of garlic. [Matsuura H, Slowing K, Tejerina T, Graham J, Fransworth NR; Cholesterol lowering effects of saponins from garlic, *Phytomedicine* **7**(Suppl II), 48-49 (2000)].

In cholesterol-fed rabbits, effect of garlic on aortic mechanical properties and plaque formation was investigated. Administration of garlic did not reduce plasma lipid. It also did not prevent aortic plaque formation. Aortic endothelial function and contractile properties were not significantly affected by garlic. However, garlic slightly increased the viscoelasticity of the atherosclerotic vessel wall. [Brehme U, Emmerich M, Hafner HM, Polligkeit J, Wolf AT, Frey JC, Altepeter HK, Muller BM, Schmahl FW, Junger M, Heinle H; Effect of garlic (*Allium sativum* L.) on aortic mechanical properties and plaque formation in cholesterol-fed rabbits, *Phytomedicine* **7**(Suppl II), 48-(2000)].

In cholesterol-induced hyperlipidemic rabbits, changes in lipid profile and atherosclerotic plaque formation were investigated following treatment with garlic extract. Total, HDL and LDL-cholesterol levels were decreased after feeding of garlic extract (1.5ml/kg/d) for three months. A significant reduction in the plaque surface area in the aorta of garlic treated rabbits was also evident. The treated animals exhibited relatively higher antioxidant potential. [Durak I, Ozturk HS, Olcay E, Guven C; Effects of garlic extract supplementation on blood lipids and antioxidant parameters and atherosclerotic plaque formation process in cholesterol-fed rabbits, *J Herb Pharmacother* **2**(2), 19-32 (2000)].

The hypocholesterolemic effect of dietary garlic was studied using male rats. The serum cholesterol level was significantly lower in the group receiving diet supplemented with 10% fresh garlic than the control group. Hypercholesterolemia induced by cholesterol feeding was also significantly reduced by garlic. Garlic supplementation increased high density lipoprotein and decreased low density lipoprotein in normal and hypercholesterolemic rats. The reduction in the plasma cholesterol by feeding garlic was in low density lipoprotein and very low density lipoprotein cholesterol fractions. Feeding the garlic diet decreased liver weight compared to the control group. The results demonstrate that garlic exerts hypocholesterolemic effects in normal or cholesterol-fed rats and reduces the liver weight. [Aouadi R, Aouidet A, Elkadhi A, Rayana CB, Jaafoura H, Tritar B, Nagati K; Effect of fresh garlic (*Allium sativum*) on lipid metabolism in male rats, *Nutr-Res* **20**(2), 273-80 (2000)].

See *Allium cepa:* [Kumar *et al.*; *Indian J Poultry Sci* **35**(1), 95-98 (2000)].

Diet (2% cholesterol or 40% cocoanut kernel or ground nut) induced alterations in serum and tissue lipids, lipid peroxidations and enzyme activities (HMG CoA reductase, AST, ALT or ALP) were significantly decreased by incorporation of garlic (5%) in any of the above mentioned high fat diets. [Augusti KT, Narayanan A, Pillai LS, Ebrahim RS, Sivsdasan R, Sindhu KR, Subba I, Abdeen S, Nair SS; Beneficial effect of garlic (*Allium sativum* Linn.) on rats fed with diets containing cholesterol and either of the oil seeds *Indian, J Exp Biol* **39**(7), 660-67 (2001)].

Serum and tissue lipids, lipid peroxidation and certain enzyme activities were significantly increased following 3 months feeding of butter fat and beef separately as dietary components (21%) to albino rats. On incorporation of 5% garlic in the above diet, the deleterious effects of the animal fats were ameliorated. Similar effect was also observed by amla (*Emblica officinalis* Gaertn) and onion (*Allium cepa* Linn). However, garlic was most active followed by amla and onion. [Augusti KT, Arathy SL, Asha R, Ramakrishnan J, Zaira J, Lekha V, Smitha S, George S, Vijayasree VM; A comparative study on the beneficial effects of garlic (*Allium sativum* Linn), amla (*Emblica officinalis* Gaertn) and onion (*Allium cepa* Linn) on the hyperlipidemia induced by butter fat and beef fat in rats, *Indian J Exp Biol* **39**(8), 760-66 (2001)].

It is well known that hypercholesterolemia is a major risk factor for atherosclerosis and that lowering of cholesterol can significantly reduce risk for cardiovascular diseases. Recently, oxidation of LDL has been recognized as playing an important role in the initiation and progression of atherosclerosis. Experimental evidence has been presented to show that several garlic compounds can effectively suppress LDL oxidation *in vitro*. Short-term supplementation of garlic in human subjects has demonstrated an increased resistance of LDL to oxidation. The antiatherosclerotic properties of garlic are considered to be due to its ability to suppress LDL oxidation. [Lau BH; Suppression of LDL oxidation by garlic, *J Nutr* **131**(3S), 985S-8S (2001)].

In addition to hypolipidemic, antiplatelet and procirculatory effects, some garlic preparations are claimed to possess hepatoprotective, immune-enhancing, anticancer and chemopreventive activities. These additional biological effects, attributed to aged garlic extract, may be due to compounds, such as S-allylcysteine, S-allylmercaptocysteine, N(α)-fructosyl arginine and others, formed during the extraction process. [Amagase H, Petesch BL, Matsuura H, Kasuga S, Itakura Y; Intake of garlic and its bioactive components, *J Nutr* **131**(3S), 955S- 62S (2001)].

It has been shown that the cholesterol-lowering effects of aged garlic extract stem, in part, from inhibition of hepatic cholesterol synthesis by water-soluble sulphur compounds, especially S-allylcysteine. [Yeh YY, Liu L; Cholesterol-lowering effect of garlic extracts and organosulfur compounds: Human and animal studies, *J Nutr.* **131**(3S), 989S-93S (2001)].

In order to ascertain the putative hypolipidemic effect of garlic, the inhibitory effects of water-soluble organosulphur compounds, present in garlic, on triglyceride (TG) and fatty acid synthesis were studied in cultured rat hepatocytes. The results of the investigation indicated inhibition of lipid biosynthesis by S-allyl cysteine and other S-alkyl cysteins in cultured rat hepatocytes, and further suggested that these S-alk(en)yl cysteines of garlic impair triglyceride synthesis in part due to decreased *de novo* fatty acid synthesis resulting from inhibition of lipogenic enzyme, fatty acid synthase. Whether tissue concentrations of active garlic components can achieve levels required to inhibit TG synthesis *in vivo* warrants further investigation. [Liu L, Yeh YY; Water-soluble organosulfur compounds of garlic inhibit fatty acid and triglyceride syntheses in cultured rat hepatocytes, *Lipids* **36**(4), 395-400 (2001)].

The hypocholesterolemic effect of an enteric-coated garlic supplement, standardised for allicin-releasing potential, in mild to moderate hypercholesterolemic patients was evaluated. The study suggests that garlic supplementation has a cholesterol-lowering-effect, which may be mediated by direct action of a biologically active compound or compounds and in part through the effect on food and nutrient intake. [Kannar D, Wattanapenpaiboon N, Savige GS, Wahlqvist ML; Hypocholesterolemic effect of an enteric-coated garlic supplement, *J Am College Nutr* **20**(3), 225-31 (2001)].

Clinical trials using garlic powder tablets to assess any effect of garlic that might be related to allicin cannot be considered valid for garlic when the trial shows no effect, unless the expected allicin release from the tablets has at least been determined under standardised drug release conditions (USP 724A). [Lawson LD, Wang ZJ, Papadimitriou D; Allicin release under simulated gastrointestinal conditions from garlic powder tablets employed in clinical trials on serum cholesterol, *Planta Med.* **67**(1), 13-18 (2001)].

The duration of the hypocholesterolemic effect of garlic supplements was studied. [Lawson LD; Duration of the hypocholesterolemic effect of garlic supplements, *Arch Internal Med* **161**(20), 2505 (2001)].

Hypolipidemic, antioxidant and hypoglycemic activity of a compound herbal preparation (SBC) containing *Allium sativum, Terminalia belerica, Terminalia chebula, Andrographis peniculata* and *Gymnema sylvestre* was studied in triton WR-1339-induced hyperlipidemic rats. This drug (200mg/kg) caused significant lowering of total cholesterol, phospholipids and triglycerides. Hypolipidemic effects were comparable with that of Gemifibrozil. Superoxide anions and hydroxyl radical generation was also inhibited in treated animals in a dose dependant manner. Non-enzymic and enzymic system-induced microsomal lipid peroxide formation was also prevented by this drug. [Chander R, Khanna AK, Mathur S, Kar A, Rastogi AK;

Antidyslipemic and antioxidant activities of SBC: A herbal preparation, *Ethnobotany* **14**(1-2), 123-28 (2001)].

Fresh garlic extract reduced microsomal triglyceride transfer protein mRNA levels in both the human hepatoma HepG2 and intestinal carcinoma Caco-2 cells in dose-dependent fashion; significant reductions were detected with 3 g/l fresh garlic extract. A new mechanism for the hypolipidemic effect of fresh garlic extract has been advanced. [Lin MC, Wang EJ, Lee C, Chin KT, Liu D, Chiu JF, Kung HF; Garlic inhibits microsomal triglyceride transfer protein gene expression in human liver and intestinal cell lines and in rat intestine, *J Nutr.* **132**(6), 1165-68 (2002)].

A critical examination of scientific literature claiming cardiovascular benefits from regular consumption of garlic or garlic preparations was made. While there are indications of its antiatherosclerotic effects there are insufficient data in humans. [Brace LD; Cardiovascular benefits of garlic (*Allium sativum* L), *J Cardiovasc Nurs* **16**(4), 33-49 (2002)].

Inclusion of garlic powder (2%) or curcumin, the active principle of *Curcuma longa* (0.2%) or capsaicin, a constituent of *Capsicum annuum* (0.015%) in the diet, produced hypolipidemic effect in rats rendered hypercholesterolemic by maintaining them on a cholesterol-enriched diet (0.5%) for 8 weeks. Plasma cholesterol in hypercholesterolemic rats was decreased by these dietary spice principles and garlic by 25-39%. Dietary curcumin, capsaicin and garlic also produced a significant (10-14%) decrease in membrane cholesterol content. [Kempaiah RK, Srinivasan K; Integrity of erythrocytes of hypercholesterolemic rats during spices treatment, *Mol Cell Biochem* **236**(1-2), 155-61 (2002)].

It is still not certain whether garlic or garlic preparations can be used as a lipid-lowering agent. It is important to characterise the active components in garlic and their bioavailability after ingestion. [Kerckhoffs DA, Brouns F, Hornstra G, Mensink RP; Effects on the human serum lipoprotein profile of β- glucan, soy protein and isoflavones, plant sterols and stanols, garlic and tocotrienols, *J Nutr* **132**(9), 2494-505 (2002)].

Short-term garlic therapy in adults with mild to moderate hypercholesterolemia does not affect either lipid levels or various psychopathologic parameters. [Peleg A, Hershcovici T, Lipa R, Anbar R, Redler M, Beigel Y; Effect of garlic on lipid profile and psychopathologic parameters in people with mild to moderate hypercholesterolemia, *Isr Med Assoc J* **5**(9), 637- 40 (2003)].

Chemical composition of garlic and hypolipidemic, antioxidative, antibacterial and antitumorogenic properties of garlic preparations has been reviewed. [Ryzhenkov VE, Makarov VG; Biologically active substances in garlic (*Allium sativum* L.) and their application in nutrition for humans, *Vopr Pitan* **72**(4), 42-6 (2003) [Article in Russian].

The effect of garlic supplementation on cholesteryl ester transfer protein activity (CETP) along with its anti-atherosclerotic effect in cholesterol-fed rabbits was examined. The garlic-supplemented group exhibited significantly lower CETP activity than the control group during the experimental period. Among the atherogenic parameters, the total cholesterol, triglyceride, LDL-c, VLDL-c, and atherogenic index were all significantly lower in the garlic treated group than in the control group during the experimental period ($P < 0.05$), whereas HDL-c concentration was significantly higher in the garlic group than in the control group after 12 weeks. The results of the invesigation suggest that garlic exerts hypocholesterolemic and/or antiatherogenic activity. The inhibitory activity of garlic supplementation against CETP may delay the progression of atherosclerosis. [Kwon MJ, Song YS, Choi MS, Park SJ, Jeong KS, Song YO; Cholesteryl ester transfer protein activity and atherogenic parameters in rabbits supplemented with cholesterol and garlic powder, *Life Sci* **72**(26), 2953-64 (2003)].

After a thorough search of the literature for randomized controlled trials addressing the efficacy of garlic as an antihyperlipidemic agent and a critical appraisal of these studies, it is best not to recommend garlic to treat mild to moderate hyperlipidemia until larger randomized controlled trials of longer duration, which correct the existing methodological flaws, are designed and carried out. [Alder R, Lookinland S, Berry JA, Williams M; A systematic review of the effectiveness of garlic as an anti-hyperlipidemic agent, *J Am Acad Nurse Pract* **15**(3), 120-29 (2003)].

See *Allium cepa:* [Kumar et al.; *Indian J Exp Biol* **44**(1), 88-90 (2003)].

See *Commiphora mukul:* [Mary et al.; *Phytomedicine* **10** (6-7), 474-82 (2003)].

See *Zingibar officinale :* [Singh VK, Singh S, Singh DK; Pharmacological effects of spices. Recent progress in medicinal plants: Phytochemistry and pharmacology, JN Govil, VK Singh (eds.), Studium press, LLC, Houston, Texas, USA. 2, p 321-353(2003)].

The knowledge on the antihyperlipidemic effect of garlic, its formulations and of its individual components has been summarized. Varying opinions based on experimental results concerning the mechanisms by means of which the effect takes place have also been presented in the paper. *In vitro* experiments were carried out mainly on the cultures of rat hepatocytes and an inhibitory effect on important enzymic activities in the biosynthesis of cholesterol and fatty acids was demonstrated. The most frequently employed *in vivo* models were rabbits. The antiatherogenic effect was markedly manifested by a reduction of lipid plaques in the arteries in hypercholesterolemic animals, decreased accumulation of cholesterol in vascular walls, and other positive interventions. [Sovova M, Sova P; Pharmaceutical importance of *Allium sativum* L.; Hypolipemic effects *in vitro* and *in vivo, Ceska Slov Farm* **53**(3), 117-23 (2004) [Article in Czech].

The reported beneficial effects of garlic on risk factors associated with cardiovascular disease, including normalisation of plasma lipid levels have been questioned by numerous studies. As this contradiction might result from the use of different garlic-derived materials, experimental designs, and/or animal models, the hypolipidemic effect of garlic-derived materials was studied in APOE*3-Leiden mice, a model well suited for drug and dietary intervention studies of hyperlipidemia. Mice were fed a nonpurified diet for 4 weeks, followed by a western diet for 8 weeks, both supplemented with the garlic-derived materials (allicin. or diallyldisulfide or powdered garlic). The amounts of garlic-derived materials allowed free intake of allicin or allicin equivalents at 44 mg/kg bw/d. These diets had no consistent effect on plasma lipids and did not affect lipoprotein profiles, which are markers for wholebody cholesterol synthesis and intestinal sterol absorption. The data indicated that the postulated effects of garlic on cardiovascular disease are not caused *via* modulation of plasma lipid levels. [Santo SM, van Vlijmen BJ, Buytenhek R, van Duyvenvoorde W, Havekes LM, Arnault I, Auger J, Princen HM; Well-characterized garlic-derived materials are not hypolipidemic in APOE*3-Leiden transgenic mice, *J Nutr* **134**(6), 1500-03 (2004)].

The reported protective effect of garlic against atherosclerosis has been questioned. In order to settle the controversy, the effect of the chemically well-characterized and production-controlled garlic powder, printanor, was studied on atherosclerosis in the APOE*3-Leiden transgenic mouse, a mouse model well suited for evaluating anti-atherosclerotic properties of drugs and food components under human-like conditions. Commercially available fermented garlic kyolic was included as reference. After 28 weeks of treatment, printanor and kyolic did not affect atherosclerotic lesion type, area or composition. Under conditions relevant to the human situation, the well-characterised and production-controlled garlic powder, printanor, does not display hypolipidemic, anti-inflammatory or anti-atherosclerotic properties. [Santo SM, van Vlijmen BJ, van Duyvenvoorde W, Offerman EH, Havekes LM, Arnault I, Auger J, Princen HM; Absence of an atheroprotective effect of the garlic powder printanor in APOE*3- Leiden transgenic mice, *Atherosclerosis* **177**(2), 291-97 (2004)].

Allicor, a long-acting garlic powder tablet, was found to lower total cholesterol and LDL-c and raise HDL-c in a double-blind placebo-controlled study. [Andrianova IV, Demidova OM, Medvedeva LA, Latyshev OA; Correction of hyperlipidemia with Allicor, *Klin Med* (Mosk) **82**(4), 56-58 (2004) [Article in Russian].

The transcription factor NF-kappaB is suggested to play a pivotal role in atherogenesis by regulating the expression of proinflammatory gene products such as adhesion molecules. Garlic is consumed as food or dietary supplement in order to benefit from its antiatherogenic effect. The answer to the question whether garlic metabolites diallyldisulfide and allylmercaptane influence the TNF- α.induced activation of NF-*kappa*B and the NF-*kappa*B-regulated endothelial gene product E-selectin in human umbilical endothelial cells was sought. From the results of the investigation it has been concluded that NF-kappaB is not a major target of garlic metabolites such as diallyldisulfide or allylmercaptane. [Dirsch VM, Keiss HP, Vollmar AM; Garlic metabolites fail to inhibit the activation of the transcription factor NF-kappaB and subsequent expression of the adhesion molecule E-selectin in human endothelial cells, *Euro J Nutr* **43**(1), 55-59 (2004).

The effect of garlic on arteriosclerotic nanoplaque formation and size was studied. The experiments clearly proved that garlic extract strongly inhibits Ca^{2+} binding to proteoheparan sulphate. In consequence, the formation of the ternary proteoheparan sulfate/LDL/Ca^{2+} complex, initially responsible for the nanoplaque composition and ultimately for the arteriosclerotic plaque generation, is decisively blunted. [Siegel G, Malmsten M, Pietzsch J, Schmidt A, Buddecke E, Michel F, Ploch M, Schneider W; The effect of garlic on arteriosclerotic nanoplaque formation and size, *Phytomedicine* (Jena) **11**(1), 24-35 (2004)].

See *Curcuma longa* (Turmeric): [Kempaiah & Srinivasan; *Ann Nutr Metab* **48**(5), 314-20 (2004)].

***Allium suworowii*:** See Polysaccharides in Appendix [Khushbaktova *et al.*, *Khim-Farm-Z* **21**(11), 1348-52 (1987)].

Aloe barbadensis (H. Gwarpatha, S. Ghritakumari)**:** In triton (WR-1339)-induced hyperlipidemic Presbytis monkeys, administration of aqueous extract of *A. barbadensis* significantly lowered the serum total cholesterol, triglycerides, phospholipids and nonesterified free fatty acid levels.. LDL and VLDL-cholesterols were also significantly decreased in treated group of monkeys. HDL cholesterol / total cholesterol ratio in *A. barbedensis* treated animals was significantly increased as compared to their initial levels. [Dixit VP, Joshi S; Effect of *Aloe barbedensis* and clofibrate on serum lipids in triton induced hyperlipidemia in Presbytis monkeys, *Ind J Med Res* **78**(Sept.), 417-21 (1983)].

Aloe vera (syn. *Aloe barbadensis*)**:** The hypolipidemic and hypoglycemic action of a polyherbal compound containing *Aloe vera, Lupinus termis, Trigonella foenum-graecum, Commiphora myrrha, Bryonia critica* and *Rheum officinale* was studied in alloxanised male rats. Administration of this herbal preparation (1g/kg) to diabetic rats, for a period of 8 weeks, significantly decreased serum cholesterol and triglyceride levels. This drug also produced a sharp decline in blood glucose levels at the end of 2, 4 and 8 weeks of treatment of these animals. [Nada SA, Bashandy SAE, Negm SA; Evaluation of the hypoglycemic activity of a traditional herbal preparation in male diabetic rats, *Fitoterapia* **68**(3), 240-44 (1997)].

Alpinia galanga (H. Barakulanjan, S. Sugandha vacha): Oral administration of ethanolic extract of *A. galanga* and *Kaemferia galanga* (20mg/d) to cholesterol-rich diet fed rats for 4 weeks reduced serum and tissue levels of total cholesterol, triglycerides, and phospholipids along with enhancement of serum HDL-cholesterol. It was suggested that these plant drugs might be effectively used in various lipid disorders like atherosclerosis etc. [Achuthan CR, Padikkala J; Hypolpidemic effect of *Alpinia galanga* (Rasna) and *Kaemeferia galanga* (Kachoori), *Amla Res Bull* **15**, 53-56, (1995)].

The hypocholesterolemic action of ethanolic extracts of rhizomes of *A. galanga* and

Kaempferia galanga was investigated in high cholesterol diet fed rats. Administration of these extracts (20 mg/d, po) caused a significant lowering of serum and tissue levels of total cholesterol, triglycerides and phospholipids alongwith enhancement of HDL cholesterol levels. [Achuthan CR, Padikkala J; Hypolipidemic effect of *Alpinia galanga* (Rasna) and *Kaemeferia galanga* (Kachoori), *Indian J Clin Biochem* **12**(1), 55-58 (1997)].

Alpinia officinarum (H. Kulinjan): Galangin-3-methyl ether, isolated from the ethyl acetate-soluble fraction of the aqueous extract of *A. officinarum* rhizomes, was found to be an inhibitor of pancreatic lipase with an IC_{50} value of 1.3 mg/ml (triolein as a substrate). Aqueous extract of the rhizomes of the plant and its ethyl acetate soluble fraction significantly inhibited the serum triglyceride level in corn oil feeding-induced triglyceridemic mice, and serum triglyceride and cholesterol in Triton WR-1339-induced hyperlipidemic mice. However, neither galangin-3-methyl ether nor the ethyl acetate fraction showed any hypolipidemic activity in high cholesterol diet-induced hyperlipidemic mice. The results of the investigation suggested that the hypolipidemic activity of the plant and its constituent, galangin 3-methylether, was due to the inhibition of pancreatic lipase. [Shin JE, Joo Han M, Kim DH; 3-Methylethergalangin isolated from *Alpinia officinarum* inhibits pancreatic lipase, *Biol Pharm Bull* **26**(6), 854-57 (2003)].

Antihyperlipidemic activity of 5-hydroxy-7-(4'-hydroxy-3'-methoxyphenyl)-1-phenyl-3- heptanone, a pancreatic lipase inhibitor, isolated from the rhizome of *A. officinarum*, was measured. The heptanone derivative significantly lowered the serum triglyceride level in corn oil feeding-induced triglyceridemic mice, and reduced serum triglyceride and cholesterol in Triton induced hyperlipidemic mice. However, the compound did not show hypolipidemic activity in high cholesterol diet-induced hyperlipidemic mice. Based on these findings, it was proposed that pancreatic lipase inhibitors may be effective as hypolipidemic agents. [Shin JE, Han MJ, Song MC, Baek NI, Kim DH; 5-Hydroxy-7- (4'-hydroxy-3'-methoxyphenyl)-1- phenyl-3-heptanone: A pancreatic lipase inhibitor isolated from *Alpinia officinarum, Biol Pharm Bull* **27**(1), 138-40 (2004)].

***Amaranthus esculantus*:** Hypocholesterolemic effect of amaranth seeds was studied in male Wistar strain albino rats. Feeding with amaranth seed showed a definite hypocholesterolemic effect. [Chaturvedi A, Sarojini G, Devi N; Hypocholesterolemic effect of amaranth seeds (*Amaranthus esculantus*), *Plant Foods Hum Nutr* **44**(1), 63-70 (1993)].

***Amaranthus* species:** The effect of amaranth and oat bran on the lipids of blood and liver in rats depending on the kind of fats in diet was studied. The influence of amaranth and oat bran on the concentration of triglycerides in the blood serum depended on the kind of fats in a diet. The diets containing amaranth or oat bran with lard did not decrease the concentration of lipids, however, the same diets with sunflower oil decreased this concentration significantly (by 22%). In liver, significant hypotriglyceridemic effect of amaranth and oat bran was observed for both of the diets; based on lard and sunflower. The decrease of triglycerides concentration under the influence of amaranth amounted to 10% (diet with lard) and 15% (diet with sunflower oil). Oat bran decreased the concentration of triglycerides in liver by 15% (diet with lard) and 20% (diet with sunflower oil). Sunflower oil added to the diets augmented the hypolipemic effect of amaranth and oat bran. [Grajeta H; Effect of amaranth and oat bran on blood serum and liver lipids in rats depending on the kind of dietary fats, *Nahrung* **43**(2), 114-17 (1999)].

The hypocholesterolemic effects of amaranth grain, amaranth oil and amaranth squalene were examined. Both amaranth grain and amaranth oil lowered serum and hepatic cholesterol and triglyceride levels. Faecal excretion of cholesterol and bile acid in the amaranth oil group increased, while amaranth grain affected only bile acid excretion. To study the effect of amaranth squalene, rats were fed the cholesterol diet for four weeks and injected (i.p.) with saline (control), amaranth squalene or shark liver squalene (200 mg/kg) for seven days. The hypolipidaemic effects of amaranth squalene were evident in both serum and liver. Amaranth squalene also markedly increased faecal excretions of cholesterol and bile acid and slightly inhibited HMG-CoA reductase activity. None of these effects were observed in the shark liver squalene group. The cholesterol-lowering effect of amaranth squalene may be mediated by increased faecal elimination of steroids through interference with cholesterol absorption and that plant and animal squalenes may affect cholesterol metabolism differently. [Shin DH, Heo HJ, Lee YJ, Kim HK; Amaranth squalene reduces serum and liver lipid levels in rats fed a cholesterol diet, *Brit J Biomed Sci* **61**(1), 11-14 (2004)].

Ammi visnaga: In cynomologous monkeys, administration of khellin and khelloside, isolated from *Ammi visnaga*, at a dose of 20mg/kg/d for 2 weeks significantly lowered the total cholesterol, LDL-cholesterol and HDL-cholesterol levels. The hypocholesterolemic effect was relatively more marked in case of khellin compared to khelloside. However, the triglyceride and VLDL-cholesterol levels did not change. Similar results were obtained even at lower doses of khellin (5mg/kg) and khelloside (10mg/kg). These cmpounds did not show any toxic effects. [Stevens IJ, Jones BW, Widmar IJ, Moran JJ, Manni DS, Day CE; Hypocholesterolemic effect of khellin and khelloside in female cyanomologous monkeys, *Arzneimittel Forsch* **35** II (8), 1257-60 (1985)].

Ammothamnus species: See Flavonoids in Appendix: [Khushbaktova *et al.*; *Khim Farma Zh* **25**(4), 53-57 (1991)].

Amorphophallus konjac: Hypocholesterolemic activity of crude konjac mannans, prepared from different *Amorphophallus* species, was studied in rats fed on a hypercholesterolemic diet. Konjac mannans, prepared from the tuber of *A. konjac*, depressed more significantly the elevation of serum cholesterol level due to dietary cholesterol than that prepared from the tuber of *Amorphophallus oncophyllus*. The quality of konjac mannans from *A. konjac* tubers also varied with the race and the area of cultivation of the plant. For example, Konjac Mannans from Shina (Chinese) race were superior to those from Zairai (domestic) race. Again, Mannans from the tuber of *A. konjac,* harvested in Gunma prefecture, were found to be most active. Of the different methods used for extraction of Konjac Mannans, ethanol extraction yielded samples of superior activity. [Tsuji K, Tsuji E, Suzuki S, Umemoto SI, Irie Y; Effect of polysaccharides on cholesterol metabolism. Part **5:** Effect of various crude Konjac Mannans on serum cholesterol levels in hypercholesterolemic rats, *Annual Report National Inst Nutr* (24), 75-82 (1975)].

See Polysaccharides in Appendix: [Tsuji *et al.*; *Annual Report National Inst Nutr* (24), 83- 91 (1975)].

The lipotropic effect of refined konjac meal (RKM), containing about 80% glucomannan and prepared from the tubers of *A. konjac,* was confirmed by histopathologic examination of the livers. In addition to the hypocholesterolemic effects, RKM diets also increased stool bulk. Minor effects on the absorption and utilization of Ca, Fe, Zn, and Cu were also found. [Hou YH, Zhang LS, Zhou HM, Wang RS, Zhang YZ; Influences of refined konjac meal on the levels of tissue lipids and the absorption of four minerals in rats, *Biomed Environ Sci* **3**(3), 306- 14 S (1990)].

The effects of refined konjac meal (containing 80% of glucomannan) on the level of serum and liver lipids, hepatic histopathology and on the composition and output of faecal bile acids in comparison with pectin, algin and agar were studied. All four kinds of dietary fibre were given at a level of 5% in the diet to the young male Wistar rats fed on a lipid-rich diet containing 5% lard, 1% cholesterol and 0.25% cholate. The control group was fed on a lipid rich diet alone without fibre. All the dietary fibres tested showed similar effects on serum lipid composition. At the end of 2-week of the experiment, the serum total cholesterol levels of the four experimental groups were only 62% to 75% of that of the control group but at the end of 7-week they were lowered to the same level of the normal group. The effects of these fibres on the level of the triglyceride in serum and on liver weights were also studied. The concentrations of total cholesterol and triglyceride in liver in refined konjac meal group were lower than those in control group as well as other three experimental groups. From the results of the detailed experiment, it could be concluded that refined konjac meal has the same significant hypocholesterolemic effect as the pectin, algin and agar, but its lipotropic effect is more potent. [Wu J, Peng S; Comparison of the hypolipidemic effects of refined konjac meal with several common dietary fibres and their mechanisms of action, *Acta Nutr Sin* **15**(2), 130-36 (1993) [Article in Chinese].

See Plant Fibres in Appendix: [Wu Jie; *Biomed Environ Sci* **10**(1), 27-37 (1997)].

The effect of konjac (*Amorphophallus konjac*) flour on the plasmatic lipids (TC, TG, LDL-c, HDL-c), as well as on the hepatic lipids (TC and TG) was studied and its hypocholesterolemic effect was compareed with cholestyramine and pravastatin, using Wistar rats with neonatal diabetes and induced hypercholesterolemia. All the diabetic hypercholesterolemic animals showed a reduction in the level of plama cholesterol as a consequence of different treatments, the degree of reduction varying between 25% and 35% due to konjac flour, which also showed a high hypotriglyceridemic activity. The results indicated a high therapeutical potential of konjac flour for the control and treatment of the lipids in diabetic hyperlipidemic individuals consuming atherogenic diet. [Gregorio SR, Areas MA, Reyes FGR; Effect of the konjac fibre on plasmatic lipids in Wistar rats with neonatal diabetes and induced hypercholesterolemia, *Alimentaria* **40**(347), 29-38 (2003)].

Glucomannan is the main polysaccharide of the tubers of *A. konjac,* a plant of the family Araceae. Of the known dietary fibres, it has the highest molecular weight and viscosity. It has been demonstrated to be highly effective in the treatment of obesity due to the satiety sensation that it produces. It has been found to be a remedy for constipation, because it increases the faeces volume. It is a hypocholesterolemic agent and it interferes in the transport of cholesterol and of bile acids. The different properties of this dietary fibre have been reviewed. [Gonzalez Canga A, Fernandez Martinez N, Sahagun AM, Garcia Vieitez JJ, Diez Liebana MJ, Calle Pardo AP, Castro Robles LJ, Sierra Vega M, Glucomannan; Properties and therapeutic applications. *Nutr Hosp.* **19**(1), 45-50 (2004) [Article in Spanish].

***Amorphophallus oncophyllus*:** See *Amorphophallus konjac*: [Tsuji *et al.*; *Annual Report National Inst Nutr* (24), 75-82 (1975)].

***Amphypterygium adstringens*:** Subcutaneous administration of the hexane extract of the stem bark of *A. adstringens* at a dose of 100 mg/kg exhibited significant hypocholesterolemic effect on 24 h fasted rats, lowering the cholesterol levels by 31%, an effect similar to 15 mg/kg estrone given by the same route. [Mata R, Calzada F, Navarrete A, del Rio F, Delgado G; Long-chain phenols from the bark of *Amphypterygium adstringens, J Ethnopharmacol* **34**(2- 3), 147-54 (1991)].

Ananas comosus (H. Anannas)**:** Hypoglycemic and hypolipidemic activities of the ethanolic extract of *A. comosus* leaves were evaluated in normal and alloxan-induced diabetic rats by oral glucose tolerance test and an olive oil load test. The leaf extract, at the dose of 0.40 g/kg, significantly inhibited the increase in blood glucose in diabetic rats in oral glucose tolerance test, but did not cause any hypoglycemic activity in normal rats. It also significantly inhibited the increase in post-prandial triglycerides levels in both normal and diabetic rats in olive oil load test. After 15 days of treatment of diabetic dyslipidemic rats, the ethanolic extract of *A. comosus* leaves significantly decreased blood glucose and LDL-c levels, significantly increased serum high density lipoprotein cholesterol levels and significantly lowered lipid peroxidation productions of blood, brain and kidneys. The data suggest that *A. comosus* leaf extract has antidiabetic, anti-dyslipidemic and anti-oxidative activities, which may be developed into a new plant medicine for treatment of diabetes and its complications. [Xie W, Xing D, Sun H, Wang W, Ding Y, Du L; The effects of *Ananas* *comosus* L. leaves on diabetic-dyslipidemic rats induced by alloxan and a high-fat/high-cholesterol diet, *Am J Chin Med* **33**(1), 95-105 (2005)].

Andrographis peniculata (H. Kiryat, S. Bhunimba): The ethanolic extract of *A paniculata* caused 49.8% reduction of fasting serum triglyceride levels, compared to 27.7% with metformin. Its hypotriglyceridemic effect is also beneficial in the diabetic state. [Zhang XF, Tan BK; Anti-diabetic property of ethanolic extract of *Andrographis paniculata* in streptozotocin-diabetic rats, *Acta Pharmacol Sin* **21**(12), 1157-64 (2000)].

See *Allium sativum* (Garlic): [Chander *et al.*; *Ethnobotany* **14**(1-2), 123-28 (2001)].

Angelica keiskei: Flavone glycosides, luteolin-7-O-β-glucoside and luteolin 7-O-β-rutinoside were isolated from methanolic extract of aerial parts of *A. keiskei*. Administration of methanolic extract of the plant (100mg/kg i.p.) and luteolin-7-O-β- D-glucoside (5mg/kg i.p.) exhibited significant antihyperlipidemic activity in rats [Park JC, Choys, Park SY, Park JR, Chun SS, K. KD, Choi JW; Isolation of flavone-7-O-glycosides from the aerial parts of *Angelica keiskei* and its antihyperlipidemic effect, *Korean J Pharmacogn* **26**(4), 337-43 (1995)].

Anisomeles malabarica (S. Vaikuntha): The plant belonging to family Labiatae has been selected for its hypocholesterolemic activity. The ethanolic extract of the aerial parts of this plant has been studied against the standard drug lipocor tablets and rabbits have been used as experimental animals. [Kalhoro MA, Kapadia Z, Badar Y; Comparative study of hypocholesterolemic activity in *Anisomeles malabarica* R.Bc., *J Faculty Pharm*, Gazi Univ **14**(1), 37-50 (1997)].

Annona squamosa (H. Sharifa, S. Sitaphala): Administration of aqueous extract of *A. squamosa* leaves (350 mg/kg bw) to streptozotocin-induced diabetic rats significantly lowered serum cholesterol, triglycerides, LDL- and VLDL-cholesterol levels alongwith enhancement of HDL-cholesterol. The extract also decreased lipid peroxidation with a significant increase in the activity of antioxidant enzymes (superoxide dismutase and catalase). [Gupta RK, Tyagi A, Watal G, Tandon V; Antioxidant and hypolipidemic effect of aqueous extract of *Annona squamosa* leaves in normal and STZ-induced diabetic rats, *Chemistry Biology Interface*: *Synergistics New Frontiers,* New Delhi, India, p. 25, November 21-26, 2004].

Apium graveolens (Celery, H. Ajmud, S. Ajamoda)): Incorporation of an aqueous extract of celery in high fat diet fed to rats, significantly reduced serum total cholesterol, LDL-cholesterol and triglyceride levels compared to rats given high fat diet without celery extract. However, celery treated rats exhibited significantly higher hepatic triglyceride contents. Hepatic triacylglycerol lipase activity was significantly decreased in celery treated rats. [Tsi D, Das NP, Tan BKH; Effect of aqueous celery (*Apium graveolens*) extract on lipid parameters of rats fed high fat diet, *Planta Med* **61**(1), 18-21 (1995)].

In genetically hyperchoesterolemic rats and triton-induced hypercholesterolemic mice, celery extract significantly lowered the serum total cholesterol levels without affecting serum triglyceride levels. [Tsi D, Tan BKH; Effect of aqueous celery extract on lipid profile in hypocholesterolemic rats and mice, *Phytomedicine* **3**(Suppl 1), 173 (1996/97)].

Drinking aqueous celery extract for 8 weeks caused a significant reduction in serum total cholesterol level in growing genetically hypercholesterolaemic (RICO) rats. In addition, administration of butanol and aqueous fractions of celery extract for 7 days by intraperitoneal infusion effectively decreased the serum total cholesterol and high-density lipoprotein cholesterol (HDL-c) levels of adult RICO rats. The butanol and aqueous fractions of celery extract lowered serum total cholesterol level mainly through increased bile acid excretion but not by modulating the activity of the rate-limiting enzyme for cholesterol biosynthesis, HMGCoA reductase. The presence of sugars and amino acids were detected in celery extract and there is a possibility that polar compounds with sugar or amino acid side chain(s) could contribute to the hypocholesterolaemic action of celery extract. [Tsi D; Tan BKH; The mechanism underlying the hypocholesterolaemic activity of aqueous celery extract, its butanol and aqueous fractions in genetically hypercholesterolaemic RICO rats, *Life Sci* **66**(8), 755-67 (2000)].

Arachis hypogaea (Peanut, Groundnut, H. Mungphali, S. Buchanaka)**:** See *Oryza sativa* [Seetharamaiah & Chandrasekhara, *Atherosclerosis*, **78**(2-3), 219-23 (1989)].

See *Glycine max* (Soya bean, soybean): [Jacques *et al.*, *Nutr-Res* **13**(8), 969-77 (1993)].

Aqueous extract of the plant caused a significant decrease in serum triglyceride, total cholesterol, HDL-cholesterol and LDL-cholesterol in both normal and alloxan-induced diabetic rats. [Bilbis LS, Shehu RA, Abubakar MG; Hypoglycemic and hypolipidemic effects of aqueous extract of *Arachis hypogaea* in normal and alloxan-induced diabetic rats, *Phytomedicine* **9**(6), 553-55 (2002)].

***Aralia elata*:** *A. elata* is an edible mountain vegetable in Korea. Ethanol extract of the plant was found to exert antioxidant and strong hypocholesterolemic and hypolipidemic effects *in vivo* with the administration of benzo-(α)-pyrene. [Chung CK, Jung ME; Ethanol fraction of *Aralia elata* Seemann enhances antioxidant activity and lowers serum lipids in rats when administered with benzo-(α)-pyrene, *Biol Pharm Bull* **26**(10), 1502-04 (2003)].

Aralia mandshurica (Manchurian aralia)**:** Saponosides of *A. mandshurica* and *Calendula officinalis* exhibited hypolipidemic activity in experimental normolipidemic and hyperlipidemic rats. [Wojcicki J, Samochowiec L; Comparative evaluation of *Aralia mandshuria Rupr, et maxim* and *Calendula officinalis* L saponosides effect on blood serum and liver homogenate, *Herba Pol* **26**(4), 233-37 (1980)].

In rats and rabbits the hypocholesterolemic activity of separal (a mixture of aralosides A, B and C with oleanolic acid) and oleanolic acid, isolated from *Aralia mandshurica* (Manchurian Aralia) was examined. These phytochemicals exhibited marked hypocholesterolemic activity alongwith lowering of β-lipoprotein contents. In liver and aortic tissue, there occurred a marked shift in the lipid metabolism parameters following administration of the phytochemicals. These compounds also reduced the cholesterol uptake in the blood. [Voskanyan VL, Vasilenko YK, Ponomarev VD; Hypolipidemic properties of separol and oleanolic acid, *Khim Farma Zh* **17**(2), 123-26 (1983)].

***Argania sideroxylon*:** The chronic ingestion of 5 ml/kg/d of argan oil (oil of *A. sideroxylon*) to spontaneously hypertensive rats restored normal blood pressure and induced hypocholesterolemia. The effect was verified by use of Meriones shawi, a rodent of the Gerbillideae family, as a second animal model. The action of polyunsatured fatty acids of the Argan oil is predominant, but in addition, other constituents play an active part. [Berrada Y, Settaf A, Baddouri K, Cherrah A, Hassar M; Experimental evidence of an antihypertensive and hypocholesterolemic effect of oil of argan, *Argania sideroxylon, Therapie* (London) **55**(3), 375-78 (2000) [Article in French].

***Argania spinosa*:** Significant reduction in blood lipoproteins was observed in rats receiving high calorie cholesterol-rich diet by administration of argan oil (1ml/100g bw) daily by oral route during 7 weeks. The beneficial effect of argan oil (oil from seeds of *Argania spinosa*) in the treatment of hyperlipidemia and hypercholesterolemia was shown. [Berrougui H, Ettaib A, Herrera Gonzalez MD, Alvarez de Sotomayor M, Bennani Kabchi N, Hmamouchi M; Hypolipidemic and hypocholesterolemic effect of argan oil (*Argania spinosa* L.) in Meriones shawi rats, *J Ethnopharmacol* **89**(1), 15-18 (2003)].

Aristolochia bracteata (H. Kiramar, S. Dhumrapatra)**:** See *Saccharum officinarum* [Tarvady & Dhar; *Biomedicine* **9** (1) 39-42 (1989); *Indian J Exp Biol* **28**(7), 657-60 (1990)].

***Artemisia* species:** Hypolipidemic effect of "Jianzhilin", a traditional chineese drug containing *Artemisia* spp, *Gardenia jasminoides*, *Psoralea corrylifolia* and *Phellodendron amurense* was investigated in 100 patients of hyperlipidemia. This compound drug significantly lowered the blood cholesterol, β- lipoprotein and triglycerides. The drug did not show any toxic effect. [Jing W, Fu G, Chen Y; Clinical observation of 100 patients with hyperlipidemia treated with traditional drug Jianzhilin, *Chin J Integ Trad West Med* **6**(1), 21-23 (1986)].

***Aster* species:** See Plant Fibres in Appendix: [Kim & Han; *Korean J Animal Sci* **27**(6), 374- 80 (1985)].

Avena sativa (Oat)**:** Male and female volunteers were paired in two groups based on similar cholesterol levels and each individual in group I, ate 43 g of oatmeal daily in the form of porridge for six weeks, while the corresponding individuals in the control group were given 43g of cornflakes daily. Serum cholesterol levels and. α-lipoprotein fractions were measured twice at three-week intervals during the experimental period and no significant differences were found between the groups. Porridge apparently did not have a hypocholesterolemic effect in the quantities consumed for the time period of this experiment. [Gormley TR, Kevany J, O'Donnell B, McFarlane R; Potential of porridge as a hypocholesterolemic agent, *Irish J Food Sci Technol* **2**(2), 85-92 (1979)].

See Plant fibres in Appendix: [Chen and Anderson; *Am J Clin Nutr* **34**(6), 1077-82 (1981)].

Oat bran products, rich in water-soluble fibre, have distinct hypocholesterolemic effects in humans. Oat-bran diets decreased serum cholesterol concentrations by 19%, low density lipoprotein cholesterol by 23%, increased faecal weight by 43% and also increased faecal bile acid excretion. Oat bran supplements may have an important role in nutritional management of selected hypercholesterolemic patients. [Anderson JW, Story L, Sieling B, Chen WJ, Petro MS, Story J; Hypocholesterolemic effects of oat bran or bean intake for hypercholesterolemic men, *Am J Clin Nutr* **40**(6), 1146-55 (1984)].

The hypocholesterolemic effects of dietary oat bran and its effects on gastrointestinal function and macromorphology were investigated. Plasma total cholesterol, the ratio of total to high-density lipoprotein cholesterol, liver cholesterol and liver lipid were decreased by diets containing 10-40% oat bran. Growth was consistently reduced only on 40% oat bran diets. Dietary oat bran level was consistently associated with progressive reductions in plasma total cholesterol, liver cholesterol and liver lipid but not with growth and thus the hypocholesterolemic effects of oat bran could not be attributed to reductions in weight gain. Chicks fed 30% oat bran also showed macromorphological gastrointestinal adaptations with enlarged stomachs and longer small intestines. [Welch RW, Peterson DM, Schramka B; Hypocholesterolemic gastrointestinal and associated responses to oat bran in chicks, *Nutr Res* **6**(8), 957-66 (1986)].

Dietary fibre has important hypocholesterolemic effects and may reduce risk for coronary artery disease. Foods such as oat bran or beans, rich in water-soluble fibre, can decrease serum total cholesterol by 19% while decreasing serum low density lipoprotein cholesterol by 22%. Food supplements rich in soluble fibre such as psyllium mucilloid are well tolerated and may lower serum cholesterol by 15%. [Anderson JW; Dietary fibre: Lipids and atherosclerosis, *Am J Cardiol* **60**(12), 17G-22G (1987)].

The effect of oat fibre on VLDL, LDL and HDL composition was investigated by feeding male Sprague-Dawley rat diets containing 1.0% cholesterol and 0.2% cholic acid, and 6% dietary fibre from oat bran, high-fibre oat flour or a processed oat product for 20 days. Compared to cholesterol-fed cellulose controls, all oat fibres altered the response to cholesterol feeding as indicated by 25-45% lower total lipoprotein cholesterol, 40-60% lower VLDL + LDL-cholesterol, and 25-40% higher HDL cholesterol contents. The effect of the oat fibres on VLDL composition was especially pronounced as demonstrated by 30-65% lower VLDL protein, VLDL apo E and plasma apo B concentrations. The processed oat product, which contained 40% more soluble fibre than oat bran or oat flour, normalised the lipoprotein profile associated with ingestion of the atherogenic diet significantly more than oat bran or oat flour. It was thus inferred that ingestion of oat fibre tends to normalise the lipoprotein profile induced by feeding an atherogenic diet in the rat. [Ney DM, Lasekan JB, Shinnick FL; Soluble oat fibre tends to normalise lipoprotein composition in cholesterol-fed rats, *J Nutr* **118**(12), 1455-62 (1988)].

Oat and bean products, which contain large amounts of water-soluble fibre, are particularly effective hypocholesterolemic agents. Recent experiments with human subjects using these products as supplements to the diet were reviewed. [Anderson JW, Gustafson NJ; Hypocholesterolemic effects of oat and bean products, *Am J Clin Nutr* **48**(3 Suppl), 749-53 (1988)].

Experiments were conducted on chicks to determine which of the five components (oil, starch and insoluble fibre, protein, gum, and soluble residue), separated from oat bran is responsible for the hypocholesterolemic and gastrointestinal effects of oat bran. Compared to the control, only the diets containing oat bran or the gum or protein fractions significantly reduced plasma total cholesterol. Only oat bran and gum diets significantly lowered liver cholesterol. Intestinal transit times were not significantly different between the control and each experimental diet. Small intestine length was significantly increased only by oat bran or oat gum diets. Native oat bran and the remixed fractions gave similar responses indicating that the effects of oat bran were not influenced by the fractionation procedure. Although the protein fraction contributed to the hypocholesterolemic properties of oat bran, gum is the main cholesterol-lowering agent in oat bran, and its effect appears to be associated with increases in small intestine length. [Welch RW, Peterson DM, Schramka B; Hypocholesterolemic and gastrointestinal effects of oat bran fractions in chicks, *Nutr Reports International* **38**(3), 551-62 (1988)].

See *Oryza sativa:* [Haumann BF; *J Am Oil Chem Soc* **66**(5), 615-18 (1989)].

Because of the similarities in the responses of humans and of the cholesterol-fed rats to oat fibre ingestion, it was suggested that larger intakes of soluble oat fibre might be accompanied by greater reduction in serum cholesterol levels in humans. [Shinnick FL, Ink SL, Marlett JA; Dose response to a dietary oat bran fraction in cholesterol-fed rats, *J Nutr* **120**(6), 561-68 (1990).].

Hypocholesterolemic effects of oat products have been reviewed. [Anderson JW, Siesel AE; Hypocholesterolemic effects of oat products. *Adv Exp Med Biol* **270**,17-36 (1990)].

Oat cereals are rich in water-soluble fibre, β-glucan and a dose-dependent reduction in LDLc levels with oat cereals supports the independent hypocholesterolemic effects of β- glucan. [Davidson MH, Dugan LD, Burns JH, Bova J, Story K, Drennan KB; The hypocholesterolemic effects of β-glucan in oatmeal and oat bran: A dose-controlled study, *J Am Med Assoc* **265**(14), 1833-39 (1991)].

To carefully document the hypocholesterolemic effects of oat bran, which have been recently challenged, 20 hypercholesterolemic men were randomly allocated to either oat bran or wheat bran for 21 days after a seven-day control-diet period. Control and treatment diets were designed to be identical in energy content and nutrients, differing only in the amount of soluble fibre. After 21 days, oat bran significantly decreased total cholesterol by 12.8%, low density lipoprotein cholesterol by 12.1%, and apolipoprotein B-100 by 13.7% whereas wheat bran had no significant effect. High density lipoprotein cholesterol and apolipoprotein A-I did not change significantly in either group. Serum triglycerides decreased by 10% in both groups. [Anderson JW, Gilinsky NH, Deakins DA, Smith SF, O'Neal DS, Dillon DW, Oeltgen PR; Lipid responses of hypercholesterolemic men to oat bran and wheat bran intake, *Am J Clin Nutr* **54**(4), 678-83 (1991)].

Triton WR 1339 - induced hypercholesterolemic rats were treated with *A. sativa* hydroalcoholic extract (15 ml/kg bw/d; the extract containing 0.533 mg water-soluble fibres and 0.64 mg saponins/ml) for three weeks. A significant decrease of cholesterolemia in hypercholesterolemic rats receiving *A.sativa* hydroalcoholic extract was obtained. [Coprean D, Giurgea R, Hodisan V, Coprean D; Hypocholesterolemic effect of oat bran hydroalcoholic extract, *Revue Roumaine de Biologie Serie de Biologie Animale* **36**(1-2), 85-87 (1991)].

In adult male rats fed on a cholesterol-free synthetic diet, plasma cholesterol concentrations were lowest with oat bran, intermediate with cellulose and highest with wheat bran. Plasma triacylglycerols were similar with wheat bran and cellulose but higher with oat bran. Feeding oat bran after extraction with n-pentane gave plasma cholesterol concentrations similar to that found with wheat bran. Reconstitution of oat bran with extracted lipids did not restore the cholesterol-lowering effect. It is concluded that oat bran affects cholesterol metabolism through a pentane-soluble component as well as non-starch polysaccharides. It appears that the activity of this lipid is not transferable by simple addition of the solvent extract to the whole diet. [Illman RJ, Topping DL, Dowling K, Trimble RP, Russell GR, Storer GB; Effects of solvent extraction on the hypocholesterolemic action of oat bran in the rat, *Brit J Nutr* **65**(3), 435-44 (1991)].

To determine whether oat bran possesses greater cholesterol-lowering activity than wheat bran, the effects of breads of similar total fibre content containing either oat bran or wheat bran were compared. Twelve hyperlipidaemic subjects were stabilised on lipid-lowering diets for at least three months prior to the study. Subjects were given each type of bread for four-week periods in a single blind, crossover design. Cholesterol, triglyceride and LDL-cholesterol levels did not change significantly during the oat and wheat bread periods. HDL-cholesterol rose equivalently but only to a just significant level during the oat bran diet. Both diet treatments lowered serum cholesterol approximately 4%. The findings indicate that oat bran bread consumed as part of a lipid-correcting diet does not influence lipoproteins to any greater extent than wheat bread of similar total fibre content. [Bremer JM, Scott RS, Lintott CJ; Oat bran and cholesterol reduction: Evidence against specific effect, *Australian New Zealand J Med* **21**(4), 422-26 (1991)].

See *Cyamopsis tetragonoloba:* [Spiller *et al.; Arterioscler Thromb.* **11**(5), 1204-8 (1991)].

A higher excretion of dry matter, fat, nitrogen and total bile acids in ileal effluents; a lower plasma low density lipoprotein (LDL) and total cholesterols but no change in plasma highdensity lipoprotein (HDL) cholesterol or apolipoproteins A-I and B were observed in nine subjects with ileostomies when they consumed an oat bran bread-based high-fibre diet as compared with a wheat-flour bread-based low-fibre diet for 3 weeks. Total cholesterol, LDL-cholesterol, and apolipoprotein B in plasma decreased by 11.3%, 15.3%, and 10.7%, respectively, after consumption of the oat bran-based high-fibre diet for 3 weeks. [Zhang JX, Hallmans G, Andersson H, Bosaeus I, Aman P, Tidehag P, Stenling R, Lundin E, Dahlgren S; Effect of oat bran on plasma cholesterol and bile acid excretion in nine subjects with ileostomies, *Am J Clin Nutr* **56**(1), 99-105 (1992)].

Oat bran decreased serum cholesterol 12.8% whereas wheat bran had no effect. Mechanisms for the hypocholesterolemic effects of oat bran remain unclear. Soluble fibres such as oat bran are fermented in the colon to short-chain fatty acids, which may enter the portal vein and attenuate hepatic cholesterol synthesis. Serum acetate values were significantly higher in subjects fed with oat bran compared to those receiving wheat bran diets. [Bridges SR, Anderson JW, Deakins DA, Dillon DW, Wood CL; Oat bran increases serum acetate of hypercholesterolemic men, *Am J Clin Nutr* **56**(2), 455-59 (1992)].

The effect of replacement of conventional continental breakfast by a single oat bran cereal muesli containing 60 g of oat bran on serum lipids in 13 patients with hypercholesterolemia type IIa was studied. In the first, second, and third week of oat bran ingestion, the total serum cholesterol level was reduced by 10.9, 8.4 and 9.7%, respectively. High density lipoprotein and low density lipoprotein cholesterol as well as apolipoprotein A1 decreased to the same extent (8 to 11%) during the oat bran period, whereas a pronounced reduction of 25.8% was seen for apolipoprotein B100, which is a major component of low density lipoprotein. [Bartram P, Gerlach S, Scheppach W, Keller F, Kasper H; Effect of a single oat bran cereal breakfast on serum cholesterol, lipoproteins, and apolipoproteins in patients with hyperlipoproteinemia type IIa, *JPEN* **16**(6), 533-7 (1992)].

The effects of β-glucan-rich oat bran on serum lipids and lipoproteins were examined in a randomized 8-week study. After a 4-week run-in phase, subjects with mild to moderate hypercholesterolemia on cholesterol-lowering diets were randomly allocated to an oat bran (10.3 g β-glucan/d) or wheat bran group. Serum total cholesterol (TC) and low density lipoprotein cholesterol (LDL-c) significantly declined in the oat bran group during the first 4 weeks but at 8 weeks the values were not significantly different from baseline. Changes in serum TC were mainly confined to those who ate at least two-thirds of the planned daily dose of oat bran. In wheat bran group no changes were observed in serum TC or LDL-c levels. Apolipoprotein A1 and B did not change significantly in either group. Only subjects with apolipoprotein E 3/3 phenotype had hypocholesterolemic response to oat bran at 4 weeks [Uusitupa MI, Ruuskanen E, Makinen E, Laitinen J, Toskala E, Kervinen K, Kesaniemi YA; A controlled study on the effect of β- glucan-rich oat bran on serum lipids in hypercholesterolemic subjects: relation to apolipoprotein E phenotype, *J Am Coll Nutr* **11**(6), 651-59 (1992)].

The hypocholesterolemic activity of oat bran concentrate depends upon the method of extraction, viscosity, hydrodynamic properties, and molecular weight of β-glucan present in the bran. The diet containing untreated oat bran was found ineffective. The factors influencing the hypocholesterolemic activity of oat bran concentrate have been discussed. [Malkki Y, Autio K, Hanninen O, Myllymaki O, Pelkonen K, Suortti T, TorronenR; Oat bran concentrates: Physical properties of β- glucan and hypocholesterolemic effects in rats, *Cereal Chem* **69**(6), 647-53 (1992)].

High fibre muffins, prepared by replacing traditionally used wheat flour with oat bran, a high β-glucan barley fraction or rice bran, provided relatively more total dietary fibres compared to commercial oat bran muffins and contained more moisture, proteins and fewer calories with low glycemic properties than the commercial muffins. [Hudson CA, Chiu MM, Knuckles BB; Development and characteristics of high fibres muffins with oat bran, rice bran or barley fibre fractions, *Cereal Foods World* **37** (5) 373-376 (1992)].

See *Plantago psyllium* (Psyllium): [Arjmandi *et al; J Nutr* **122**(2), 246-53 (1992)].

See Tocotrienols in Appendix: [Pearce *et al.; J Med Chem* **35**(2), 3595-606 (1992)].

The effect of dietary fibres on plasma lipids, liver cholesterol and faecal cholesterol excretion was investigated in hamsters. After 4 weeks of fibre diet consumption, the plasma total cholesterol concentrations of diet-induced hypercholesterolemic hamsters were significantly decreased in the oat bran, guar gum and xylan groups. Plasma HDL-cholesterol concentration was significantly decreased only in the guar gum group. The combined plasma VLDL+LDL-cholesterol concentrations were significantly lowered by the oat bran, xylan and cellulose diets. [Jonnalagadda SS, Thye FW, Robertson JL; Plasma total and lipoprotein cholesterol, liver cholesterol and faecal cholesterol excretion in hamsters-fed fibre diets, *J Nutr* **123**(8), 1377-82 (1993)].

Ethanolic extract of legumes of *A. sativa* exhibited cholesterol-lowering activity. [Gorecki P, Mseisz A, Segiet Kujawa E, Kedzia B; Phytochemical analytical microbiological and pharmacological investigations of a polish *Avena sativa* sort, *Planta Med* **59**(Suplement), A 674 (1993)].

See *Hordeum vulgare* (Barley) [Wang and Klopfenstein; *Cereal Chem* **70**(6), 712-15 (1993)].

Amylodextrins with soluble β- glucan contents from 1 to 10% were prepared from oats and the hypocholesterolemic properties of the preparation (OATRIM) were evaluated. It lowered blood cholesterol. In the chick model, it decreased total blood cholesterol and LDL-cholesterol and increased HDL-cholesterol. [Inglett GE, Newman RK, Oat β- glucan-amylodextrins: Preliminary preparations and biological properties, *Plant Foods Hum Nutr* **45**(1), 53-61 (1994)].

Despite beneficial hypocholesterolemic effects associated with β-glucan, the water-soluble fibre component of oat, β-glucan content in oat grain is variable and it depends on environment, especially soil nitrogen and year-to-year climatic variability. [Brunner BR, Freed RD; Oat grain β-glucan content as affected by nitrogen level, location, and year, *Crop Sci* **34**(2), 473-76 (1994)].

A nutritional evaluation of oatrim (an oat product) in chicks showed a very significant reduction in total and low density lipoprotein cholesterol levels. [Inglett GE, Warner K, Newman RK; Sensory and nutritional evaluations of oatrim, *Cereal Foods World* **39**(10), 755- 56, 758-59 (1994)].

Untreated oat bran and hydrolysed oat bran (hydrolysed by endo-β-D-glucanases from *Bacillus subtilis*) were incorporated into hypercholesterolemic purified diets and fed to rats for 4 weeks; a diet containing cellulose was used as a control. Hepatic cholesterol accumulation was affected by dietary treatment and this was less in the oat bran group than in the enzyme-treated oat bran or cellulose groups. Thus, functional properties of β-D-glucan, such as viscosity, appear to be related to its hypocholesterolemic potential. [Tietyen JL, Nevins DJ, Shoemaker CF, Schneeman BO; Hypocholesterolemic potential of oat bran treated with an endo-β-Dglucanase from *Bacillus subtilis, J Food Sci* **60**(3), 558-60, 579 (1995)].

See *Plantago psyllium* [Matheson *et al.*; *J Nutr* **125**(3), 454-8 (1995)].

See Plant Fibres in Appendix: [Ismail *et al.*; *Biochem Arch* **13**(3), 161-70 (1997)].

See *Oryza sativa* (Rice): [Gerhardt and Gallo; *J Nutr* **128**(5), 865-9 (1998)].

See *Oryza sativa* (Rice): [Kahlon *et al.*; *Cereal Chem* **75**(6), 897-903 (1998)].

The oat bran was processed by means of extrusion and the hyperlipidemic rats were fed with extruded oat bran for 4 weeks. The hypocholesterolemic effect of extruded oat bran was better than control group. Extrusion is an effective method of increasing the biological action of dietary fibre and improving the quality of oat bran. [Anonymous; The effect of extruded oat bran on level of serum lipid in rats and analysis of nutrients composition, *Acta Nutr Sinica* **21**(2), 196-99 (1999) Article in Chinese].

See *Amaranthus* species: [Grajeta H; *Nahrung* **43**(2), 114-7 (1999)].

The effects of β-glucan from oat bran in bread, cookies and in orange juice on serum lipoproteins in mildly hypercholesterolemic subjects were studied. From the study, it was concluded that the food matrix or the food processing, or both, could have adverse effects on the hypocholesterolemic properties of oat β-glucan. [Kerckhoffs DA, Hornstra G, Mensink RP; Cholesterol-lowering effect of β-glucan from oat bran in mildly hypercholesterolemic subjects may decrease when β-glucan is incorporated into bread and cookies, *Am J Clin Nutr* **78**(2), 221-7 (2003)].

Averrhoa bilimbi (H. Bilimbi)**:** To study the hypoglycemic and hypolipidemic effect of an ethanolic extract of leaves of the plant, streptozotocin-induced diabetic rats were treated with vehicle (distilled water), the plant extract (125 mg/kg) or metformin (500 mg/kg) twice a day for 2 weeks. Like metformin, leaf extract of the plant significantly lowered blood glucose and blood triglyceride when compared with the vehicle. The plant extract also significantly increased the HDL-cholesterol concentrations, the antiatherogenic index and HDL-cholesterol/ total cholesterol ratio. The plant extract was thus proved to have hypoglycemic, hypotriglyceridemic, anti-lipid peroxidative and anti-atherogenic properties in STZ-diabetic rats. [Pushparaj P, Tan CH, Tan BK; Effects of *Averrhoa bilimbi* leaf extract on blood glucose and lipids in streptozotocin-diabetic rats, *J Ethnopharmacol* **72**(1-2), 69-76 (2000)].

Water-soluble fraction of the ethanol extract of *Averrhoa bilimbi* leaves showed significant potency in the amelioration of hyperglycemia and hyperlipidemia in high fat diet -fed streptozotocin-induced diabetic rats. Aqueous fraction was found to be more potent than butanol-soluble fraction. Aqueous fraction is considered to be a potential source for the isolation of active principle(s) for oral anti-diabetic therapy. [Tan BK, Tan CH, Pushparaj PN; Anti-diabetic activity of the semi-purified fractions of *Averrhoa bilimbi* in high fat diet-fed streptozotocin- induced diabetic rats, *Life Sci* **76**(24), 2827-39 (2005)].

Azadirachta indica (H. Neem, S. Nimba)**:** Effect of intraperetoneal adminstration of an extract of *A. indica* on some biological constituents of rat blood was studied. The leaf extract significantly decreased serum cholesterol but the levels of serum protien, blood urea and uric acid remained unchanged. [Chattopadhyay RR, Sarkar SK, Ganguli S, Banerjee RN; Active effects of *A. indica* leaves on some biochemical constituents of blood in rats, *Sci Cult* **58**(182), 39-40 (1992)].

Effect of Neem oil on hyperlipidemia was studied in chicks. Administration of Neem oil to cholesterol-fed chicks lowered the serum total cholesterol, triglycerides, phospholipids and LDL-cholesterol levels. Hyperlipidemia induced aortic lesions also regressed following neem oil treatment. In addition, neem oil and the bark extract of neem showed antihyperglycemic and anti-androgenic activity. [Dixit VP, Jain Prabha, Purohit AK; Medicinal uses of neem (*Azadirachta indica*) in fertility regulation, diabetes and atherosclerosis, *Recent Advances in Medicinal, Aromatic and Spice crops, Today and Tomorrow,* New Delhi India, 2, 463-71 (1992)].

Administration of *A. indica* leaf extract to atherogenic diet-fed rats significantly lowered the serum and liver cholesterol, total lipids and triglycerides. [Chattopadhyay RR; Hypolipidemic activity of *Azadirachta indica* leaf extract in rats, *Proc Ind Natl Sci Acad* B **61**(4), 281-84 (1995)].

Ethanolic extract of neem (*A. indica*) flowers caused lowering of cholesterol, phospholipids, and triglyceride levels in hyperlipidemic rabbits. Liver and heart lipid contents were also decreased following treatment with neem flower extract in these animals. [Purohit A, Daradka HMM; Hypolipidemic effects of neem flower (*Azadirachta indica* A.Juss) in rabbits, *Geobios* **26**(2-3), 146-48 (1999)].

In hyperlipidemic rabbits, 50% ethanolic extract of *A. indica* barks normalised the cholesterol levels. The bark extract also decreased the serum phospholipids and triglycerides levels in these animals. Liver and heart tissue lipid contents were also reduced following treatment with neem bark extract. [Purohit A, Purohit Y, Vyas KK; Hypolipidemic effect of neem bark (*Azadirachta indica* A.Juss) in rabbits, *Indian J Nutr Diet* **36**(2), 53-57 (1999)].

In alloxan-induced diabetic rabbits, effect of neem (*A. indica*) leaf extract (100, 200 and 400 mg/kg) on lipid profile was studied. At the end of 7, 14 and 28 days, neem leaf extract significantly lowered blood cholesterol, triglyceride and sugar levels in diabetic animals. HDL-cholesterol level was enhanced in treated animals. Maximum decrease in blood cholesterol, triglycerides and sugar levels and increase in the HDL cholesterol level was noted in the rabbits that received neem leaf extract with tolbutamide. It was suggested that in view of the potent hypoglycemic and antihyperlipidemic activity, neem leaf extract might be effective in cases of atherosclerosis. [Gosain R, Devi I; Effect of *Azadirachta indica* on blood glucose and lipid profile in alloxan induced diabetes in rabbits, *J Med Arom Plant Sci* **22**(Suppl I), 32-33 (2000)].

Administration of aqueous extract of *A. indica* fresh leaves (250mg/kg) for 16 weeks to streptozotocin-induced diabetic rats significantly lowered the levels of serum cholesterol, triglyceride, LDL-cholesterol and blood glucose levels. This extract also improved the body weight and diabetes-induced retinopathy. [Ali Hussain HEM; Reversal of diabetic retinopathy in streptozotocin induced diabetic rats using traditional Indian antidiabetic plant, *Azadirachta indica, Indian J Clin Biochem* **17**(2), 115-23 (2002)].

See *Commiphora mukul:* [Raut et al.; *J Mahatma Gandhi Inst Med Sci* **7**(2), 10-16 (2002)].

B

Balanites aegyptiaca (H. Hingan, S. Ingudi)**:** Whole and extracted pulps of *B. aegyptiaca* fruits were tested as a hypocholesterolemic agent using adult albino rats. The addition of 10% whole or extracted pulp to the diet at the expense of starch caused a highly significant decrease in the serum and liver cholesterol and serum protein levels when compared with a positive control (hypocholesterolemic diet). The fruit pulp was thus proved to contain powerful hypocholesterolemic agent(s). [Abdel Rahim EA, El Saadany SS, Wasif MM; Biochemical dynamics of hypocholesterolemic action of *Balanites aegyptiaca* fruit, *Food Chemi* **20**(1), 69- 78 (1986)].

Balduina angustifolia**:** Administration of halenalin, isolated from *B. angustifolia*, to mice at a dose of 20mg/kg/d significantly lowered serum cholesterol and serum triglycerides. Similar results were also obtained by tenulin and aromaticin, isolated from *Helenium amarum* and eupahyssopin from *Eupatorium hyssopifolium* and some of their synthetic analogues. Hypolipidemic activity of these compounds was attributed to the presence of α-methylene-γ- lactone moiety, β-unsubstituted cyclopentenone ring and α-epoxycyclopentenone system. [Hall IH, Lee KH, Starnes CO, Muraoka O, Simida Y, Wadddell TG; Antihyperlipidemic activity of sesquiterpene lactones and related compounds, *J Pharm Sci* **69**(6), 694-97 (1980)].

Bambusa arundinacea (H. Bans, S. Vansh)**:** See *Saccharum officinarum:* [Tarvady & Dhar; *Biomedicine* **9** (1) 39-42 (1989) and *Indian J Exp Biol* **28**(7), 657-60 (1990)].

Barbarea orthoceras (Winter cress): See *Brassica campestris:* [Garbuzov *et al.*; *Vopr Pitan* (4), 46-8 (1986)].

***Bauhinia candicans*:** Phytochemical analysis of the leaves and flowers of *B. candicans* revealed the presence of steroids, flavonoids and protoalkaloids. Trigonelline, isolated from its aqueous extract, elicited hypocholesterolemic and hypoglycemic effects. [Iribarren AM, Pomilio AB; Components of *Bauhinia candicans*, *J Nat Prod* **46**(5), 752-53 (1983)].

Berberis aristata (H. Dar haldi, S. Daru haridra)**:** Hypolipidemic effect of a decoction of a mixture of *B. aristata, Nymphaea lotus, Prunus bokharensis* and *Rosa indica* was evaluated in cholesterol-fed and normal rabbits. The decoction (1g or 2g/kg bw) significantly reduced serum cholesterol levels in hypercholesterolemic rabbits after one week. However, the formulation did not affect the serum cholesterol levels in normal rabbits. [Kamran MAJ, Ahmad Q R; Hypocholesterimic effect of a crude drug mixture of Pakistani herbs in rabbits, *Int J Pharmacogn* **30**(1), 5-8 (1992)].

Beta vulgaris (Sugar beet, H. Chukandar, S. Palanki): The effects of coarse and fine sugar beet fibre and coarse wheat bran were compared with those of cellulose on rat weight gains, serum and liver lipids, and faecal weight and water-holding capacity. No significant differences were found in overall weight gains or feed efficiencies with diets containing various fibres at the 5% level of supplementation. By the end of the sixth week, total serum cholesterol levels were lower in animals fed beet fibre diets than in those fed with the cellulose diet, and the lowering effect was not at the expense of high density lipoprotein cholesterol. Animals fed with 5% wheat bran diet had cholesterol levels intermediate between those of animals fed with cellulose and beet fibre. Increasing levels of beet fibre also resulted in reduced liver cholesterol pools. At the end of week 6, serum triglyceride concentrations did not differ significantly among groups, but rats fed with sugar beet fibre had lower liver triglyceride concentrations. Coarse beet fibre appeared to have a greater effect than fine beet fibre. The results indicate that sugar beet fibre has potential as a dietary aid in the treatment of hypercholesterolemia and constipation. [Klopfenstein CF; Nutritional properties of coarse and fine sugar beet fibre, hard and red wheat bran: **I**: Effects on rat serum and liver cholesterol and triglycerides and on faecal characteristics, *Cereal Chem* **67**(6), 538-41 (1990)].

The effects of beet dietary fibre were examined in rats fed with acholesterol-free feed containing sucrose and 25% casein for 45 weeks. The addition of beet dietary fibre to the level of 5% prevented the elevation of serum cholesterol and triglyceride levels in rats fed the 25% casein basal diet. Beet fibre lowered the lipid levels in the liver and the weight of epididymal fat tissues. Pectin did not affect lipid levels but increased faecal sterol excretion and beet fibre did not. Therefore, the effect of beet dietary fibre in helping to make serum lipids normal was related to factors other than changes in faecal sterol excretion. The hypocholesterolemic activity of beet fibre was independent of changes in the concentrations of short-chain fatty acids in the cecum. Based on this observation and the fact that cecectomy prevented beet dietary fibre having any of these effects, it was suggested that its effect in helping to make serum cholesterol levels normal was associated with its fermentation or to changes in other cecal functions. [Aritsuka T, Tanaka K, Kiriyama S; Long-term effects of serum cholesterol concentration of beet dietary fibre in normal cecectomized rats fed a cholesterol-free casein diet, *Nippon Nogeikagaku Kaishi* **66**(5), 881-89 (1992) Article in Japanese].

Dietary beet fibre lowers plasma cholesterol concentrations in rats, and the lower digestive tract, especially the cecum, seems to be necessary for this effect. [Nishimura N, Nishikawa H, Kiriyama S; Ileorectostomy or cecectomy but not colectomy abolishes the plasma cholesterol lowering effect of dietary beet fibre in rats, *J Nutr* **123**(7), 1260-69 (1993)].

Experiments revealed that the hypocholesterolemic effect of dietary beet fibre is associated with diminished expression of the hepatic apolipoprotein A-I gene. [Sonoyama K, Nishikawa H, Kiriyama S, Niki R; Apolipoprotein mRNA in liver and intestine of rats is affected by dietary beet fibre or cholestyramine, *J Nutr* **125**(1), 13-19 (1995)].

It has been suggested that the cecum plays an important role in the regulation of hepatic apolipoprotein A-I expression, which seems to be responsible for the hypocholesterolemic effect of dietary beet fibre. [Sonoyama K, Kiriyama S, Niki R; Expression of apolipoprotein AI mRNA in liver and intestine of cecectomized rats fed with beet fibre, *J Nutr Biochem* **6**(7), 380-84 (1995)].

See Plant Fibres in Appendix: [Ismail *et al.*; *Biochem Arch* **13**(3), 161-70 (1997)].

The effect of diets supplemented with sugar beet pulp fibre (10%) and apple pomace fibre (10%) on lipids and lipids peroxides was investigated in male Wistar rats. The results of the investigation demonstrate that sugar beet pulp fibre and to a lesser degree apple pomace fibre possess hypolipidemic properties. These properties are more evident when sugar beet pulp fibre or apple pomace fibre is added to the diet of rats fed with cholesterol. The hypolipidemic effects of both sugar beet pulp fibre and apple pomace fibre can be attributed to their water-soluble parts. The sugar beet pulp and apple pomace fibres have no antioxidant properties. [Leontowicz M; Gorinstein S, Bartnikowska E, Leontowicz H, Kulasek G, Trakhtenberg S; Sugar beet pulp and apple pomace dietary fibres improve lipid metabolism in rats fed with cholesterol, *Food Chem* **72**(1), 73-78 (2001)].

***Betula* species** (Birch tree): The triterpene betulenol, isolated from birch bark, and its diacetate showed hypolipidemic, cholagogic, antilithogenic and hepatoprotective activities. [Vasilenko IuK, Semenchenko VF, Frolova LM, Konopleva GE, Parfent'eva EP, Skul'te IV; The pharmacological properties of the triterpenoids from birch bark, *Eksp Klin Farmakol* **56**(4), 53-5 (1993) [Article in Russian].

***Bidens pilosa*:** Feeding of 10 % fructose solution for 3-6 weeks to Wistar rats increased the blood levels of cholesterol and insulin alongwith enhancement of systolic blood pressure. Administration of *B. pilosa* leaf extract to these rats caused significant reduction of insulin and cholesterol levels. This drug also lowered the blood pressure. [Dimo T, Rakotonirina SV, Tan VP, Azay J, Dongo E, Cros G; Leaf methanol extract of *Bidens pilosa* prevents and attenuates the hypertension induced by high fructose diet in Wistar rats, *J Ethnopharmacol* **83**(3), 183-91 (2002)].

Biophytum sensitivum (H. Lajalu, S. Lajjaluka): The possible hypocholesterolemic effect of water extract of leaves of *B. sensitivum* was examined on male albino rabbits. The treatment of hypercholesterolemic rabbits with the plant extract not only prevented the elevation of serum triglycerides, very low density lipoprotein plus low density lipoprotein cholesterol (VLDL-c + LDL-c), and the ratios of total cholesterol to high density lipoprotein cholesterol (TC/HDL-c) and (VLDL-c + LDL-c)/HDL-c, but also brought down most of these values. The plant extract thus showed significant hypocholesterolemic effect. [Puri D; Hypocholesterolemic effect of *Biophytum sensitivum* leaf water extract, *Pharm Biol* **41**(4), 253-58 (2003)].

Bombax mori: Hypolipidemic effect of the unani formulation containing *Bombax mori*, *Nepeta hindostana* and *Terminalia arjuna* was examined on 50 human volunteers. This compound drug significantly lowered the serum cholesterol, triglyceride and VLDL-cholesterol levels as compared to placebo treated volunteers. No side effects were noted. [Ahmad N, Tajuddin, Saba Z, Ahmad S; Hypolipidemic effect of a non-pharmacopial unani formulation, *National Symposium on Emerging Trends in Indian Medicinal Plants*, Lucknow p 89 (8- 0/8)10-12 October, 2003].

Borago officinalis: In hyperlipidemic rats, feeding of oil of *Borago officinalis* led to significant lowering of serum total lipid, triglycerides and LDL-cholesterol along with enhancement of HDL-cholesterol levels. Similarly, liver tissue lipid contents were also reduced in treated hyperlipidemic rats. Hypolipidemic activity of Borago oil was attributed to its high γ -linolenic acid contents. Cholesterol induced plasma LDL-receptor activity was also diminished by this oil. [El-Gengaihi S, Salem A, Bashandi Ibrahim N, Abdel Hamid S; Chemical and biological evaluation of *Borago officinalis* L., *Phytomedicine* **7**(Suppl. II), 116 (2000)]

Borassus flabellifer (Palmyra Palm, H. Tar, S. Tal): Ethanolic extract of female palm exhibited hypocholesterolemic and hypoglycemic activity. [Ravishanker B, Sasikala CK, Sasaswathy VN, Sulochana S; Some pharmacological studies on female palm of *Borassus flabellifer* Linn (Palmyra palm), *J Res Ayur Siddha* **10**(1-2), 75-86 (1989)].

Boswellia serrata (H. Luban, S. Shallaki): Experimental study revealed that *Boswellia serrata* affected the cholesterol biosynthesis in a dose dependant manner. [Zutshi U, Rao PG, Kaur S, Singh GB, Surjeet singh, Atal CK; Mechanism of cholesterol lowering effect of salai guggulu ex. *Boswellia serrata* Roxb, *Ind J Pharmacol* **18**(3), 182-83 (1986)].

Brassica campestris (Rapeseed, H. Sarson, S. Sarshap): Rapeseed and Linden (*Tilia cordata*) pollens significantly decreased the serum lipid concentration in high lipid diet-fed rats. Both these pollens also significantly reduced the hepatic lipid contents. In addition, the pollens lowered the blood glucose levels in these animals. [Samochowiee L, Wojcicki J; Effect of pollen on serum and liver lipids in rats fed on high lipid diet, *Herba Pol* **27**(4), 333-39 (1981)].

The capacity of rape and winter cress (*Barbarea orthoceras*) oils to decrease a high cholesterol level in the blood and liver was studied in cholesterol-fed rats. Based on the data obtained it is suggested that rape oil and winter cress oil initiate the lipid transport in the blood and tissues leading to the reduction of the cholesterol level in the blood and liver tissue in cholesterol-fed rats. [Garbuzov AG, Kalinina TI, Nazarova NA, Levachev MM; Hypocholesterolemic action of oils from the seeds of new selection varieties of winter rape and winter cress in trials on rats, *Vopr Pitan* (4), 46-8 (1986) Article in Russian].

The effects of different monounsaturated fatty acid (MUFA)-rich oils (18:1-rich sunflower oil, rapeseed oil, olive oil) in comparison to polyunsaturated (PUFA)-rich oils (18:2-rich sunflower oil) and saturated fat (palm stearin) on cholesterol and bile acid metabolism were studied using Syrian golden hamsters. After 5 weeks, plasma total cholesterol (TC) was highest with palm stearin while the MUFA- or PUFA-rich fats significantly lowered TC. The lowest TC concentrations were found with refined rapeseed, cold pressed rapeseed and 18:2-rich sunflower oil, whereas TC was 10-15% higher with 18:1-rich sunflower, virgin and refined olive oil. Liver cholesterol concentrations were lowest in hamsters, fed palm stearin or 18:2-rich sunflower oil while MUFA-rich fats increased hepatic cholesteryl ester accumulation, especially of cholesteryl oleate. There were no significant differences in the faecal neutral sterol and bile acid excretion. The data demonstrated that MUFA-rich dietary fats, e.g. rapeseed, olive and 18:1-rich sunflower oil, are comparable in their hypocholesterolemic potential and cause similar effects on plasma cholesterol as 18:2-rich sunflower oil in hamsters when the dietary cholesterol intake is moderate. [Trautwein EA, Rieckhoff D, Kunath-Rau A, Erbersdobler HF; Replacing saturated fat with PUFA-rich (sunflower oil) or MUFA-rich (rapeseed, olive and high-oleic sunflower oil) fats resulted in comparable hypocholesterolemic effects in cholesterol-fed hamsters, *Ann Nutr Metab* **43**(3), 159-72 (1999)].

Fatty acids, sterols, antioxidant compounds, stability and total radical-trapping antoxidative potential (TRAP) of four different seed oils (sunflower, sunflower high oleic, rapeseed and grapeseed oils) were determined with an objective to find atherosclerosis preventing diets. The highest stability and the highest TRAP and the lowest stability and the lowest TRAP were in rapeseed and sunflower oils, respectively. Rapeseed oil has high organoleptic properties and the highest antioxidant capacity. Its influence on plasma lipid levels and antioxidant potential is significantly higher than of oils with relatively low antioxidant capacity. The above-mentioned properties make rapeseed oil a preferable choice for atherosclerosis preventing diets. [Gorinstein S, Leontowicz H, Leontowicz M, Lojek A, Ciz M, Krzeminski R, Zachwieja Z,

Jastrzebski Z, Delgado Licon E, Martin Belloso O, Trakhtenberg S; Seed oils improve lipid metabolism and increase antioxidant potential in rats fed diets containing cholesterol, *Nutr Res* **23**(3), 317-30 (2003)].

Brassica juncea (Mustard, H. Rai, S. Rajika): See *Murraya koenigii:* [Khan *et al.*; *Plant Foods for Human Nutr* **49**(4), 295-99 (1996)].

See *Murraya koenigii* [Khan *et al.*; *J Food Sci Technol* **35**(1), 66-68 (1998)].

The hypolipidemic effects of *Brassica juncea, Brassica rapa, Brassica oleacea* and Yamagata-midorina (*Brassica* spp.) were studied on human subjects. Serum total cholesterol level in human decreased significantly by intaking *B. juncea* and Yamagata-midorina diet (100 g/d) for 2 weeks. HDL-cholesterol level increased by taking *B. rapa* and *B. oleacea* 2 weeks after the start of the diet but the triglyceride levels were not affected by taking these vegetables. Intake of *B. juncea, B. oleacea* and Yamagata-midorina lowered atherogenic index but the last one was most effective. The findings of the present study indicate that the new vegetable, Yamagata-midorina, may be useful for treatment of hyperlipidemia. [Kasahara Y; Aoki Y; Decrease effect of Yamagata-midorina, *Burassica juncea* spp. on serum cholesterol level in humans, *Report of the Yamagata: Prefectural Institute of Public Health* (34), 15-22 (2001)].

Brassica napus (Canola, H. Kali sarson): The effect of dietary fatty acid composition on plasma lipids was studied in normolipidemic men. The canola oil and sunflower oil diets produced similar decreases in plasma total and low density lipoprotein cholesterol. Plasma high density lipoprotein cholesterol and triglyceride concentrations were not altered by either fat source. The hypocholesterolemic effects of the canola oil diet were equivalent to those of the sunflower oil diet. [McDonald BE, Gerrard JM, Bruce VM, Corner EJ; Comparison of the effect of canola oil and sunflower oil on plasma lipids and lipoproteins and on *in vivo* thromboxane A2 and prostacyclin production in healthy young men, *Am J Clin Nutr* **50**(6), 1382-88 (1989)].

See *Cocos nucifera* (Cocoanut): [Nicolosi *et al.*; *Med Sci Sports Exerc* **29**(11), 1422-28 (1997)].

Brassica nigra (Mustard, H. Aslrai, S. Madhurika): Incorporation of mustard oil into high cholesterol diet did not prevent high fat diet-induced increase in the serum cholesterol or atherosclerosis in experimental rabbits, [Thakur CP, Kumar SC; Influence of mustard oil on cholesterol induced atherosclerosis in albino rabbits. *Atherosclerosis* **39**(3), 437-38 (1981)].

Feeding mustard and tamarind to experimental rats produced marked increase in the bile flow rate. The bile acids output was noticeably higher in animals fed mustard, tamarind, onion or curry powder, and this was accompanied by similar increases in biliary phospholipid and cholesterol. The results of the investigation suggest increased hepatic conversion of cholesterol to bile acids under the influence of dietary mustard, tamarind, onion and curry powder. [Sambaiah K, Srinivasan K; Secretion and composition of bile in rats fed diets containing spices, *J Food Sci Technol* **28**(1), 35-38 (1991)].

See *Curcuma longa* (Turmeric): [Srinivasan & Sambaiah; *Int J Vitamin Nutr Res* **61**(4), 364-69 (1991)].

Feeding of crude mustard oil for 6 months significantly raised HDL –cholesterol levels without affecting cholesterol and triglycerides as compared to base line. It also significantly lowered the systolic and diastolic blood pressure. [Prakash S, Bharadwaj P, Arora M, Joshi YK, Tandon RK; Effects of mustard oil with and without erueic acid and glucosinolate on lipid profile and blood pressure, *Nutrition Society of India, 35th Annual Meeting* NIN Hyderabad p.66, Dec 12-13,2003].

Brassica oleracea (Cabbage, H. Pattagobi, S. Dalamalini): Ethanol feeding increased the triglycerides and total cholesterol levels in serum, liver and kidneys and total lipids in the liver of rats. When ethanol-fed rats were given cabbage oil (10 mg/100 g bw) as oral drops, all the above lipid levels were significantly reduced. Serum albumin, serum total proteins and blood glucose levels were not affected either by feeding ethanol or cabbage oil. [Umar I, Augusti KT, Joseph PK; Hypolipidemic action of cabbage oil in ethanol-fed rats, *Indian J Biochem Biophys* **24**(4), 241-43 (1987)].

Antihypercholesterolemic and antihyperlipidemic effects of cabbage extracts were studied. [Jahodar L, Opletal L, Lukes J, Zdansky P, Solichova D; A study on the antihypercholesterolemic and antihyperlipidemic effects of cabbage extracts and their phytochemical evaluation, *Pharmazie* **50**(12), 833-34 (1995)].

In rats fed with the cholesterol enriched diet with cabbage leaf protein concentrate, total cholesterol, triacylglycerol and phospholipid concentrations in both the serum and liver, as well as the atherogenic index were significantly lower than those of the rats fed a casein diet. A supplement of methionine to the cabbage leaf protein diet raised serum HDL-cholesterol and body weight gain. [Igarashi K, Satoh A, Numazawa S, Takahashi E; Effects of cabbage leaf protein concentrate on the serum and liver lipid concentrations in rats, *J Nutr Sci Vitaminol* **43**(2), 261-70 (1997)].

See *Brassica juncea*: [Kasahara & Aoki, *Report of the Yamagata: Prefectural Institute of Public Health* (34), 15-22 (2001)].

Brassica oleracea* var *botrytis (Cauliflower, H. Phoolgobhi): In hypercholesterolemic patients, the effect of canned mixed green vegetable and fruit beverage, which mainly contained *B. oleracea* var *botrytis* and *B. oleracea* var *capitata,* on serum lipid level was studied. Consumption of this beverage (310 ml/d) for three weeks resulted in significant lowering of total serum cholesterol and LDL-cholesterol levels. However, after nine weeks of withdrawl of this beverage, the levels of cholesterol and LDL-cholesterol reversed back to pretreatment levels. [Suido H, Tanaka T, Tabei T, Takeuchi A, Okita M, Kaishimoto T, Kasayama S, Higashino K; A mixed green vegetable and fruit beverage decreased the serum levels of low density lipoprotein cholesterol in hypercholesterolemic patients, *J Agric Food Chem* **50**(11), 3346-50 (2002)].

Brassica oleracea var. capitata (Cabbage, H. Pattagobi) Administration of cabbage oil prepared from fresh sliced vegetable to streptozotocin diabetic rats significantly reduced blood sugar, serum and liver cholesterol and total liver lipids. Serum, liver and kidney glycerides were also significantly decreased in these animals. The hypocholesterolemic activity of this plant was attributed to the presence of sulphur compounds. [Tarfa SP, Joseph PK, Augusti KT; Preliminary studies on the antidiabetic effects of cabbage (*Brassica oleracea var. capitata*) oil in streptozotocin diabetic rats, *Curr Sci* **57**(1), 32-33 (1988)].

See *Brassica oleracea var botrytis:* [Suido et *al.*; *J Agric Food Chem* **50**(11), 3346-50 (2002)].

Brassica rapa (Hakusai)**:** See *Brassica juncea*: [Kasahara & Aoki; *Report of the-Yamagata: Prefectural Institute of Public Health* (34), 15-22 (2001)].

Breynia officinalis**:** Breynins A and B, the two sulphur-containing glycosides isolated from *B. officinalis*, showed significant hypocholesterolemic activity in rats at a daily dose of 0.005 mg/kg and 0.025 mg/kg, respectively. [Koshiyama H, Hatori M, Ohkuma H, Sakai F, Imanishi H, Ohbayashi M, Kawaguchi H; Breynins: New sulfur-containing glycosides with hypocholesterolemic activity, *Chem Pharm Bull* (Tokyo) **24**(1), 169-72 (1976)].

The complete structures of breynins A and B, isolated from *Breynia officinalis*, were established by spectroscopic analysis and chemical degradation. Both these compounds elicited hypocholesterolemic activity. [Ohkuma H, Tsuno T, Konishi M, Naito T, Kawaguchi H; Complete structures of Breynin A and B, *Chem Pharm Bull* (Tokyo) **39**(4), 942-44 (1991)].

Breynia spiroketal glycosides have been reported to exhibit hypocholesterolemic activity. [Smith AB III, Keenan TP, Gallagher RT, Furst GT, Dorman PG; Structure of Breynin A and B architecturally complex, orally active hypocholesterolemic spiroketal glycosides, *J Org Chem* **57**(19), 5115-20 (1992)].

Bryonia critica**:** See *Aloe vera:* [Nada et *al.*; *Fitoterapia* **68**(3), 240-44 (1997)].

C

Caesalpinia bonducella (H. Kat karanja, S. Kuberakshi): Hypoglycemic and hypolipidemic activities of the aqueous and 50% ethanolic extracts of *C. bonducella* seeds were studied in normal and streptozotocin - induced diabetic rats. In addition to hypoglycemic activity, aqueous extract of *C. bonducella* seeds exhibited antihypercholesterolemic and antihypertriglyceridemic effects in streptozotocin -diabetic rats. [Sharma SR, Dwivedi SK, Swarup D; Hypoglycemic, antihyperglycemic and hypolipidemic activities of *Caesalpinia bonducella* seeds in rats, *J Ethnopharmacol* **58**(1), 39-44 (1997)].

Cajanus cajan (Pigeon pea, H. Arhar, S. Adhaki): Administration of protein fraction of *C. cajan* (5%, 7.5% and 10 %) to high fat diet-fed rats, significantly decreased serum, liver and aortic total and free cholesterol, phospholipids and triglyceride contents. Choletserol absorption was increased in protein fraction-fed rats along with enhancement of bile acid excretion. The 10% protein-fed hypercholesterolemic rats exhibited more marked lowering of serum, hepatic and aortic cholesterol, phospholipids and triglyceride levels as compared to untreated hypercholesterolemic animals. [Prema L, Kurup PA; Hypolipidemic activity of protein isolated from *Cajanas cajan* in high fat cholesterol diet-fed rats, *Indian J Biochem Biophys* 10(4), 293-96 (1973)].

See *Phaseolus mungo:* [Joshi & Singhal; *Indian J Nutr Dietet,* **19**(11), 337-41 (1982)].

Administration of filtered juice of fresh raw seeds of *Cajanus cajan* (2 ml) to alloxan-induced diabetic albino rats produced lowering of cholesterol, blood sugar and blood urea levels. The treated animals did not show any toxic or adverse effect of the juice. [Giri J,

Suganthi B, Kowsalya S; Effect of red gram (*Cajanus cajan*) on blood glucose levels in diabetic rats, *Indian J Nutr Diet* **23**(4), 82-87 (1986)].

See *Phaseolus aconitifolius* [Mayilvaganan *et al.*; *Indian J Exp Biol* **42**(9), 904-08 (2004)].

***Calendula officinalis*:** See *Aralia mandshuria* [Wojcicki and Samochowiec; *Herba Pol* **26**(4), 233-37 (1980)].

Calotropis gigantea (H. Ak, S. Arka): See *Saccharum officinarum* [Tarvady & Dhar; *Biomedicine* **9** (1) 39-42 (1989); *Indian J Exp Biol* **28**(7), 657-60 (1990)].

Camelia sinensis (Tea, H. Cha): Effects of tea catechins on lipid metabolism were studied in male weanling rats, fed a 25% casein diet containing 15% lard and 1% cholesterol, for 28 days. The addition of 2% tea catechins (prepared from green tea powder) to the lard-cholesterol diet slightly depressed growth but was without any effect at the 1% level. Tea catechins decreased plasma total cholesterol, cholesterol ester, (total cholesterol + HDL-cholesterol), (VIDL-+ LDL-cholesterol) and atherogenic index (VLDL- + LDL-cholesterol) / HDL-cholesterol). Tea catechin supplementation increased faecal excretion of total lipids and cholesterol. The results demonstrate that tea catechins exert a hypocholesterolemic effect in cholesterol-fed rats. [Muramatsu K, Fukuyo M, Hara Y; Effect of green tea catechins on plasma cholesteol level in cholesterol fed rats, *J Nutr Sci Vitaminol* **32**(6), 613-22 (1986)].

Tea pigment significantly decreased aortic wall cholesterol contents and prevented platelet adhesion and aggregation, as revealed by pharmacological and clinical studies. It also reduced blood coagulability and enhanced fibrinolysis. These observations suggested that tea pigment could be effectively used to prevent atherosclerosis. [Lou FQ, Liu JM, Zhang JMF, Zhang XG, Yuar WL; A study on tea pigment in prevention of atherosclerosis, *Chinese Med J* **102**(8), 579-83 (1989)].

Feeding of purified tea polyphenols from green tea for 6 weeks to experimental hyperlipidemic rats markedly lowered both serum total cholesterol and triglyceride levels and significantly enhanced serum high density lipoprotein cholesterol level compared to the control group. Tea polyphenols could also improve the red cell deformability and reduce the thrombus formation *in vitro*. The results of this study suggested that the tea polyphenols might be useful in the prevention and treatment of hyperlipidemia and thrombosis. [Shen X, Lu R, Tang J, Chen R; A study on the the hypolipidemic and anticoagulant effects of tea polyphenols in rats, *Acta Nutrimenta Sinica* 15(2), 147-51 (1993)].

C. sinensis exhibited hypocholesterolemic, antiatherosclerotic, anticancer, antimutagenic, hypotensive and antiageing activity. Catechin present in tea may also inhibit HIV reverse transcriptase and DNA polymerase. [Agnihothrudu V; Tea- a herbal drink for health, *International Conference on Current Progress in Medicinal and Aromatic Plant Research*, Calcutta , (India) 74-75, Dec30, 1994 –Jan 1, 1995].

Feeding of green or black tea *ad libitum* to high cholesterol diet-fed hamsters significantly improved the lipid profile compared to control animals. Consumption of tea also significantly decreased plasma lipid peroxide and LDL and VLDL oxidizability. Green tea was found to be relatively more effective than black tea. [Vinson JA, Dabbajh YA; Effect of green and black tea supplementation on lipids, lipid peroxidation and fibrinogen in hamsters: Mechanism for the epidemiological benefits of tea drinking, *FEBS Letters* **433** (1,2), 44-46(1998)].

The influence of black tea polyphenols on plasma lipid levels was investigated in rats and it was observed that only a high dose of black tea polyphenols (1%) exerts a hypocholesterolemic effect in cholesterol-fed rats. [Matsumoto N, Okushio K; Hara Y; Effect of black tea polyphenols on plasma lipids in cholesterol-fed rats, *J Nutr Sci Vitaminol* **44**(2), 337-42 (1998)].

The antioxidative and hypolipidemic effects of green tea polyphenols in mice fed with a fish oil-supplemented diet were investigated. Administration of the fish oil-supplemented diet with tea polyphenols inhibited the increase of lipid peroxide levels caused by fish oil in the liver and serum of mice. The decrease of vitamin E content in the biological samples caused by fish oil feeding was also suppressed by additional tea polyphenols administration. Addition of 0.5% tea polyphenols to the fish oil-supplemented diet was found to have significant hypolipidemic and antioxidative effects in mice. [Yoshino K, Goto T, Kuribayashi H, Tamura M, Sano M, Murata H, Tomita I; Antioxidative and hypolipidemic effects of dietary green tea polyphenols in ddY mice fed fish oil-rich diet, *J Food Hyg Soc Japan* **39**(3), 192-98 (1998)].

Wistar rats were fed 2.5% green tea (longjing) leaves for 27 and 63 weeks and the changes of GOT, GPT, γ -GT, and creatinine were compared with the control. The results suggested that long-term feeding of green tea leaves was not toxic to the liver or kidney. Serum total cholesterol, triglyceride, and LDL-c were decreased in the test group. The activities of antioxidant enzymes (SOD and catalase) and phase II enzyme (GST) and glutathione concentration in the liver of Wistar rats were significantly higher in the treated group. The biological significance of these results can be implicated in relation to the hypolipidemic effect as well as the cancer chemopreventive action of green tea. [Lin YL, Cheng CY, Lin YP, Lau YW, Juan IM, Lin JK; Hypolipidemic effect of green tea leaves through induction of antioxidant and phase II enzymes including superoxide dismutase, catalase, and glutathione S-transferase in rats, *J Agric Food Chem* **46**(5), 1893-99 (1998)].

The hypolipidemic activity of green tea epicatechins, isolated from jasmine green tea, was tested in hamsters. The hypolipidemic effects of dietary green tea epicatechins were evident after feeding for 2 weeks. Green tea epicatechins did not affect liver fatty acid synthase but induced higher faecal excretions of total fatty acids, neutral sterols and acidic sterols compared with the control group. No differences in activities of HMG-CoA reductase and intestinal acyl CoA: cholesterol acyltransferase were observed between the control and experimental group of hamsters. It is suggested that the hypolipidemic activity of green tea epicatechins is not due to inhibition of synthesis of cholesterol or fatty acid but is most likely mediated by its influence on absorption of dietary fat and cholesterol. [Chan PT, Fong WP, Cheung YL, Huang Y, Ho WKK, Chen ZY; Jasmine green tea epicatechins are hypolipidemic in hamsters (*Mesocricetus auratus*) fed a high fat diet, *J Nutr* **129**(6), 1094-101 (1999)].

See *Quillaja saponaria:* [Ueda & Tanoue; *Animal Sci J* **71**(4), 393-99 (2000)].

In view of the hypocholesterolemic activity of *C. sinensis*, its effect on the expression of LDL receptor, a cell surface protein involved in the regulation of plasma cholesterol, was investigated. Green tea enhanced the LDL receptor binding activity of human Hep. G2 liver cells *in vitro*. An ethyl acetate extract of *C. sinensis* containing 70% catechins also increased the LDL binding proteins and mRNA indicating that green tea works at gene transcription level and catechins are the main constituents responsible for this action. A decrease of cell cholesterol concentration alongwith an increase of HMG CoA reductase activity was observed following administration of green tea. [Bursill C, Roach PD, Bottema CDK, Pal S; Green tea upregulates the low density lipoprotein receptors through the sterol, regulated element binding protein in Hep G2 liver cells, *J Agric Food Chem* **49**(11), 5639-645 (2001)].

See *Quillaja saponaria*: [Ueda and Yokoyama; *J Poultry-Sci* **38**(3), 225-33 (2001)].

In order to understand the hypocholesterolemic activity of green tea, the relative efficacy of two structurally distinct green tea catechins, epicatechin and epigallocatechin gallate on apolipoprotein B-100 (apoB) and lipid production was studied *in vitro* using human hepatoma cell-line, Hep G2, as the model system. The study showed that HepG2 cells pretreated with epicatechin and epigallocatechin gallate for 8 h exerted a dose-dependent inhibitory effect on apoB secretion. Under lipid-rich conditions, apoB secretion was markedly reduced by epigallocatechin gallate and to a lesser extent by epicatechin at 50 μM. The effect on apoB secretion was also found to be independent of lipid biosynthesis. The data suggest that epigallocatechin gallate, in contrast to epicatechin, is a potent inhibitor of apoB secretion and that the gallate moiety in the catechin molecule may result in a beneficial effect on lipid metabolism in terms of apoB secretion. [Yee WL, Wang Qi, Agdinaoay T, Dang K, Chang H, Grandinetti A; Franke AA, Theriault A; Green tea catechins decrease apolipoprotein B-100 secretion from HepG2 cells, *Mol Cell Biochem* **229**(1-2), 85-92 (2002)].

In cholesterol-fed rats, antioxidative and hypolipidemic activity of green tea polyphenol was compared with probucol. Administration of green tea polyphenol significantly inhibited LDL oxidation and enhanced serum antioxidative activity similar to probucol. However, relatively higher doses of polyphenol, compared to probucol, were required to decrease total, free and LDL cholesterol levels. Unlike probucol, green tea polyphenol effectively enhanced HDL-cholesterol levels and improved the atherogenic index in a dose dependent manner. In view of its antioxidative and HDL-cholesterol increasing action, it was suggested that green tea polyphenol might be used as potential antiatherosclerotic agent. [Yokozawa T, Nakagawa T, Kitani K; Antioxidative activity of green tea polyphenol in cholesterol fed rats, *J Agric Food Chem* **50**(12), 3549-52 (2002)].

The effects of dietary powdered green tea and theanine on *in vivo* hepatoma growth and cancerous hyperlipidemia were investigated in rats that had been implanted with a rat ascites hepatoma cell line of AH109A cells. The hepatoma-bearing rats were fed with a 20% casein diet, supplemented either with 2% powdered green tea or with 0.1% theanine for 14 days. Dietary green tea powder significantly and time-dependently reduced the solid tumor volume and weight, as did dietary theanine. The hepatoma-induced endogenous hyperlipidemia, which was characterised by rises in the serum cholesterol and triglyceride levels, was significantly suppressed by green tea powder and theanine supplementation. Bile acid excretion into the faeces was significantly higher in the green tea powder and theanine-fed rats than in the control rats. This inhibition of hypercholesterolemia may have resulted from tumor growth suppression as well as increased excretion of steroids from the body. These results suggest that powdered green tea had both anti-proliferative activity toward hepatoma cells and hypolipidemic activity in the hepatoma bearing rats. Theanine, at least in part, was considered responsible for the actions exhibited by green tea powder. [Zhang G, Miura Y, Yagasaki K; Effects of dietary powdered green tea and theanine on tumor growth and endogenous hyperlipidemia in hepatoma-bearing rats, *Biosci Biotechnol Biochem* **66**(4), 711-16 (2002)].

The effect of powdered green tea on the lipid metabolism was studied in male Zucker rats fed on 50% sucrose diet containing 15% butter. Oral administration of 130 mg powdered green tea per day depressed body weight increase and various adipose tissue weights but food intake remained unaffected. Powdered green tea lowered the plasma total cholesterol but liver total cholesterol was unaffected. It has been inferred that powdered green tea probably inhibits the synthesis of cholesterol in the liver. [Hasegawa N, Yamda N, Mori M; Powdered green tea has antilipogenic effect on Zucker rats fed a high fat diet, *Phytother Res* **17**(5), 477-80 (2003)].

In an oxidative model using human LDL, antioxidant activity of oolong tea, a semifermented tea made from *Camelia sinensis,* was investigated. 2, 2'-Azobis 4-methoxy-2,4- dimethylvaleronitrile (V70) induced LDL oxidation was suppressed by oolong tea in a dose-dependant manner. Using electron spin resonance (ESR), the active oxygen radical scavenging effect of oolong tea was also studied. At 19.9μg/ml (IC_{50}), the oolong tea decreased the ESR signals formed by hypoxanthine/ xanthine oxidase reaction with 5,5-dimethyl-1-pyrroline Noxide (DMPO). [Kurihara H, Fukami H, Toyda Y, Kageyama N, Tsuruoka N, Shibata H, Kiso Y, Tanaka T; Inhibitory effect of oolong tea on the oxidative state of low density lipoprotein (LDL), *Biol Pharm Bull*

26(5), 739-42 (2003)].

The catechins isolated from *C. sinensis* and heat-epimerized catechin both reduced lymphatic recovery of cholesterol in rats. However, epimerised catechins were more effective than the tea catechins. Purified catechins lowered micellar solubility of cholesterol by precipitating it from bile salts micelles. In precipitating cholesterol, gallo-catechins gallate and catechin-gallate were relatively more effective than epicatechin gallate and epi-gallo-catechin gallate respectively. It was suggested that heat epimerised catechins were more effective as hypocholesterolemic agents than the tea catechins. [Ikada I, Kobayashi M, Hamada T, Tsuda K, Goto H, Imaizumi K, Nozawa A, Sugimoto A, Kakuda T; Heat epimerized tea catechins rich in gallo-catechin gallate and catechin gallate are more effective to inhibit cholesterol absorption than the tea catechins rich in epigallo catechins gallate and epicatechin gallate, *J Agric Food Chem* **51**(25), 7303-07 (2003)].

The effect of fermented black tea {prepared by fermenting black tea (0.5%) decoction containing sugar (10%) with symbiotic culture of *Candida* and *Acetobacter* sp.} on lipids and hypertension was investigated in human subjects. Consumption of fermented black tea (60ml/d) for 90 days caused a significant reduction in blood cholesterol, triglycerides, LDL and VLDL cholesterol levels. A slight increase in HDL-cholesterol was also noted following consumption of fermented tea. Blood pressure was reduced in these treated patients. [Hiremath US, Vaidehi MP; Fermented tea: A value added nutraceutical for the management of hypertension and hypercholesterolemia, *Proceedings of First National Interactive Meet on Medicinal and Aromatic plants* (eds. AK Mathur et al.) CIMAP Lucknow, India p 282-87 (2003)].

The protective effects of green tea polyphenols on the cytotoxic effects of hypolipidemic agent fenofibrate, a peroxisome proliferator, in human HepG2 cells were investigated. Fenofibrate, in high concentrations, induced human HepG2 cell death through a mechanism involving an increase of reactive oxygen species and intracellular reduced glutathione depletion. These effects were partially prevented by antioxidant green tea polyphenols. The result of the investigation demonstrates that oxidative stress and PPAR α (Peroxisomeproliferator activated receptor *alpha*) are involved in fenofibrate cytotoxicity and green tea polyphenols have a protective effect against fenofibrate-induced cellular injury. [Jiao HL, Ye P, Zhao BL; Protective effects of green tea polyphenols on human HepG2 cells against oxidative damage of fenofibrate, *Free Radical Biol Med* **35**(9), 1121-28 (2003)].

The effects of black tea on coronary flow velocity reserve (CFVR), using transthoracic Doppler echocardiography (TTDE), were studied and it was observed that acute black tea consumption improved coronary vessel function, as determined by CFVR. [Hirata K, Shimada K, Watanabe H, Otsuka R, Tokai K, Yoshiyama M, Homma S, Yoshikawa J; Black tea increases coronary flow velocity reserve in healthy male subjects, *Am J Cardiol* **93**(11), 1384- 8, A6 (2004)].

Of the four major commercial teas (oolong, black, pu-erh, and green teas), pu-erh and oolong teas could lower the levels of triglyceride more significantly than green and black teas, but pu-erh tea and green tea were more efficient than oolong tea and black tea in lowering the level of total cholesterol. In lipoprotein, 4% pu-erh tea could increase the level of HDL-c and decrease the level of LDL-c, but other teas simply decrease the levels of both. The activity of antioxidant enzyme super-oxide dismutase increased in all tea-fed groups. From the results of the investigation, it appeared that the fully fermented pu-erh and black tea leaves and partially fermented oolong tea leaves were more effective in growth suppressive and hypolipidemic effects as compared to the nonfermented green tea leaves. [Kuo KL, Weng MS, Chiang CT, Tsai YJ, Lin-Shiau SY, Lin JK; Comparative studies on the hypolipidemic and growth suppressive effects of oolong, black, pu-erh, and green tea leaves in rats, *J Agric Food Chem* **53**(2), 480-89 (2005)].

Campanula lactiflora (bellflower)**:** See Plant Fibres in Appendix: [Kim & Han; *Korean J Animal Sci* **27**(6), 374-80 (1985)].

Cannabis sativa (H. Bhang, S. Bhanga)**:** Intraperitoneal administration of a chloroform extract of cannabinoids from *Cannabis sativa* (100mg/kg) to albino mice for three days significantly increased the adrenal total and free cholesterol contents. However, a slight decrease of the adrenal esrterified cholesterol content was noted in treated mice as compared to controls. [Khan TH, Cheema AM; Effect of crude chloroform extracted cannabinoids on cholesterol fractions of adrenal glands, *Philipp J Sci* **115**(4), 347-51 (1986)].

Capparis deciduas (Teent, H. Karer, S. Karira)**:** Fibre from *C. deciduas, Ficus bengalensis, F. glomerata, F. religiosa* and *Prosopis cineraria* fed at the 10% dietary level to rats, induced a greater resistance to hyperlipidemia than cellulose. Teent had the most pronounced hypocholesterolemic effect, which appeared to operate through increased faecal excretion of cholesterol as well as bile acids. [Agarwal V, Chauhan BM; A study on composition and hypolipidemic effect of dietary fibre from some plant foods, *Plant Foods Hum Nutr* **38**(2), 189- 97 (1988)].

Administration of 50% alcoholic extract of *C. deciduas* fruits to cholesterol-fed rabbits inhibited the development of atheroma. The deposition of cholesterol and triglycerides in liver and aorta was also prevented in treated animals. [Sharma I, Gusain D, Sharma A, Dixit VP; Hypolipidemic effect of *Capparis deciduas* fruit extract (50% EtOH) in cholesterol-fed rabbits, *Indian drugs* **28**(9), 412-16 (1991)].

Capsicum annuum (Red pepper, H. Lal-mircih)**:** Effect of red pepper and capsaicin on serum and liver cholesterol was investigated in rats. Both significantly prevented the increase in hepatic cholesterol contents. However, red pepper partially inhibited rise of serum cholesterol levels. [Sambaiah K, Satyanarayanan MN; Hypocholesterolemic effect of red pepper and capsaicin, *Indian J Exp Biol* **18**(8), 898-99 (1980)].

See *Curcuma longa:* (Turmeric) [Srinivasan & Satyanarayana; *J Biosci* **12**(2), 143-52 (1987)].

See *Curcuma longa* (Turmeric): [Srinivasan & Sambaiah; *Int J Vitamin Nutr Res* **61**(4), 364-69 (1991)].

See *Allium cepa* (Onion): [Babu & Srinivasan; *Mol Cell Biochem.* **175**(1-2), 49-57 (1997)].

See *Allium sativum* (Garlic): [Kempaiah et al.; *Mol Cell Biochem* **236**(1-2), 155-61 (2002)].

See *Curcuma longa* (Turmeric): [Kempaiah & Srinivasan; *Ann Nutr Metab* **48**(5), 314-20 (2004)].

Carica papaya (H. Papaya): See Pectin in Appendix: [Prasanna Kumar *et al.*; *J Food Sci Technol* **34**(2), 103-07 (1997)].

Carthamus tinctorius (Safflower, H. Kusum, S. Kusumbha): See *Oenothera biennis* (Evening primrose): [Sugano *et al.*; *Agric Biol Chem* **50**(9), 2335-40 (1986)].

The hypolipidemic effect of feeding of linoleate (safflower oil) or α-linoleate (Perilla oil)-rich diet to mice for five months was investigated. The whole body cholesterol was significantly lower (28%) in groups of mice, which consumed high α-linoleate diet compared to linoleate-fed mice. However, total lipid, plasma lipoprotein and neutral lipids did not differ much between these two groups of mice. These observations indicate that high α-linoleate diet produced more pronounced lipid lowering effect than the high linoleate diet. [Sakai K, Shimokawa T, Kobayashi T, Okuyama H; Lipid lowering effect of high linoleate and high α linoleate diets in rats and mice: Consequence of long-term feeding, *Chem Pharm Bull* (Tokyo) **40**(8), 2129-32 (1992)].

Some clinical studies have shown that dietary supplementation of safflower oil reduced serum cholesterol levels. However, changes in lipid profile induced by safflower oil were not considered important as suggested earlier in terms of reducing the risk of cardiovascular disorders. [Liberti L; Safflower- a monograph, *Lawrence Review of Natural Products* p1-2 Nov. (1992)].

The hypolipidemic effect of *C. tinctorius* extract was studied in nomal and hyperlipidemic mice. A methanol extract of *C. tinctorius* lowered the total cholesterol and triglyceride level of normal and cholesterol-fed mice. The therapeutic effect was not observed but the preventive effect was recognised on the hyperlipidemic mice. [Kasahara Y, Suzuki M; Effect of *Carthamus tinctorius* L. on blood components, *Report of theYamagata Prefectural Institute of Public Health* (32), 12-16 (1999)].

The hypolipidemic activity of powdered safflower seed and its ethanol and hot water extracts was studied in male rats. All the safflower seed preparations significantly lowered the plasma cholesterol concentration, whereas the plasma triglyceride concentration was only lowered by the ethanol and aqueous extracts. While aqueous extract significantly lowered hepatic total cholesterol contents both the solvent extracts significantly lowered the hepatic triglyceride contents. Again, hepatic HMG-CoA reductase activities were significantly higher in both the solvent extract groups compared with the other group. The hepatic ACAT activities were significantly lower in the ethanol extract group compared to all the other groups. These results indicate that the solvent extracts are more effective than powdered safflower seed in improving the atherogenic risk factors in high-cholesterol fed rats. [Moon KD, Back SS, Kim JH, Jeon SM, Lee MK, Choi MS, Safflower seed extract lowers plasma and hepatic lipids in rats fed high-cholesterol diet, *Nutr Res* **21**(6), 895-904 (2001)].

See *Typha angustifolia*: [Park *et al.*; *Phytother Res* **18**(3), 224-29 (2004).].

Carum copticum (H. Ajwan, S. Ajamoda): When *C. copticum* seed powder (1% mixed with powdered rabbit feed) was fed for four weeks to normal albino rabbits, hypocholesterolemic, hypotriglyceridemic and hypophospholipidemic effects were observed from the first week itself. The serum cholesterol binding reserve and highdensity lipoprotein levels, on the other hand, showed an increase in the corresponding periods. [Agrewalas JN, Pant MC; Effect of feeding *Carum copticum* seeds on serum lipids, high-density lipoproteins and serum cholesterol binding reserve in albino rabbits, *Indian J Med Res* **83**(Jan), 93-95 (1986)].

Cassia tora (H. Chakunda, S. Chakramarda): Ethanolic extract of seeds of the plant and its fractions were investigated for hypolipidemic activity on triton-induced hyperlipidemic profile. Ethanolic extract and its ether soluble and water soluble fractions decreased serum total cholesterol level by 42.07, 40.77 and 71.25%, increased the serum HDL-cholesterol level by 6.72, 17.20 and 19.18%, decreased triglyceride level by 26.84, 35.74 and 38.46%, and reduced LDL-cholesterol level by 69.25, 72.06 and 76.12%, respectively. [Patil UK, Saraf S, Dixit VK; Hypolipidemic activity of seeds of *Cassia tora* Linn, *J Ethnopharmacol* **90**(2-3), 249-52. (2004)]

Catharanthus lanceus: 3,4-Dimethoxyphenylacetamide, isolated from *C. lanceus*, exhibited hypocholesterolemic effect. The compound showed a tendency to lower blood sugar levels. It also caused CNS depression. [Safia Duane R, Segelman AB, Farnsworth NR, Buckley JP; Pharmacological evaluation of 3,4-dimethoxyphenyl acetamide, *J Pharm Sci* **60**(8), 1240-42 (1971)].

Catharanthus roseus (Sadabahar): Aqueous and methanolic extracts of leaves of *C. roseus* significantly decreased total cholesterol, triglycerides and low density lipoprotein cholesterol along with an increase in the HDL-c levels. Atherogenic index was also lowered in treated mice. The aqueous extract was found to be more effective than the methanolic extract. [Kulkarni S, Ghosh R, Chatterjee M; Hypolipidemic activity of *Catharanthus roseus* leaf extract in mice, *Indian J Pharm Sci* **56**(4), 162 (1994)].

Oral administration of aqueous and methanolic extracts of fresh leaves of *C. roseus* to hyperlipidemic mice for 3 weeks, significantly lowered serum cholesterol, triglycerides and LDL-cholesterol levels alongwith an enhancement of HDL-cholesterol. Aqueous extract was found to be more effective than methanolic extract in terms of their hypolipidemic activitry. Aqueous extract-treated mice also exhibited relatively lower atherogenic index. [Muckerjee B, Sarkar A, Kulkarni S, Chatterjee M; Hypolipidemic activity of *Catharanthus roseus* leaf extracts in mice, *Fitoterapia* **66**(6), 483-87 (1995)].

See *Coccinia indica:* [Annapurna *et al.*; *Indian J Exp Biol* **39**(5), 500-02 (2001)].

Celastrus paniculatus (H. Malkangni, S. Kanguni)**:** The extract of *C. paniculatus* seeds decreased serum cholesterol and LDL-cholesterol in hyperlipidemic rabbits. Treated animals also exhibited a reduction in cholesterol / phospholipid ratio with a significant increase in the total cholesterol / HDL-cholesterol ratio. The extract inhibited deposition of cholesterol and triglycerides in liver and aorta, enhanced faecal excretion of cholesterol and prevented atherogenesis [Mathur NT, Verma M, Dixit VP; Hypolipidemic and antiatherosclerotic effect of *Celastrus paniculatus* seed extract (50% EtOH) in cholesterol-fed rabbits, *Indian Drugs* **30**(2), 76-82 (1993)].

Cephalandra indica (Syn. *Coccinia indica*, H. Kanduri, S. Bimba)**:** See *Saccharum officinarum:* [Tarvady & Dhar; *Biomedicine* **9** (1) 39-42 (1989); *Indian J Exp Biol* **28**(7), 657- 60 (1990)].

The effect of oral administration of *C. indica* was studied in hundred hyperlipidemic human subjects of 25-70 years age. The drug significantly lowered serum total cholesterol, low density lipoprotein cholesterol and triglycerides alongwith enhancement of high density lipoprotein cholesterol levels in these subjects. [Ghoshal J, Roy A, Ray R; Influence of *Cephalandra indica,* Naud (Telakucha) on serum lipids and lipoproteins in humans of different age groups, *International Seminar –Traditional Medicine, Calcutta* p 110-11, Nov7-9, 1992].

See *Cyamopsis tetragonoloba* (Cluster bean, Guar gum): [Bharadwaj *et al.*; *J Indian Med Assoc* **92**(3), 80-81 (1994)].

Cicer arietinum (Bengal gram, chickpea, H. Chana, S. Chanaka): Two isoflavones, biochanin-A and formononetin isolated from *C. arietinum*, have been shown to possess hypolipidemic properties [Siddiqui MT, Siddiqi M; Hypolipidemic principles of *Cicer arietinum*: biochanin-A and formononetin, *Lipids* **11**(3), 243-46 (1976)].

Glycosaminoglycans (acid mucopolysaccharide) content of the aorta in egg yolk-induced atherosclerosis in rabbits showed a highly significant increase compared to untreated controls. Animals receiving 40% of their diet as Bengal gram showed decreased glycosaminoglycans content and the same was observed in estrogen treated animals. The hypocholesterolemic and antiatherogenic properties of the Bengal gram may be due to the isoflavone, biochanin A, which shows some structural similiarity with estrogen. [Madhavan M; The effect of Bengal gram on acid mucopolysaccharide content of aorta in experimental atherosclerosis, *Indian J Med Res* **64**(10), 1504-08 (1976)].

Incorporation of isoflavones, biochanin A and formononetin, from *C. arietinum*, into hypercholesterolemia-inducing diet, produced lipid lowering effect, Another isoflavone was found to be devoid of such a hypolipidemic activity. However, *p*-coumaric acid exhibited hypocholesterolemic effect. [Sharma RD, Isoflavones and hypercholesterolemia in rats, *Lipids* **14**(6), 535-40 (1978)].

In egg yolk-fed rabbits, aortic glycosaminoglycans and its fractions, especially chondroitin– 4-sulphate and chondroitin-6-sulphate contents, were consistently increased during atherogenesis. Incorporation of Bengal gram (40%) in the diet, fed to hyperlipidemic rabbits, lowered above mentioned fractions leading to reduction of total aortic glycosaminoglycans contents. It was suggested that beneficial effects of Bengal gram on egg yolk-induced atherosclerosis appears to be due to its effect on glycosaminoglycans contents of the aorta. [Madhavan M, Ramkrishnan S, Rao Venugopal, Ramlingam G; Effect of Bengal gram supplementation on glycosaminoglycans fractions in egg yolk induced atherosclerosis in rabbits, *Indian J Exp Biol* **16**(July), 828-30 (1978)].

Isoflavones isolated from three commonly used pulses such as Bengal gram (*Cicer arietinum*), greengram (*Phaseolus aureus*) and blackgram (*P. mungo*) and p-coumaric acid were tested for their antihypercholesterolemic activity. Among isoflavones, biochanin A and formononetin showed hypolipidemic activity but diadzein did not; p-coumaric acid also produced a significant reduction in serum cholesterol levels. [Sharma RD; Isoflavones and hypercholesterolemia in rats, *Lipids* **14**(6), 535-39 (1979)].

Adminstration of isoflavones biochanin A, formononetin and pratensein, isolated from *C. arietinum* to triton-induced hyperlipidemic rats, led to significant hypolipidemic activity. However, diadzein did not exhibit such an activity. [Sharma RD; Effect of various isoflavones on lipid levels in triton treated rats, *Atherosclerosis* **33**(3), 371-75 (1979).].

Chickpea and greengram (*Phaseolus aureus*) in ungerminated and germinated form were tested for their hypocholesterolemic property by feeding them to hypercholesterolemic rats along with cholesterol and bile acids. Both legumes were effective in lowering the serum and liver cholesterol levels with chickpea being more effective than greengram. Germinated legumes were more effective than the corresponding ungerminated ones in lowering the cholesterol levels. The excretion of bile acids was more in rats, fed with the legume-based diet, than those fed the hypercholesterolemic diet. The activities of hepatic enzymes like succinic dehydrogenase, transferases and glucose-6-phosphatase lowered with higher levels of cholesterol in liver and serum. [Jaya TV, Venkataraman LV, Krishnamurthy KS;

Influence of germinated legumes on the levels of tissue cholesterol and liver enzymes of hypercholesterolemic rats: Influence of ungerminated and geminated chickpea (*Cicer arietinum*) and greengram (*Phaseolus aureus*) whole, *Nutr Reports International* **20**(3), 371-82 (1979)].

Germinated and ungerminated chickpea and greengram (*Phaseolus aurus*]. and the different constituents of these legumes were tested for their hypocholesterolemic property by feeding them along with cholesterol to rats. Both legumes were effective in lowering the cholesterol levels; germinated ones were more effective. The rats were fed protein concentrate, lipid fraction (from ungerminated chickpea) and the carbohydrate fractions of ungerminated and germinated legumes. The lipid and carbohydrate fractions-fed rats showed lower serum cholesterol levels compared to those fed whole legumes. Liver sections of rats fed with a hypercholesterolemic diet showed heavy fatty infiltration and cholesterol deposition. Livers of rats fed legume-based diets did not show any abnormality. [Jaya TV, Venkataraman LV; Germinated legumes and their influence on liver and serum cholesterol levels in rats: Influence of different components of chickpea (*Cicer arietinum*) and greengram (*Phaseolus aureus*) on tissue cholesterol levels, *Nutr Reports International* **20**(3), 383-92 (1979)].

Feeding of whole pulses and fibres isolated from *C. arietinum, Phaseolus aureus, P. mungo, Pisum sativum* and *Lens esculenta* to atherogenic diet-fed rats significantly lowered cholesterol levels. Of all the above mentioned pulses, *C. arietinum* exhibited maximum hypocholesterolemic activity. [Soni GL, George M, Rattan Singh; Role of common Indian pulses as hypocholesterolemic agents, *Indian J Nutr Dietet* **19**(6), 184-90 (1982)].

The hypocholesterolemic effect of tannin, phytate and pectin given in amounts equal to those present in Bengal gram was studied in cholesterol-fed hyperlipidemic rats and compared with the effect of Bengal gram *per se*. All the compounds showed a tendency to lower serum and tissue lipids but pectin was more effective than the other two but none was as effective as Bengal gram. Tannin, phytic acid and non-cellulosic polysaccharides, which are quite common in commonly used pulses, can render them hypocholesterolemic. [Sharma RD; Hypocholesterolemic effect of hydroxy acid components of Bengal gram (*Cicer arietinum*), *Nutr Reports International* **29**(6), 1315-22 (1984)].

Three different varieties of *Cicer arietinum*, viz., Bengal gram (brown), Kabligram (white) and green seeded gram were evaluated for their hypocholesterolemic action as well as for their nutritional status. All these varieties showed considerable hypolipidemic and hypocholesterolemic effects. Green seeded gram and Kabligram had a considerably higher hypocholesterolemic and hypolipidemic effect as compared to Bengal gram, which had the highest protein content (25 per cent). The apparent protein digestibility of Kabli gram was the highest and that of green seeded gram was the least [Birender K, Soni GL, Singh R; Nutritional evaluation of gram (*Cicer arietinum*) varieties, *Human Nutr Food Sci Nutr* **41F**(2), 121-28 (1987)].

Introduction of dietary fibre from Bengal gram in hypercholesterolaemic diets caused the lowering of plasma as well as membrane cholesterol. There seems to be a direct relationship between the increase in membrane cholesterol level and the increase in the osmotic fragility of erythrocyte membrane and this was also reflected in packed cell volume, and erythrocyte count. A direct relationship between the increased membrane cholesterol level and the increase/decrease in the activities of allosteric enzymes (Na+-K+)-ATPase and acetyl cholinesterase, respectively, has also been observed. [Thomas A, Soni GL, Singh R; Role of dietary fibre from Bengal gram (*Cicer* arietinum) as hypocholesterolemic agent: Effect on erythrocyte membrane-bound enzymes and hematological parameters, *Human Nutr Food Sci Nutr* **41F**(3-4), 193-202 (1987)].

Inclusion of legumes such as Bengal gram (*Cicer arietinum*), soya bean (*Glycine max*), winged bean (*Psophocarpus tetragonolobus*), rajmah (*Phaseolus vulgaris*) and khesari dhal (*Lathyrus sativus*) in the hypercholesterolemia-inducing diet of rats, prevented the elevation of serum lipids. Amino acids, saponins and the fibre profile of these legumes were correlated with their serum lipid-lowering effect. Lysine, serine and tyrosine showed a positive correlation, while arginine, alanine, glycine and threonine had a negative correlation. A significant correlationship was observed also with lysine/arginine ratio. Saponins showed a negative correlation. [Sharma RD; An evaluation of hypocholesterolemic activity of some uncommon legumes, *Nutr Res* **7**(4), 351-64 (1987)].

Seed coat of Bengal gram appeared to be a potent hypocholesterolemic/hypolipidemic agent in rabbits. When fed to hypercholesterolemic rabbits, it lowered hepatic cholesterol/lipid much more than in the control group. It failed to prevent the development of atherosclerosis in hypercholesterolemic rabbits, but certainly slowed down the process of its development. The hypocholesterolemic action of Bengal gram seed coat appeared to be due to the increased catabolism and excretion of cholesterol. [Mand JK, Soni GL, Gupta PP, Vadhera S, Singh R; Role of Bengal gram (*Cicer arietinum*) seed coat as an antiatherogenic agent in rabbits, *Indian Heart J* **43**(5), 347-50 (1991)].

Rabbits maintained on hypercholesterolemic diet for 12 weeks showed gradual increase in the blood lipids and cholesterol levels. Such an increase in the lipid levels was comparatively less in the animals fed with Bengal gram (*C. arietinum*) fibre. Hepatic lipids were also decreased in these animals. However, the atherosclerosis was not affected by Bengal gram fibre. Hypolipidemic effect of Bengal gram seed coat seems to be due to enhanced excretion of bile acids. [Mand JK, Soni GL, Vadhera S, Rattan Singh; Hypocholesterolemic and hypolipidemic action of Bengal gram seed coat fibre in rabbits, *Bioved* **3**(1)), 13-16 (1992)].

Effects of Bengal gram on the egg yolk-induced atherosclerosis were investigated in rabbits. Egg yolk feeding significantly increased the serum, liver, heart and aortic cholesterol, triglycerides and phospholipid levels. These rabbits also showed well-defined atherosclerotic plaques. Supplementation of diet with Bengal gram significantly lowered various fractions of serum and tissue lipids levels and caused flattening of atherosclerotic plaques. [Gracias D, Gopalan R, Maruthi K, Madhavan M; Studies on serum and tissue lipid fractions in Bengal gram induced retardation of experimental atherosclerosis, *Indian Heart J* **43**(5), 341-45 (1992)].

A differential hypocholesterolemic effect between dietary casein and chickpea intake in a model of diet-induced hypercholesterolemia was found with beneficial effects on the lipid metabolism when chickpea legume was included in the diet as compared to casein. This suggests that chickpea consumption may have a corrective effect in some alterations of the lipid profile. [Zulet MA, Martinez JA; Corrective role of chickpea intake on a dietary-induced model of hypercholesterolemia, *Plant Foods Hum Nutr* **48**(3), 269-77 (1995)].

See *Allium sativum* (Garlic): [Dwivedi S; *Ann Natl Acad Med Sci* (India) 32(3&4) 159- 175(1996)].

See *Allium sativum* (Garlic): [Sharma & Dwivedi; *Indian Drugs* **34**(5), 242-51 (1997)].
See *Glycine max* (Soya bean, soybean): [Park *et al.*; *Cardiol Rev* **13**(1), 13-17 (2005)].

***Cicer moglotavicum*:** See Flavonoids in Appendix: [Khushbaktova *et al.*; *Khim Farma Zh* **25**(4), 53-57 (1991)].

***Cimicifuga dahurica*:** Administration of cimicilen (85-90% cycloartenic triterpenoids), isolated from rhizomes of *C. dahurica*, elicited hypolipidemic activity in different experimental models of hyperlipidemia. [Muravyov IA, Vasilenko Yu K, Bagariv A ya, Parfentieva EP, Sukulte IV; Hypolipidemic properties of cimicilen the drug, isolated from *Cimicifuga dahurica* (Tirez) *Maxim Farmatsiya* (Moscow) **34**(4), 38-42 (1985)].

Cinnamomum tamala (H. Tejput, S. Tamalaka)**:** Oral feeding of ethanolic extract of *C. tamala* leaves to streptozotocin-induced diabetic rats significantly lowered serum cholesterol and triglyceride levels. This extract also significantly decreased blood glucose levels in normoglycemic and streptozotocin-induced hyperglycemic rats. [Sharma SR, Dwivedi SK, Swarrop D; Hypoglycemic and hypolipidemic effect of *Cinnamomum tamala* Nees leaves, *Indian J Exp Biol* **34**(4), 372-74 (1996)].

Citrus aurantium (Syn. *C. reticulata*, Orange, H. Sangtara, S. Airavata)**:** Preliminary studies showed that in mildly hypercholesterolemic rats with chemically induced breast cancer, dietary orange juice reduced total plasma cholesterol and dietary grapefruit juice tended to reduce VLDL + LDL-cholesterol. In rabbits fed with the experimental diet for 3 weeks, replacement of drinking water with either orange juice or grapefruit juice reduced serum LDL-cholesterol by 43% and 32%, respectively. This was associated with total liver cholesterol reduction in the orange juice group and with hepatic cholesterol ester reduction in both juice groups. The juices were not acting as intestinal sequestrants since neither increased faecal cholesterol or bile acid excretion. In fact, cholesterol excretion was decreased in both orange juice and grapefruit juice groups. These results suggest that the reduction of LDL-cholesterol, induced by dietary citrus juices, could be due to`endogenous effects of juice components, possibly flavonoids. [Kurowska EM, Borradaile NM, Spence JD, Carroll KK; Hypocholesterolemic effects of dietary citrus juices in rabbits, *Nutr Res* **20**(1), 121-29 (2000)].

Consumption of 750 ml orange juice daily, increased HDL-cholesterol, triacylglycerol and folate concentrations with a decreas of the LDL/HDL-cholesterol ratio. [Kurowska EM, Spence JD, Jordan J, Wetmore S, Freeman DJ, Piche LA, Serratore P; HDL-cholesterol raising effect of orange juice in subjects with hypercholesterolemia, *Am J Clin Nutr* **72**(5), 1095-100 (2000)].

In obese women volunteers, the effect of dried orange peel compound (30ml/twice daily) on blood lipid parameters was compared with the group of volunteers who participated in an exercise program (70minutes/day, 3 times/week) for 12 weeks. Intake of dried orange peel compound or exercise positively influenced blood HDL-cholesterol, LDL-cholesterol, triglyceride levels, body weight and body fat per cent almost in a similar manner. However, intake of dried orange peel compound with exercise training was more effective on thr above mentioned parameters. It was suggested that dry orange peel compound might be quite useful in the management of obesity. [Choi J, Lee KM, Kim HJ, Kim SH, Kim HS, Ro JS, Oh KW, Lee KS; The effect of dried orange peel compound intaking and exercise training on the physique, body fat and concentration of blood lipids in obese women, *Korean J Pharmacogn* **33**(1), 57-63 (2002)].

Citrus paradisi (Grapefruit): See *Citrus aurantium* (Orange): [Kurowska *et al.*; *Nutr Res* **20**(1), 121-29 (2000)].

The grapefruit flavonoid, naringenin, is hypocholesterolemic *in vivo*, and inhibits basal apolipoprotein B (apoB) secretion and the expression and activities of both acyl CoA: Cholesterol acyl transferase (ACAT) and microsomal triglyceride transfer protein (MTP) in human hepatoma cells (HepG2). The effects of naringenin on apoB kinetics in oleate-stimulated-HepG2 cells were examined and the contribution of microsomal lumen cholesteryl ester availability to apoB secretion was determined. Naringenin was shown to inhibit apoB secretion in oleate-stimulated HepG2 cells and selectively increase intracellular degradation *via* a largely proteasomal, rapid kinetic pathway. [Borradaile NM, de Dreu LE, Barrett PHR, Huff MW; Inhibition of hepatocyte apoB secretion by naringenin: Enhanced rapid intracellular degradation independent of reduced microsomal cholesteryl esters, *J Lipid Res* **43**(9), 1544-54 (2002)].

Citrus sinensis cv. Liucheng (H. Musambi): The effects of diet containing a water-insoluble fibre-rich fraction, isolated from the peels of *C. sinensis* cv. Liucheng, on lipid and cholesterol absorption in hamsters were investigated and compared with those of a cellulose-containing diet and fibre-free diet, as controls. The water-insoluble fibre-rich fraction of *C. sinensis* significantly decreased the levels of serum triglyceride, serum total cholesterol, liver total lipids, and liver cholesterol, and significantly increaseed the levels of faecal total lipids, faecal cholesterol, and faecal bile acids, as well as the faecal bulk and moisture. The pronounced hypocholesterolemic and hypolipidemic effects of water-insoluble fibre-rich fraction of *C. sinensis* might be attributed to its ability to enhance cholesterol and bile acids excretion. [Chau CF, Huang YL, Lin CY; Investigation of the cholesterol-lowering action of insoluble fibre derived from the peel of *Citrus sinensis* L. cv. Liucheng, *Food Chem* **87**(3), 361-66 (2004)].

***Citrus* species:** Hesperidin, the most important flavanone of *Citrus* sp., was found to significantly increase HDL and lower cholesterol, LDL, total lipid and triglyceride plasma levels in normolipidemic and triton-induced hyperlipidemic rats. [Monforte MT, Trovato A, Kirjavainen S, Forestieri AM, Galati EM, Lo Curto RB; Biological effects of hesperidin, a citrus flavonoid (note II): Hypolipidemic activity on experimental hypercholesterolemia in rat *Farmaco* (Rome) **50**(9), 595-99 (1995].

Following one month feeding of a citrus fruit extract with ascorbic acid to hypercholesterolemic hamsters, significantly decreased plasma total cholesterol, LDL + VLDL, and triglycerides. In another group of hamsters administration of citrus fruit extract with ascorbate for 10 weeks, significantly lowered plasma lipids, lipid peroxides and ex *vivo* LDL and VLDL oxidizability. Citrus fruit extract with ascorbate also prevented atherosclerosis. [Vinson JA, Hu SJ, Jung S, Stanski AM; A citrus extract plus ascorbic acid decrease lipids, lipid peroxide, lipoprotein oxidative susceptibility and atherosclerosis in hypercholesterolemic hamsters, *J Agric Food Chem* **46**(4), 1453-459 (1998)].

The effects of the citrus bioflavonoid naringin were tested using it as a supplement in a high cholesterol diet. Male rats were fed for 42 days with a 1% (wt/wt) high-cholesterol diet either with or without naringin-supplementation. Naringin did not significantly alter the levels of plasma triglycerides, however, the levels of plasma cholesterol and hepatic cholesterol were significantly lowered compared to those of the control. HMG-CoA reductase and ACAT activities were both substantially lower in the naringin-supplemented group than in the control. The naringin supplementation markedly decreased the excretion of faecal neutral sterols compared to the control. The combination of the inhibited HMG-CoA reductase and ACAT activities as a result of naringin supplementation could account for the decrease of faecal neutral sterols. [Shin YW, Bok SH, Jeong TS, Bae KH, Jeoung NH, Choi MS, Lee SH, Park YB; Hypocholesterolemic effect of naringin associated with hepatic cholesterol regulating enzyme changes in rats, *Int J Vit Nutr Res* **69**(5), 341-47 (1999)].

Citrus flavonoids, naringenin and hesperetin, were found to lower plasma cholesterol *in vivo*. With the objective to understand the underlying mechanisms, the ability of these flavonoids to modulate apolipoprotein B (apoB) secretion and cellular cholesterol homeostasis was determined in the human hepatoma cell line, HepG2 and it was concluded that both naringenin and hesperetin decrease the availability of lipids for assembly of apoB-containing lipoproteins, an effect mediated by reduced activities of acyl CoA cholesterol acyltransferase (ACAT1 and ACAT2), a selective decrease in ACAT2 expression, and reduced microsomal triglyceride transfer protein (MTP) activity. [Wilcox LJ, Borradaile NM, de Dreu LE, Huff MW; Secretion of hepatocyte apoB is inhibited by the flavonoids, naringenin and hesperetin, *via* reduced activity and expression of ACAT2 and MTP, *J Lipid Res* **42**(5), 725-34 (2001)].

In a preliminary study with hamsters, citrus peels were found to have a cholesterol lowering effect comparable to that of pectin extracted from these peels. The results of an investigation, aimed at ascertaining whether the activity was solely due to pectins present in the peels, revealed that lemon peels and the waste stream of the lemon peels are as effective in lowering plasma and liver cholesterol in hamsters as the pectin extracted from the peels and that compounds other than pectin are probably responsible for the cholesterol lowering effect of the citrus peels. [Terpstra AH, Lapre JA, de Vries HT, Beynen AC; The hypocholesterolemic effect of lemon peels, lemon pectin, and the waste stream material of lemon peels in hybrid F1B hamsters. *Eur J Nutr* **41**(1), 19-26 (2002)].

See Pectin in Appendix: [Terpstra *et al.*; *Nahrung* **46**(2), 83-86 (2002)].

Naringin, a flavonoid found in *Citrus* species and grapes, is known to have anti-inflammatory and anti-oxidative properties. A study was undertaken to ascertain whether naringin protects vascular smooth muscle cells from the mitogenic effect of lysophosphatidylcholine, an atherogenic lysophospholipid of oxidized low density lipoprotein (LDL), known to impair endothelial release of nitric oxide, up-regulate the expression of adhesion molecules, and promote the proliferation of vascular smooth muscle cells. . The study demonstrates that naringin suppresses the mitogenic effect of lysophosphatidylcholine on vascular smooth muscle cells, whereas lysophosphatidylcholine promotes the proliferation of vascular smooth muscle cells. [Kim SH, Zo JH, Kim MA, Hwang KK, Chae IH, Kim HS, Kim CH, Sohn DW, Oh BH, Lee MM, Park YB; Naringin suppresses the mitogenic effect of lysophosphatidylcholine on vascular smooth muscle cells, *Nutr Res* **23**(12), 1671-83 (2003)].

Naringenin 7-O-oleic ester and naringenin 7-O-cetyl ether inhibited the formation of aortic atherosclerotic lesions in high cholesterol-fed rabbits. [Lee S, Lee CH, Moon SS, Kim E, Kim CT, Kim BH, Bok SH, Jeong TS; Naringenin derivatives as anti-atherogenic agents, *Bioorganic Med Chem Lett* **13**(22), 3901-03 (2003)].

The preventive effects of diets supplemented with a new kind of citrus fruit pummelo grapefruit hybrid (sweetie fruits), in hypercholesterolemic patients suffering from coronary artery disease were investigated. Peeled sweeties have high contents of dietary fibres and antioxidant compounds. Diets supplemented with peeled sweeties positively influence plasma lipid metabolism and plasma antioxidant capacity in patients suffering from coronary artery disease and hypercholesterolemia. Therefore, the addition of peeled sweeties to a generally accepted antiatherosclerotic diet may be beneficial in prevention of atherosclerosis, mainly in hypercholesterolemic patients. [Gorinstein S, Caspi A, Libman I, Katrich E, Lerner HT, Trakhtenberg S; Preventive effects of diets supplemented with sweetie fruits in hypercholesterolemic patients suffering from coronary artery disease, *Prev Med* **38**(6), 841-7 (2004)].

Formulations containing polymethoxylated flavones (PMFs) or flavanone glucosides, isolated from *Citrus* species (mainly tangeretin, hesperidin and naringin) were evaluated for cholesterol-lowering potential in hamsters with diet-induced hypercholesterolemia. Diets containing 1% PMFs significantly reduced serum total and VLDL + LDL-cholesterol and either reduced or tended to reduce serum triacylglycerols. Comparable reductions were achieved by feeding a 3% mixture of hesperidin and naringin (1:1, w/w), implying lower hypolipidemic potency of the hesperidin-naringin mixture in comparison to PMFs. PMFs were thus regarded as novel flavonoids with cholesterol and triacylglycerollowering potential. [Kurowska EM, Manthey JA; Hypolipidemic effects and absorption of citrus polymethoxylated flavones in hamsters with diet-induced hypercholesterolemia, *J Agric Food Chem* **52**(10), 2879-86 (2004)].

Clementsia semenovii: Oligomeric proanthocyanidins rhodichimoside and rhodichin, isolated from the roots of *C. semenovii,* have been shown to possess hypocholesterolemic, hypolipidemic and antiinflammatory activities. The structures of these compounds have been established by using chemical and spectral data [Kuliev ZA, Kim KK, Vdovin AD, Abdullaev ND, Khushbaktova ZA, Syrov VN; Oligomeric proanthocyanidin glycosides of *Clementsia semenovii* and their biological activity III, *Chem Nat Comp* **36**(1), 60-67 (2000); Translated from *Khim Prir Soedin* No.1, 47-53 (2000)].

***Cleome droserifolia*:** In addition to a promising therapeutic value in the treatment of diabetes mellitus, the extract of the plant showed hypocholesterolemic effect more specifically on low density lipoprotein cholesterol (LDL-c), which consequently raised the (HDL-c/LDL-c) ratio. [Nicola WG, Ibrahim KM, Mikhail TH, Girgis RB, Khadr ME; Role of the hypoglycemic plant, *Cleome droserifolia,* extract in improving glucose and lipid metabolism and its relation to insulin resistance in fatty liver, *Boll Chim Farm* **135**(9), 507-17 (1996)].

***Clerodendron colebrookianum*:** With the objective of verifying the scientific basis for the use of *C. colebrookianum* by Mizo people of north eastern region of India as a cardioprotective agent, the effect of different extracts of the leaves of the plant on serum lipid profile was examined. Administration of both crude and organic solvent extracts of the leaves of the plant significantly lowered total cholesterol, triglycerides and low-density lipoprotein (LDL). Methanol extract treated rats, however, failed to show any reduction of triglycerides. Both total cholesterol and triglycerides were lowered significantly even after the administration of crude extract against high fat diet. Significant increase of cardioprotective lipid, i.e high density lipoprotein (HDL), after administration of ethyl acetate and methanol extracts was another interesting finding of this experiment. Total cholesterol/HDL and LDL/HDL ratios were also significantly lower in the experimental group. The leaves of *C. colebrookianum* were thus proved to have definite cardioprotective potentiality. [Devi R, Sharma DK; Hypolipidemic effect of different extracts of *Clerodendron colebrookianum* Walp in normal and high fat diet-fed rats, *J Ethnopharmacol* **90**(1), 63-68 (2004)].

Cnidium monnier: See *Typha angustifolia*: [Park *et al.*; *Phytother Res* **18**(3), 224-29 (2004)].

Coccinia indica (Syn. *Cephalandra indica*, H. Kanduri, S. Bimba): The effect of *C. indica* stem powder on blood sugar and lipid levels was investigated in cases of maturity onset diabetes mellitus. The drug elicited marked hypolipidemic and hypoglycemic activity in these patients. An improvement in the clinical symptoms was also noted in these treated patients. [Kupparajan K, Seshadri C, Revathi R, Venkataraghavan S; Hypoglycemic effect of *Coccinia indica* in diabetes mellitus *Nagarjun* **29**(5), 1-4 (1986)].

See Pectin in Appendix: [Prasanna Kumar *et al.*; *J Food Sci Technol* **34**(2), 103-07 (1997)].

A polyherbal formulation (tincture of leaves of *Coccinia indica, Cocculus villosus, Catharanthus roseus, Momordica charantia* and *Gymnema sylvestere*) in the dose of 1 ml/kg for 30 days decreased serum cholesterol and glucose in alloxan-induced diabetic rats. However, in normal rats this formulation failed to show any hypocholesterolemic or hypoglycemic effect. [Annapurna A, Kanaka D, Mahalakhmi D, Muralikrishna K; Antidiabetic activity of polyherbal preparation (tincture of *panchaparna*) in normal and diabetic rat, *Indian J Exp Biol* **39**(5), 500- 02 (2001)].

Cocculus villosus (H. Jamtiki-Bel, S. Garudi): See *Coccinia indica:* [Annapurna *et al.*; *Indian J Exp Biol* **39**(5), 500-02 (2001)].

Cocos nucifera (Cocoanut, H. Nariyal, S. Narikela): In high fat diet-fed rats, the effect of cocoanut and black gram fibre on lipids and lipid peroxide was studied. The cocoanut and black gram fibre-treated animals showed a significant decrease in the serum, liver, aortic and intestinal cholesterol, free fatty acid and phospholipid levels. Hepatic and intestinal malondialdehyde and conjugated dienes were also significantly decreased in these animals. These fibres enhanced the superoxide dismutase and catalase activity in liver, intestine, heart and proximal and distal colon. In liver, intestine, proximal and distal colon and heart glutathione levels were significantly decreased in fibre treated animals. [Thampi BSH, Manoj G, Leelamma S, Menon VP; Dietary fibre and lipid peroxidation: Effect of dietary fibre on lipid and lipid peroxides in high fat fed diet, *Indian J Exp Biol* **29**(6), 563-67 (1991)].

Saturated vegetable oils (cocoanut, palm, and palm kernel oil) containing predominantly saturated fatty acids— lauric (12:0) or myristic (14:0) and palmitic (16:0) acids— raise plasma total cholesterol and low density lipoprotein cholesterol (LDL-c) levels in animals and humans, presumably by decreasing LDL receptor activity and/or increasing LDL-c production rate. Unsaturated vegetable oils such as corn, soybean, olive, and canola oil, by virtue of their predominant levels of either linoleic acid (18:2) or oleic acid (18:1), are hypocholesterolemic, probably as a result of their ability to upregulate LDL receptor activity and/or decrease LDL-c production rate. [Nicolosi RJ, Rogers EJ; Regulation of plasma lipoprotein levels by dietary triglycerides enriched with different fatty acids, *Med Sci Sports Exerc* **29**(11), 1422-28 (1997)].

See *Rosa canina:* [Gonzalez *et al.; Rev Esp Fisiol* **53**(2), 199-204 (1997)].

The neutral detergent fibre, isolated from cocoanut kernel, was digested with cellulase and hemicellulase and the residual fiber rich in hemicellulose (without cellulose) and cellulose (without hemicellulose) were fed to rats and compared with a fibre-free group. The results indicate that hemicellulose-rich fibre showed decreased concentration of total cholesterol, LDL + VLDL-cholesterol and increased HDL-cholesterol, while cellulose-rich fiber showed no significant alteration. Rats fed with hemicellulose-rich cocoanut fibre produced lower concentration of triglycerides and phospholipids and lower release of lipoproteins into circulation. There was increased concentration of hepatic bile acids and increased excretion of faecal sterols and bile acids. These results indicate that the hemicellulose component of cocoanut fibre was responsible for the observed hypolipidemic effect. [Sindhurani JA, Rajamohan T; Hypolipidemic effect of hemicellulose component of cocoanut fibre, *Indian J Exp Biol.* **36**(8), 786-89 (1998)].

Male Sprague-Dawley rats, fed fibre from cocoanut kernel, showed a significant lowering of serum total cholesterol and (LDL+VLDL)-cholesterol, and an increase in HDL-cholesterol. A hypocholesterolemic effect was observed in the aorta and other tissues. There was increased cholesterogenesis in the liver, as was evident from increased incorporation of radioactive acetate into cholesterol and increased activity of HMG-CoA reductase. An increased concentration of hepatic bile acids, increased faecal excretion of neutral sterols and bile acids, and lower release of lipoproteins into the circulation were observed in rats fed cocoanut fibre. Activities of plasma lecithin: Cholesterol acyl transferase and lipoprotein lipase were increased, while glucose-6-phosphate dehydrogenase and malic enzyme showed a decrease, in rats fed with cocoanut fibre. [Sindhurani JA, Rajamohan T; Effect of dietary fibre from cocoanut kernel (*Cocos nucifera*) on cholesterol metabolism, *J Clinical Biochem Nutr* **24**(3), 125-32 (1998)].

Feeding of cocoanut kernel protein (globulin) led to lowering of serum and tissue levels of cholesterol, phospholipids and triglycerides as compared to casein fed rats. Kernel protein fed animals exhibited increased hepatic degradation of cholesterol to bile acids, enhanced hepatic cholesterol biosynthesis and decreased esterification of free cholesterol in liver. Intestinal lipogenesis was also decreased in kernel treated rats. Hypolipidemic activity of kernel protein is attributed to its very low lysine / arginine ratio. [Nair KG, Rajmohan T, Kurup PA; Cocoanut kernel protein modifies the effect of cocoanut oil on serum lipids, *Plant Foods Hum Nutr* **53**(2), 133-144 (1998)].

Effect of cocoanut protein on the metabolism of lipids and lipid peroxides was studied in rats fed with high fat cholesterol-containing diet and the results were compared with those fed L-arginine. Both cocoanut protein and L-arginine showed significantly lower levels of total cholesterol, LDL+ VLDL-cholesterol, triglycerides and phospholipids in the serum and higher levels of serum HDL-cholesterol. Increased hepatic cholesterogenesis, increased conversion of cholesterol to bile acids and increased faecal excretion of bile acids were observed. Feeding cocoanut protein resulted in decreased levels of malondialdehyde in the heart and increased activity of superoxide dismutase and catalase. Supplementation of cocoanut protein caused increased excretion of urinary nitrate, which implied higher rate of conversion of arginine into nitric oxide. L-arginine supplemented group and the cocoanut protein-fed group produced similar effects. From the results of investigation it was inferred that cocoanut protein is able to reduce hyperlipidemia and peroxidative effect induced by high fat cholesterol-containing diet and these effects are mainly mediated by the L-arginine present in it. [Salil G, Rajamohan T; Hypolipidemic and antiperoxidative effect of cocoanut protein in hypercholesterolemic rats. *Indian J Exp Biol.* **39**(10), 1028-34 (2001)].

Ethanol-induced hyperlipidemic male albino rats showed increased concentration of cholesterol and triglycerides in the serum and tissues. Inclusion of cocoanut protein and larginine into ethanol-fed rats produced lower levels of total cholesterol, LDL+ VLDL-cholesterol, triglycerides and atherogenic index in the serum. Administration of cocoanut protein and L-arginine to ethanol-fed rats caused decreased activity of HMG-CoA reductase in the liver and increased activity of lipoprotein lipase in the heart. The lower activities of malic enzyme and glucose-6-phosphate dehydrogenase and increased concentration of hepatic bile acids and faecal excretion of neutral sterols and bile acids were also observed in these groups. All these effects were discernible also in rats fed either with cocoanut protein or L-arginine. The major factor responsible for the hypolipidemic effect of cocoanut protein was thus proved to be due to its high content of L-arginine. [Mini S, Rajamohan T; Influence of cocoanut kernel protein on lipid metabolism in alcohol-fed rats, *Indian J Exp Biol* **42**(1), 53-57 (2004)].

Coix lachryma-jobi (Adlay, Adley, H. Gurlu, S. Gavedhu): Green juice extracted from adley, alfalfa (*Medicago sativa*) and Italian ryegrass (*Lolium multiflorum*) foliages were dried with a spray-drier and their hypocholesterolemic activities were compared in rats. The chemical composition of the dried green juice powders from adley, alfalfa and Italian ryegrass was different; while adley was rich in minerals, alfalfa was relatively rich in nitrogen and crude fat was rather high in Italian ryegrass. Addition of green juice powder from adley or alfalfa to the high lipid diet was effective in reducing plasma LDL-cholesterol and phospholipid levels and plasma, liver and faecal bile acid levels of rats. Italian ryegrass had no effects on any values determined in the present experiment. Results of the investigation suggested that the efficacy of adley was due to some substances other than protein. [Hwang JM, Ohshima M, Yokota HO, Okajima T; Efficient utilization of adley (*Coix lacryma*-jobi L.) foliage by the green crop fractionation method: 2. Hypocholesterolemic activity of the green juice, *J Jpn Soc Grassland Sci* **39**(1), 7-15 (1993)].

See *Hordeum vulgare:* [Yu *et al.*; *Biol Pharm Bull* **27**(6), 802-05 (2004)].

Coix lachrymajobi* var. *mayuen (Adlay): Rats, made obese by feeding high fat diet (HFD) for 8 weeks, were injected with 50 mg/100 g body weight adlay seed crude extract (ACE), daily for 4 weeks. HFD + ACE group significantly reduced food intake and body weight. Weights of epididymal and peritoneal fat were dramatically increased in HFD groups compared with those of normal diet (ND) group but significantly decreased more in HFD + ACE group than those of HFD + saline (sham) group. The sizes of white adipose tissue were markedly larger in HFD groups than ND group but considerably reduced in HFD + ACE group. Leptin and TNF- α mRNA expressions in white adipose tissue of rats were remarkably increased in sham group but significantly decreased in HFD+ACE group. From the results of the investigation, adlay seed crude extract was considered suitable for controlling obesity. [Kim SO, Yun SJ, Jung B, Lee EH, Hahm DH, Shim I, Lee HJ; Hypolipidemic effects of crude extract of adlay seed (*Coix lachrymajobi* var. *mayuen*) in obese rat-fed high fat diet: Relations of TNF- α and leptin mRNA expressions and serum lipid levels, *Life Sci* **75**(11), 1391-404 (2004)].

***Colchicum autumnale*:** Oral administration of root powder of *C. autumnale* and pure colchicines (1.5mg/kg and 0.25mg/kg respectively) to rabbits decreased serum cholesterol and uric acid levels along with an increase in lipid levels. [Alam M, Khan MTJ, Lone KP, Hasan FAI, Choudhary SA; Studies on medicinal herbs -1. Serum biochemical changes induced in rabbits by administration of *Colchicum autumnale*, *Pak J Sci Ind Res* **32**(10), 688-90 (1989)].

Colchicum luteum (H. Hirantututiya, S. Hiranyatutha): Crude *C. luteum*, its ethanol extract and colchicine, elicited highly significant hypolipidemic and hypocholesterolemic activity in rabbits. This drug also showed transitory hypoglycemic action. [Chaudhary AR, Alam M, Ahmad M, Khan FZ, Nomani N; Studies on medicinal herbs II: Effect of *Colchicum luteum* on biochemical paramaters of rabbit serum, *Fitoterapia* **64**(6), 510-15 (1993)].

Coleus froskohlii: See *Allium sativum* (Garlic): [Dwivedi S; *Ann Natl Acad Med Sci* (India) 32(3&4) 159-175(1996)].

Commiphora mukul (H. Guggul, S. Guggulu): Effects of guggulu and its alcohol soluble and insoluble fractions on serum cholesterol, serum turbidity and coagulation and prothrombin time were studied in cholesterol-induced hyperlipidemic animals. Following three weeks of guggulu treatment of hyperlipidemic animals the serum cholesterol and serum turbidity decreased significantly alongwith an increase in coagulation and prothrombin time. Administration of guggulu (12g/d) to hyperlipidemic patients suffering from obesity and cerebral thrombosis led to a significant lowering of serum turbidity and an increase of coagulation time. [Tripathi SN, Sastri VVS, Satyavati GV; Experimental and clinical studies on the effect of guggulu (*Commiphora mukul*) in hyperlipemia and thrombosis, *J Res Indian Med* **2**(2), 140-54 (1968)].

The effects of *Commiphora mukul* on lipid metabolism in pigs, fed with athergenic diet for six weeks, were investigated. *C. mukul* effectively decreased the total serum cholesterol levels in both normal and atherogenic diet-fed pigs. The drug significantly lowered serum β-lipoprotein fraction and its cholesterol contents in these animals. In treated pigs the β /α-lipoprotein ratio was also significantly altered. [Khanna DS, Agarwal OP, Gupta SK, Arora RB; Biochemical approach to antiatherosclerotic action of *Commiphora mukul*, an Indian indigenous drug in Indian domestic pigs (*Sus scrofa*), *Indian J Med. Res* **57**(May), 900-06 (1969)].

The hypocholesterolemic activity of the oleoresin fraction of *C. mukul* (gum guggulu) was studied in high cholesterol diet-induced hypercholesterolemic male albino rabbits. This investigation revealed that oleoresin of gum guggulu significantly lowered the serum cholesterol levels and prevented the development of atherosclerosis (at the fatty streaks formation stage) in hypercholestrolemic rabbits. The drug also lowered the body weight of high cholesterol diet-fed rabbits. [Satyavati GV, Dwarkanath C, Tripathi SN; Experimental studies on the hypocholestrolemic effects of *Commiphora mukul* Engl (Guggulu), *Indian J Med Res* **57**(10), 1950-62, (1969)].

In cholesterol-fed chicks, administration of alcoholic extract and terpenoid and steroid fractions, isolated from the ether extract of oleoresin of gum guggulu, exhibited significant hypolipidemic activity. Of all the fractions, steroid fraction elicited the maximum hypolipidemic activity followed by alcoholic extract and terpenoid fraction. [Malhotra CL, Agarwal YK, Mehta VL, Prasad S; The effect of various fractions of gum guggulu on experimentally produced hypercholesterolemia in chicks, *Indian J Med Res* **58**(3), 394 (1970)].

Oral administration of alcoholic extract of *C. mukul* resin (guggulu) and a pure steroid, isolated from this extract (25-50 mg/kg), to normal, triton-induced and diet-induced hyperlipidemic rats, caused a significant lowering of serum cholesterol levels. However, alcoholic extract and pure steroids slightly inhibited the cholesterol biosynthesis in liver slices by acetate-1-14C incorporation *in vitro*. [Nityanand S, Kapoor NK; Hypocholesterolemic effect of *Commiphora mukul* resin (Guggulu). *Indian J Exp Biol* **9**(3), 376-77 (1971)].

The effects of fraction "A"of gum guggulu were studied on 44 hyperlipidemic patients and the results compared with ethyl –p- cholrophenoxyisobutyrate and CIBA-13437-Su. The drugs were administered randomly for a period of six to thirty four weeks. The gum guggulu fraction A significantly decreased the serum total lipids, cholesterol phospholipids and β-lipoprotein levels. Of all the lipid parameters, serum triglycerides showed maximum lowering following the administration of these drugs. [Malhotra SC, Ahuja MM; Comparative hypolipidemic effectiveness of Gum guggulu (*Commiphora mukul*) fraction A, Ethyl–pchlorophenoxyisobuyrate and CIBA 13437-Su, *Indian J Med Res* **59**(10), 1621-31 (1971)].

A double blind clinical study was undertaken to assess the effect of crude guggulu and fraction A of its petroleum ether extract on obese patients. Guggulu and its extracts significantly reduced the serum cholesterol levels at the end of 10 and 21 days of its administration. Guggulu also decreased cholesterol / phospholipid levels in these patients. It was suggested that guggulu should be used for a longer period i.e. at least for 3 months to have an idea about its action. [Kuppurajan K, Rajgopalan SS, Koteshwara Rao T, Vijayalakshmi AN, Dwarkanath C; Effect of guggulu (*Commiphora mukul*) on serum lipids in obese subjects, *J Res Indian Med* **8**(4), 1-8 (1973)].

The effects of various fractions of guggulu on serum and liver cholesterol biosynthesis were studied. Of all the fractions, the steroid fraction was most effective in lowering cholesterol in normal and triton-treated rats. The insoluble residue fraction of gum guggulu was toxic and inactive. [Nityanad Swarn, Kapoor Narinder K; Cholesterol lowering activity of the various fractions of the guggulu, *Indian J Exp Biol*. **11**(9), 395-96 (1973)].

In experimentally induced hyperlipidemic and atherosclerotic chicks, the effects of petroleum ether extract (fraction A) and ethyl acetate extract (fraction B) of *C. mukul* on serum total cholesterol, triglycerides, phospholipids and total lipids were evaluated. Administration of fraction A of guggulu to hypercholesterolemic chicks significantly reduced serum cholesterol, triglycerides, phospholipids and lipid levels. These changes in lipid parameters were comparable to Atromid-S, an antilipidemic drug. However, fraction B of *C. mukul* was comparatively less effective. In experimental isoprenaline-induced myocardial necrosis in rats also, fraction A and the steroidal compound isolated from it were found to be effective. The extent and severity of myocardial necrosis was assessed using ^{86}Rb uptake in these rats. [Arora RB, Das D, Kapoor SC, Sharma RC; Effects of some fractions of *Commiphora mukul* on various serum lipid levels in hypercholesterolemic chicks and their effectiveness in myocardial infarction in rats, *Indian J Exp Biol* **11**(May), 166-68 (1973)].

In esterogen-induced hyperlipidemic white leghorn chicks, the effects of petroleum ether-extract of gum guggulu on blood lipids and cholesterol levels were investigated. The administration of gum guggulu extract for 15 days significantly decreased the serum lipids and cholesterol levels in hyperlipidemic chicks as compared to untreated birds. The guggulu treated chicks also exhibited stimulation of thyroid activity. These observations tend to suggest that possibly the hypolipidemic activity of guggulu is mediated through thyroid gland. [Gupta M, Tripathi SN, Prasad B; Effect of extract of gum gugglu on esterogen induced hyperlipidemia in chicks, *J Res Indian Med* **9**(2), 4-11 (1974)].

In patients of hyperlipoproteinemia (type II), hypolidemic effects of an oleoresin fraction from guggulu (*C. mukul*) and clofibrate were studied. Serum cholesterol and triglycerides levels were significantly reduced by both guggulu and clofibrate in these patients. It was suggested that hypolipidemic activity of guggulu was comparable to clofibrate. [Malhotras SC, Ahuja MMS, Sundaram KR; Long-term clinical studies on the hypolipidemic effect of *Commiphora mukul* (Guggulu) and clofibrate, *Indian J Med Res* **65**(3), 390-95 (1977)].

The hypolipidemic and anti-atherosclerotic activities of fraction A of gum guggulu (*C. mukul*) was evaluated in diet-induced hypercholesterolemic and hypertriglyceridemic male gerbils and it exhibited significant hypolipidemic activity. This drug also effectively prevented atherosclerosis. [Ahuja MMS, Malhotra SC, Tandon HD; Effect of fraction A of *Commiphora mukul* (Guggulu) on Mongolian Gerbils (*Meriones unguiculates*), *Indian J Exp Biol* **15**(Feb), 143-44 (1977)].

In a clinical study, the effect of fraction A of the petroleum ether extract of *C. mukul* on serum cholesterol and total lipids was evaluated in 120 obese, hypercholesterolemic and hyperlipidemic patients. Administration of this fraction of guggulu for 21 days significantly reduced serum cholesterol and total lipid levels in these patients. The hypocholesterolemic effects of *C. mukul* were comparable to those of clofibrate. [Kuppurajan K, Rajgopalan SS, Koteshwara Rao T, Seetaram R; Effect of guggulu (*Commiphora mukul*-Eng) on serum lipid in obese, hypercholesterolemic and hyperlipemic cases, *J Assoc Physicians India* **26**(May), 367-73 (1978)].

Oral administration of gum guggulu (*C. mukul*) in the dose of 500mg three times a day to hypercholesterolemic subjects, singnificantly reduced serum cholesterol, total lipids and nonesterified fatty acids. These observations suggested its use as an effective and safe indigenous drug in the management of hyperlipidemia. [Kotiyal JP, Bisht DB, Singh DS; Double blind crossover trial of gum guggulu (*Commiphora mukul*) fraction A in hypercholestrolemia, *J Res Indian Med Yoga Homeo* **14**(2), 11-16 (1979)].

Adrenalin, ADP and serotonin-induced platelet aggregation was markedly inhibited by purified steroidal fraction of gum resin exudate of *C. mukul*. This effect of the steroidal fraction was comparable to clofibrate. These observations may be of therapeutic value in cases of myocardial infarction and thromboembolism. [Mester L, Mester M, Nityanand S; Inhibition of platelet aggregation by guggulu steroids, *Planta Med* **37**(4), 367-69 (1979)].

Adminstration of *C. mukul* (gum guggulu) to normal healthy individuals and patients of coronary artery disease for 30 days, caused enhancement of serum fibrinolytic activity in normal volunteers as well as in patients of coronary artery disease. Platelet adhesive index also decreased in healthy volunteers and in coronary artery disease patients at the end of 15 days of treatment. However, serum cholesterol levels did not decrease significantly. [Bordia A, Chuttani SK; Effect of gum guggulu on' fibrinolysis and platelet adhesiveness in coronary heart disease, *Indian J Med Res* **70** (Dec), 992-96 (1979)].

A clinical study revealed that fraction A of gum guggulu is a safe, effective, non toxic and well tolerated hypolipidemic drug, which may be used in the treatment of hyperlipidemia and obesity. [Kotiyal JP, Singh DS, Bisht DB; Study of hypolipidemic effect of *Commiphora mukul* (gum guggulu) fraction A in obesity, *J Res Ayur Siddha* **1**(3), 335-44 (1980)].

In a clinical study, the hypolipidemic and anticoagulant effects of the oleoresin fraction of *C. mukul* (Guggulu) were investigated on 93 hyperlipidemic patients. The patients were administered guggulu (2gTDS) for 3 months and the follow-up assessment was done every month. The guggulu therapy caused a significant lowering of serum cholesterol at the end of each month and it remained low upto three months after cessation of guggulu intake. The serum triglyceride and free fatty acids levels were reduced only after 2 months of guggulu administration. However, the body weight, skin fold thickness, bleeding time and platelet count were not significantly altered during or after guggulu treatment. [Jain AP; Clinical assessment of the volume of oleoresin of *Commophora mukul* (guggul) in obesity and hyperlipidemia, *ICMR Bull* **10,** 83-84 (1980)].

In 42 cases of ischemic heart disease, fibrinolytic and antiplatelet aggregatory activity of *Commiphora mukul* was investigated. The cases of myocardial infarction exhibited relatively lower fibrinolytic activity compared to patients of angina pectoris, acute coronary insufficiency and asymptomatic coronary artery disease. However, the platelet aggregatory activity did not differ much in these disease conditions. The fibrinolytic activity was enhanced following administration of *C. mukul* in patients of ischemic heart disease. [Baldwa VS, Sharma RC, Ranka PC, Chittora MD; Effect of *Commiphora mukul* (guggulu) on fibrinolytic activity and platelet aggregation in coronary artery disease, *Rajasthan Med J* **19**(2), 84-86 (1980)].

See *Allium sativum* (Garlic): [Dixit et al.; *Biochem Exp Biol* **16**(4), 421-4.1 (1980)].

Three groups of hyperlipidemic subjects were administered guggulu (*Commiphora mukul*), garlic pearls or clofibrate. After 15 days of treatment, all the hyperlipidemic cases showed a fall in the serum cholesterol levels. However, at the end of one month a significant lowering of serum cholesterol was noted in garlic pearls and *C. mukul* extract-treated patients. *C. mukul* was found to be relatively more potent as a hypolipidemic agent than garlic. [Baldwa VS, Ranka PC, Rishi JP, Rai RR; *Commiphora mukul* (guggulu), garlic extract and clofibrate in hyperlipidemic states, *Rajasthan Med J* **20**(2), 73-76 (1981)].

In vitro, addition of petroleum ether extract of *C. mukul* to culture media containing mice thyroid gland, significantly increased the ^{131}I uptake, T3 resin uptake and free thyroxin index in the media. It was suggested that *C. mukul* might be useful in the management of hypothyroidism and associated problems like hypercholesterolemia, hyperlipoproteinemia and atherosclerosis. [Singh AK, Prasad GC, Tripathi SN; *In vitro* studies on thyrogenic effect of *Commiphora mukul* (guggulu), *Ancient Sci Life* **2**(1), 23-28 (1982)].

Hypocholesterolemic effect of *Commiphora mukul* and biological activity of several other important medicinal plants were discussed. [Ikram M; Biologically active medicinal plants, *Hamdard Medicus* **27**(3), 73-85 (1984)].

Administration of Pushkar-guggulu, a combination of *Commiphora mukul* and *Inula raecemosa,* to patients of ischemic heart disease at a dose of 6g/d for four months decreased the serum cholesterol levels. In treated patients, precardial pain, discomfort and dyspnea were also controlled. [Tripathi SN, Upadhya BN, Sharma SD, Gupta VK, Tripathi YB; Role of Pushkar-guggulu in the management of ischaemic heart disease, *Ancient Sci Life* **4**(1), 9-19 (1984)].

In monkeys (*Presbytis entellus entellus* Dufrrsne), administration of steroid fraction of *C. mukul* caused lowering of total cholesterol, triglycerides, phospholipids and non-esterified fatty acids. These changes in lipid profile were relatively more marked in comparision to clofibrate-treated animals. [Bhargava SK; Hypolipidemic activity of a steroid fraction of guggulu resin (*Commiphora mukul* Hook ex stocks) in monkeys (*Presbytis entellus entellus* Dufrrsne), *Plant Med Phytother* **18**(2), 68-73 (1984)].

The effect of chronic feeding of guggulipid, a hypocholesterolemic and a potential antiatherosclerotic agent of plant origin, on the levels of catecholamine and dopamine β– hydroxylase activity of brain and heart tissues of rhesus monkeys was studied. The levels of norepinephrine, dopamine and activity of norepinephrine biosynthetic enzyme dopamine β– hydroxylase increased progressively with increasing dose of guggulipid. The increase in catecholamine biosynthesis by guggulipid is considered to be one of the possible mechanisms to explain the lipid-lowering activity of this plant product. [Srivastava M, Nityanand S, Kapoor NK; Effect of guggulipid on norepinephrine biosynthesis of monkey tissues, *Curr Sci* (Bangalore) **53**(21), 1131-33 (1984)].

See *Allium sativum* (Garlic): [Srivastava *et al.*; *J Biosci* (Bangalore) **6**(3), 277-82 (1984)].

Guggulipid principle of *Commiphora mukul* elicited potent hypolipidemic and antiinflammatory activity. Chemical constituents of seeds, leaves, bark, stem and roots of the plant were described. [Dahodwalla AN; Natural product pharmacology: Strategies in search of leads for new drug designs, *Trends Pharmacol Sci* **6**(2), 49-53 (1985)].

In thirty patients of primary hyperlipidemia, the antihyperlipidemic effect of guggulipid and clofibrate was investigated. This clinical study revealed superiority of gugulipid over clofibrate as an antihyperlipidemic agent. [Baldwa VS, Gupta ML; Effect of *Commiphora mukul* and clofibrate on lipid profile in hyperlipidemia. A comparative and cross over study, *Rajasthan Med J* **24**(3), 90-92 (1985)].

Hypolipidemic and antiobesity activity of gum guggulu fraction 'A' was investigated in a double blind clinical study. Fraction 'A' of gum guggulu significantly lowered the serum cholesterol, total lipids and triglyceride levels. However, the body weight and skin fold thickness except triceps skins fold were not affected in these patients. [Kotiyal JP, Singh DS, Bisht DB; Gum guggulu (*Commiphora mukul*) fraction 'A'in obesity- a double blind clinical trial, *J Res Ayur Siddha* (1, 3 & 4), 20-35 (1985)].

In 22 patients of primary hyperlipidemia, the efficacy of gugulipid was studied. Administration gugulipid (500 mg TDS) for six weeks significantly lowered serum cholesterol and triglyceride levels in 59% patients. The cholesterol-reducing effect became evident after 2 weeks and maximum reduction was noted between 4 and 6 weeks. After withdrawl of the drug, the serum cholesterol and triglyceride levels reversed back to pretreatment levels after 6 weeks. This drug was well tolerated and no side effects were observed. [Gopal K, Saran RK, Nityanands, Gupta PP, Hasan M, Das M, Sinha N, Agrawal SS; Clinical trial of ethyl acetate extract of gum guggulu (guggulipid) in primary hyperlipidemia, *J Assoc Physicians India* **34**(4), 249-51 (1986)].

Phase I (safety on chronic administration) and phase II (efficacy of the drug) clinical trials of gugulipid, isolated from *Commiphora mukul*, were undertaken repectively, on 21 and 19 patients. The drug was found to be completely safe and devoid of any effect on liver function, blood sugar or blood urea levels, haematological parameters- or electrocardiogram. Patients of primary hyperlipidemia, treated with gugulipid (500 mg TDS), showed significantly lower levels of cholesterol and triglycerides after 4 weeks of treatment. [Agrawal RC, Singh SP, Saran RK, Das SK, Sinha N, Asthana OP, Gupta PP, Nityanand S, Dhawan BN, Agrawal SS; Clinical trial of gugulipid- a new hypolipidemic agent of plant origin in primary hyperlipidemia *Indian J Med Res* **84**(Dec.), 626-34 (1986)].

Description and distribution of *Commiphora mukul*, a well-known hypolipidemic plant, alongwith its chemistry and therapeutic uses have been reviewed. Methods of purification of guggulu and preparation of some more commonly used Ayurvedic formulations containing guggulu have also been described. [Bhat B; Guggulu, *Rheumatism* **22**(4), 82-100 (1987)].

Literature on gum guggulu as a commercially viable hypolipidemic agent was reviewed and presented in a chronological order. Suggestions were also made with regard to further scientific investigations on *Commiphora mukul*. [Satyavati GV; Gum guggulu (*Commiphora mukul*)- the success story of an ancient insight leading to a modern discovery, *Indian J Med Res* **87**(April), 327-35 (1988)].

Administration of purified gum gugulu (4.5g in two divided doses) to 40 hyperlipidemic patients for 16 weeks significantly reduced serum cholesterol and triglyceride levels. The HDL- c levels were increased (35%) with a decrease in LDL-c and VLDL-c levels in these cases at the end of 16 weeks. The drug was found to be fairly safe and effective in hyperliprdemia. [Verma SK, Bordia A; Effect of *Commiphora mukul*: Gum gugulu in patients of hyperlipidemia with special reference to HDL-cholesterol, *Indian J Med Res* **87** (April), 350-60 (1988)].

Administration of oleoresin of gum guggulu (3.33mg/100g bw) for 30 days to normal albino rats, led to enhancement of faecal bile acid excretion. In cholesterol-fed albino rats, relatively higher dose of gum guggulu (10mg/100g bw) increased the bile acids and cholesterol excretion. [Ahluwalia P, Amma MKP; Effect of oral ingestion of oleoresin of gum-guggal on the faecal excretioin of cholesterol and bile acids in normocholesterolemic and hypercholesterolemic rats, *Res Bull Panjab Univ Sci* **39**(1-2), 53-57 (1988)].

Clinical evaluation of four Ayurvedic compound drugs containing Guggulu (*C. mukul*) as the major constituent *i.e.* triphala guggulu, sinhanad guggulu, gokshuradi guggulu and chandraprabhavati in 48 obese subjects revealed significant reduction in serum cholesterol and triglycerides. These patients also exhibited a reduction in the body weight, skin fold thickness and circumference of hips and waistline. Some of the minor side effects noted in these cases included mild diarrhoea and nausea [Kulkarni PH, Paranjape P; Clinical assessment of Ayurvedic anti-obesity drugs. A double blind placebo controlled trial, *J Natl Integrated Med Assoc* **32**(1), 7-11 (1990)].

Administration of various preparations of guggulu i.e., Triphala guggulu (250mg TDS), Gokshuradi guggulu (250 mgTDS), Sinhad guggulu (100mgTDS) and chandraprabhavati (250 mg TDS) to different groups of obese subjects for 3 months significantly reduced their body weight, skin fold thickness and waist circumference compared to placebo treated group. Serum cholesterol and triglyceride levels were also decreased following treatment with these Ayurvedic preparations [Paranjape P, Patki P, Patwardhan B; Ayurvedic treatment of obesity: A randomized double blind placebo controlled clinical trial, *J Ethnopharmacol* **29**(1), 1-11 (1990)].

See *Inula racemosa*: [Singh *et al.*; *Int J Pharmacogn* **31**(2), 147-160 (1993)].

Administration of of guggulipid (50 mg) twice daily for 24 weeks to patients with hypercholesterolemia decreased the total cholesterol level by 11.7%, the low density lipoprotein cholesterol (LDL) by 12.5%, triglycerides by 12.0%, and the total cholesterol/high density lipoprotein (HDL) cholesterol ratio by 11.1% [Singh RB, Niaz MA, Ghosh S; Hypolipidemic and antioxidant effects of *Commiphora mukul* as an adjunct to dietary therapy in patients with hypercholesterolemia, *Cardiovasc Drugs Ther* **8**(4), 659-64 (1994)].

A comparative evaluation of hypocholesterolemic activity of three guggulu preparations (*Kaisora guggulu, Yograj guggulu and Nava guggulu*) was done in albino rats. All the three preparations (1g/kg) significantly lowered the serum and liver cholesterol levels. However, *Kaisora guggulu* elicited maximum hypocholesterolemic and anti-obesity activity and was superior to two other preparations of guggulu. [Nair RB, Pillai RP, Pillai BKR, Vijayaraj S, Nair CPR; Hypocholesterolemic action of three guggulu (*Commiphora mukul*) preparations, a comparative study, *J Res Ayur Siddha* **15**(3-4), 155-66 (1994)].

Administration of 'Triphala guggulu' (*C. mukul* as main constituent) to obese persons for 15 days decreased cholesterol (9.2%); triacylglycerol (11%), LDL–cholesterol (15.06%), VLDL– cholesterol (11%) and enhanced HDL- cholesterol (7.73%). Guggulu also inhibited hepatic cholesterol biosynthesis and catecholamine-induced lipolysis. [Patil ND, Dewoolkar, Chheda MS; Effect of the guggulu on lipid profile and glycosylated Hb.in obese subjects, *Biorhythm* 57-59 (1995)].

"Triphala guggulu", belonging to a group of drugs termed as *Lekhniya dravyas* in Ayurveda and used for the management of hyperlipidemia, was found to reduce serum cholesterol and triglycerides along with enhancement of HDL-cholesterol in hyperlipidemic patients. [Paranjape P; Secure management of hyperlipidemia, *Biorhythm* 78-81(1995)].

Histopathological studies on liver, spleen, intestine, lung, kidney, stomach and adrenal gland of rats, treated with synthetic guggulusterones (constituents of *C. mukul*) for a period of 16 weeks, revealed drug related changes in a few animals upon exposure to high dose of the drug. [Far SR, Master HE, Billimoria FR, Sane RT; Hypolipidemic effects of synthetic gugulsterones in normal rats and assessment of its long-term toxicity at cellular levels in various organs, *Indian J Med Sci.* **50**(3), 63-67 (1996)].

Commiphora mukul resin and its fractions exhibited significant lipid lowering action. The ethyl acetate soluble fraction of gum guggulu (Guggulipid) produced a significant reduction of serum and tissue lipids with regression of atheromatous lesions in rabbits and monkeys. It also prevented microsomal lipid peroxidation and Cu^{++}- induced LDL oxidation. A multicentric trial showed that guggulipid possessed effective lipid lowering activity comparable to standard hypolipidemic agents with minimal side effects. [Nityanand S; Development of hypolipidmic agents from plants and traditional remedies, *International Seminar on Free radical Mediated Diseases and Ayurveda,* Faculty of Ayurveda, IMS, BHU, Varanasi, India, (A-30), September 2-4, 1996].

The hypolipidemic activity of guggulusterone was studied in cholesterol-fed and triton-induced hyperlipidemic rats. Administration of guggulusterone (50mg/kg) to triton-induced hyperlipidemic rats significantly lowered serum lipid levels. In cholesterol (25mg/kg)-fed animals chronic administration of guggulusterone

(5mg/kg) for 30 days led to the lowering of lipids and LDL and VLDL-cholesterol levels. This drug activated lipolytic enzyme in blood and liver and stimulated receptor mediated catabolism of low density lipoprptein. The hypolipidemic action of this compound was attributed to inhibition of cholesterol biosynthesis, increased faecal bile acid excretion and enhanced lecithin cholesterol acyl transferase activity. [Ramesh Chandra, Khanna AK, Kapoor NK; Lipid lowering activity of guggulusterone from *Commiphora mukul* in hyperlipidemic rats, *Phytother Res* **10**(6), 508-11 (1996)].

See *Allium sativum* (Garlic): [Dwivedi S; *Ann Natl Acad Med Scs* (India) 32(3&4), 159- 175(1996)].

Guggulusterone, isolated from *C. mukul*, prevented lipid peroxide generation determined in terms of thiobarbituric acid reactive substances (TBARS), lipid hydroperoxides and conjugated dienes. This compound lowered cholesterol, cholesterol esters, triglycerides and phospholipids and inhibited the conversion of cholesterol into oxygenated cholesterol. Guggulsterone also protected LDL-apoprotein as measured by reversal of relative electrophoretic mobility (REM) after oxidation. Such a protective action of guggulusterone was attributed to its free radical scavenging activity as evidenced by inhibition of generation of hydroxyl radicals in a nonenzymic system. [Singh K, Ramesh chander, Kapoor NK; Guggulusterone, a potent hypolipidemic, prevents oxidation of low density lipoprotein, *Phytother Res* **11**(4), 291-94 (1997)].

See *Aloe vera:* [Nada *et al.*; *Fitoterapia* **68**(3), 240-44 (1997)].

See *Allium sativum:* [Sharma & Dwivedi; *Indian Drugs* **34**(5), 242-51 (1997)].

A high performance liquid chromatographic method has been developed and validated for the finger printing and quantitative determination of *E*- and *Z*-guggulsterones, the hypolipidemic agents in the gum-resin exudate of *C. mukul*, currently marketed worldwide as hypocholesterolemic. [Mesrob B, Nesbitt C, Misra R, Pandey RC; High performance liquid chromatographic method for fingerprinting and quantitative determination of *E*- and *Z*-guggulsterones in *Commiphora mukul* resin and its products, *J Chromatogr* B *Biomed Sci Appl* **720**(1-2), 189-96 (1998)].

Administration of guggulipid (containing guggulusterone), the main constituent of *C. mukul*, at a dose of 75 mg three times /day for 12 weeks to patients of nephrotic syndrome caused a significant increase of serum HDL-cholesterol at the end of 8 weeks. However, significant electrocardiographic changes were noted only after 12 weeks of the treatment. [Beg M, Afzal S, Akhter N; Hypolipidemic and cardioprotective effectiveness of guggulipid in patients of nephrotic syndrome, *Indian Med Gazette* **132**(2), 35-38 (1998)].

Administration of guggulipid, the main constituents of *C. mukul*, in the dose of 100mg/kg po for 21days to normal rats did not influence the lipid levels. However, physical stress (swimming for 5 hr)-induced increase the lipid levels was significanltly less in guggu lipid pretreated rats in comparison to controls. [Kumar R, Sharma NK, Puri JN, Jain IP, Singh S, Kapoor S, Ansari NA, Singh SP; Effect of guggulipid on stress induced alterations in lipid profile in rats, (XXXI Annual Conference of Pharmacological Society, Lucknow, Dec18 –20, 1998) *Indian J Pharmacol* **31**(1), 71 (1999)].

Guggulipid, the standardised product from the oleoresin fraction of *Commiphora mukul* plant, has been marketed as a hypolipidemic agent. The ketosteroids, *cis*- and *trans*-4, 17(20)- pregnadiene-3, 16-dione, known as *E*- and *Z*-guggulsterones, respectively, are the main ingredients in guggulipid. A liquid chromatographic method was developed for simultaneous determination of *E*- and *Z*-guggulusterones in guggulipid preparations using synthetic *E*- and Zguggulsterone standards. [Nagarajan M, Waszkuc TW, Sun J; Simultaneous determination of *E*- and *Z*-guggulsterones in dietary supplements containing *Commiphora mukul* extract (guggulipid) by liquid chromatography. *JAOAC Int* **84**(1), 24-28 (2001)].

Z-guggulsterone, a constituent of *C. mukul* exudates, acts as antagonists of the bile acid receptor (BAR), a member of the intracellular receptor superfamily. The mechanism by which the compound antagonize the activity of BAR has been studied. [Wu J, Xia C, Meier J, Li S, Hu X, Lala DS; The hypolipidemic natural product guggulsterone acts as an antagonist of the bile acid receptor, *Mol Endocrinol* **16**(7), 1590-97 (2002)].

In hyperlipidemic patients, comparative efficacy of *C. mukul*, Karneem (A herbal formulation containing *Azadirachta indica, Ocimum sanctum, Zingiber officilalis, Momordica charantia* and Guggul) and *Zingibar officinalis* in lowering lipids was studied. The patients treated with *C. mukul* and Karneem or *Z. officinale* showed marked improvement in the lipid profile. However, guggulu was more effective than Karneem and it was better than ginger in controlling the serum lipids. [Raut A, Tyagi NK, Tewari V; Application of generalized linear models and principle components in the study of effects of Guggulu, Karneem and ginger on serum lipids, *J Mahatma Gandhi Inst Med Sci* **7**(2), 10-16 (2002)].

Administration of *C. mukul* with *Inula racemosa* (1:1) to 250 cases of ischemic heart disease caused significant reduction of serum cholesterol, triglyceride and total lipid levels. Clinically also, these patients exhibited restoration of their ECG pattern towards normal and an improvement in dyspnoea, precardial pain etc following treatment with this drug. It was suggested that potent hypolipidemic activity of guggulu and anti-anginal potential of *Inula racemosa* combined together in the drug, which might be used as an effective measure in the treatment of ischemic heart disease. [Singh R, Upadhya BN, Batliwala PG; Evaluation of anti-ischemic potential of "Pushkar gugulu" in the treatment of ischemic heart disease, 2nd World Congress on "Biotechnological Development of Herbal Medicine", NBRI, Lucknow, India, p 163 February 20-22, (2003)].

Guggulsterones, the purported bioactive compounds of guggul, have been shown to be potent antagonists of two nuclear hormone receptors involved in cholesterol metabolism and this appears to be a plausible mechanism of action for the hypolipidemic effects of extracts from *Commiphora mukul* (guggul). In absence of a published safety or efficacy data on the use of guggul extracts in western populations, a short-term safety and efficacy of 2 doses of a standardized guggul extract (guggulipid, containing 2.5% guggulsterones) in healthy adults with hyperlipidemia eating a typical western diet was studied. It was concluded from this study that despite plausible mechanisms of action, guggulipid did not appear to improve levels of serum cholesterol over the short-term in this population of adults with hypercholesterolemia, and might in fact raise levels of LDL-c. Guggulipid also appeared to cause a dermatologic hypersensitivity reaction in some patients. [Szapary PO, Wolfe ML, Bloedon LT, Cucchiara AJ, DerMarderosian AH, Cirigliano MD, Rader DJ; Guggulipid for the treatment of hypercholesterolemia: A randomized controlled trial, *JAMA* **290**(6), 765-72 (2003)].

The antiatherogenic effect of a herbal formulation, Caps HT2, containing the methanolic extracts of selected parts of *Commiphora mukul, Allium sativum, Plumbago indica, Semecarpus anacardium, Hemidesmus indicus, Terminalia arjuna, Tinospora cordifolia, Withania somnifera* and *Ocimum sanctum*, was evaluated in rats. The formulation, Caps HT2 was found to scavenge superoxide and hydroxyl radicals. The lipid peroxidation was found inhibited (50%) by 48.5 μg/ml of Caps HT2. The intravenous administration of the formulation (5 mg/kg) delayed the plasma recalcification time in rabbits and enhanced the release of lipoprotein lipase enzyme significantly. The formulation also inhibited ADP induced platelet aggregation *in vitro*, which was comparable to commercial heparin. The hypolipidaemic effect of Caps HT2 was significant in diet-induced hyperlipidemic rats for a period of 30 days. Oral administration of the formulation (100, 200, 300 and 400 mg/kg) significantly raised HDL-cholesterol levels. The atherogenic index and the reduction in body weight were significant indicating its effectiveness against hyperlipidemia and obesity. All these results revealed the therapeutic potential of Caps HT2 against vascular intimal damage and atherogenesis leading to various types of cardiovascular problems. [Mary NK, Babu BH, Padikkala J; Antiatherogenic effect of Caps HT2, a herbal Ayurvedic medicine formulation, *Phytomedicine* **10**(6-7), 474-82 (2003)].

There is accumulating evidence that LDL oxidation is essential for atherogenesis, and the antioxidants that prevent this oxidation may either slow down or prevent atherogenesis. Appropriate experiments reveal that *Commiphora mukul* and its lipid-lowering component, guggulsterone significantly inhibit LDL oxidation. The combination of antioxidant and lipid- lowering properties of *C. mukul* and guggulsterone makes them especially beneficial against atherogenesis. [Wang X, Greilberger J, Ledinski G, Kager G, Paigen B, Jurgens G; The hypolipidemic natural product *Commiphora mukul* and its component guggulsterone inhibit oxidative modification of LDL, *Atherosclerosis* **172**(2), 239-46 (2004)].

It was earlier suggested that the activity of guggulsterone, the active substance of *Commiphora mukul,* is mediated by antagonism of the receptor for bile acids, the farnesoid X receptor. It has now been demonstrated that both stereoisomers of guggulsterone (*E* and *Z*) bind to the steroid receptors (mineralocorticoid, androgen, glucocorticoid and progesterone receptors) with a much higher affinity than to the farnesoid X receptor. Guggulsterones behaved as antagonists of androgen, glucocorticoid and mineralocorticoid receptors, but as agonists of progesterone receptor. It is now suggested that the variety of pharmacological effects exhibited by guggulsterone may be mediated by targeting several steroid receptors. [Burris TP, Montrose C, Houck KA, Osborne HE, Bocchinfuso WP, Yaden BC, Cheng CC, Zink RW, Barr RJ, Hepler CD, Krishnan V, Bullock HA, Burris LL, Galvin RJ, Bramlett KS, Stayrook KR; The Hypolipidemic natural product guggulsterone is a promiscuous steroid receptor ligand, *Mol Pharmacol* **67**(3), 948-54 (2005)].

Convolvulus microphyllus: The hypolipidaemic activities of *C. microphyllus* have been observed in domestic animals (rats, rabbits and rhesus monkeys). The 50% ethanolic extract of the whole plant, when administered to cholesterol-fed gerbils, reduced levels of serum cholesterol level, LDL-cholesterol, triglycerides and phospholipids significantly after 90 days. The possible mechanism of action has been discussed. [Chaturvedi M, Mali PC, Dixit VP; Hypolipidaemic effect of *Convolvulus microphyllus* in cholesterol-fed gerbils (*Meriones hurrianae* Jeroon), *J Phytol Res* **8**(2), 153-55 (1995)].

Coptis chinensis (*Coptis rhizome*): Oral administration of *Sam Wang Sasium –Tang* (a compound herbal preparation containing *Coptis rhizome* and *Rheum rhizome*) and Wang Ryum Haedok-Tang (a herbal preparation containing *Coptis rhizome, Phellodandrom* bark and *Gardenia* fruits) significantly reduced serum total lipids, triglycerides and total cholesterol levels in hyperlipemic rats. The β-lipoprotein contents were also reduced following treatment with these compound herbal preparations in experimentally-induced hyperlipidemic rats. [Chung MH, Han SJ; Effect of composite preparations of crude drugs on experimentally-induced hyperlipemia in rats - Sam Wang Sasium –Tang and Wang Ryum Haedok-Tang, *Korean J Pharmacogn*, **27**(1) 397-407(1996)].

Coptis japonica: Administration of methanolic extract of rhizome of *C. japonica* to rats fed with diet containing 0.12% cholesterol significantly lowered the serum cholesterol levels. Although, the serum HDL-cholesterol levels did not differ much between treated and untreated rats, the HDL/ total cholesterol ratio was found to be higher in treated rats. The hepatic tissue cholesterol and triglycerids contents were significantly decreased in treated rats. The extract also enhanced faecal bile acid excretion. [Choi YS, Lee YI, Lee SY; Effect of extract of *Coptis japonica* on lipid metabolism in rats, *Korean J Pharmacogn* **27**(3), 246-53 (1996)].

Coriandrum sativum (H. Dhanya, S. Dhanyaka): The effect of the administration of coriander seeds on the metabolism of lipids was studied in rats, fed with a high fat diet with added cholesterol. The levels of total cholesterol and triglycerides decreased significantly in the tissues of the animals of the experimental group, which received coriander seeds. Significant increases in β-hydroxy - β-methyl glutaryl CoA reductase and plasma lecithin cholesterol acyl transferase activity were noted in the experimental group. The level of LDL + VLDL-cholesterol decreased while that of HDL-cholesterol increased in the experimental group compared to the control group. [Chithra V, Leelamma S; Hypolipidemic effect of coriander seeds (*Coriandrum sativum*): mechanism of action, *Plant Foods Hum Nutr* **51**(2), 167-72 (1997)].

In the biphasic model of triton-induced hyperlipidemia, *C. sativum* at a dose of 1g/kg body weight reduced cholesterol and triglycerides levels in both synthesis and excretory phases in rats. From the results of the investigation, coriander was proved to decrease the uptake and enhance the breakdown of lipids. [Lal AA, Kumar T, Murthy PB, Pillai KS; Hypolipidemic effect of *Coriandrum sativum* L. in triton-induced hyperlipidemic rats, *Indian J Exp Biol* **42**(9), 909-12 (2004)].

Crataegus oxyacantha (Hawthorn berries, H. Ban-sangili): Administration of alcoholic extract of the berries of *C. oxyacantha* to rats, fed on hyperlipidemic diet, prevented the elevation in plasma lipid levels. The extract also showed an ameliorating effect on the degeneration of liver, caused by hyperlipidemic diet. [Shanthi S, Parasakthy K, Deepalakshmi PD, Devaraj SN; Hypolipidemic activity of tincture of *Crataegus* in rats, *Indian J Biochem Biophys* **31**(2), 143-6 (1994)].

Tincture of Crataegus (TCR), made from berries of hawthorn, *C. oxyacantha,* is a hypocholesterolemic and antiatherosclerotic drug and contains flavonoids, triterpene saponins and a few cardioactive amines as the main constituents. The hypocholesterolemic action of TCR appears to be due to an upregulation of hepatic LDL-receptors resulting in greater influx of plasma cholesterol into the liver. TCR also prevents the accumulation of cholesterol in the liver by enhancing cholesterol degradation to bile acids and by simultaneously suppressing cholesterol biosynthesis. [Rajendran S, Deepalakshmi PD, Parasakthy K, Devaraj H, Devaraj SN; Effect of tincture of Crataegus on the LDL-receptor activity of hepatic plasma membrane of rats fed an atherogenic diet, *Atherosclerosis* **123**(1-2), 235-41 (1996)].

Crataegus pinnatifida (Hawthorn fruit): Hawthorn fruit extract has been shown to have cardiovascular protective, hypotensive and hypocholesterolemic activities. The present work was carried out to characterise the antioxidants of hawthorn fruit and study their effect on the oxidation of human low density lipoprotein (LDL) and α-tocopherol. Of the different solvent extractives of hawthorn fruit, only ethyl acetate extract was effective in inhibition of Cu+2- mediated LDL oxidation and it furnished, on chromatography, a triterpene (ursolic acid) and seven phenolic compounds (hyperoside, isoquercitrin, epicatechin, chlorogenic acid, quercetin, rutin and protocatechuic acid). The phenolic compounds were protective to human LDL from

Cu+2-mediated LDL oxidation. They were also effective in preventing the peroxy free radical induced oxidation of α-tocopherol in human LDL. The inhibitory effect of these compounds on oxidation of LDL and α-tocopherol was dose-dependent at concentrations ranging from 5 to 40 μM. In addition, supplementation of 2% hawthorn fruit powder significantly elevated serum α-tocopherol by 18-20% in rats fed with a 30% polyunsaturated canola oil diet, as compared with the control. The present results suggest that part of the mechanism for cardiovascular protective effects of hawthorn fruit might also involve the direct protection to human LDL from oxidation or indirect protection via maintaining the concentration of α-tocopherol in human LDL. [Zhang Z, Chang Qi, Zhu M, Huang Yu, Ho Walter KK, Chen ZYu; Characterization of antioxidants present in hawthorn fruits, *J Nutr Biochem* **12**(3), 144-52 (2001)].

Rats receiving high cholesterol diet (1 g/100 g) supplemented with hawthorn fruit powder (2 g/100 g) for 12 weeks showed lower levels of cholesterol (23.4% less) and triglycerides (22.2% less) compared to those receiving only high cholesterol diet. The mechanism by which hawthorn fruit decreases serum cholesterol involves, at least in part, the inhibition of cholesterol absorption mediated by down-regulation of intestinal ACAT (acyl CoA: Cholesterol acyl transferase) activity. [Zhang Z, Ho WK, Huang Y, James AE, Lam LW, Chen ZY; Hawthorn fruit is hypolipidemic in rabbits fed with a high cholesterol diet, *J Nutr* **132**(1), 5-10 (2002)].

Supplementation of aqueous ethanolic extract of hawthorn fruit led to greater excretion of both neutral and acidic sterols. The mechanisms by which hawthorn fruit decreases serum cholesterol were investigated by enzymatic assays. It involves a greater excretion of bile acids mediated by up-regulation of hepatic cholesterol 7 α-hydroxylase activity, and an inhibition of cholesterol absorption mediated by down-regulation of intestinal acyl CoA: Cholesterol acyltransferase (ACAT) activity. [Zhanga Z, Ho WKK, Huang Y, Chen ZY; Hypocholesterolemic activity of hawthorn fruit is mediated by regulation of cholesterol-7 α- hydroxylase and acyl CoA: cholesterol acyltransferase, *Food Res International* **35**(9), 885-91 (2002)].

Croton cajucara: The hypolpidemic activity of hydroalcoholic extract of leaves of *C. cajucara* in high fat diet-fed rats was investigated. Oral administration of the extract (200mg/kg) to hyperlipidemic rats for 10 weeks significantly decreased serum total cholesterol and low density lipoprotein cholesterol (LDL-c) without much change in high density lipoprotein cholesterol (HDL-c) and triglyceride levels. However, significant increase in HDLc / total cholesterol ratio was noted in these rats. The atherogenic index was also decreased in treated animals. In view of these beneficial effects and absence of any toxicity, *C. cajucara* is expected to be useful in the treatment of atherosclerosis [Farias RA, Neto MFO, Viana GSB, Rao VSN; Effect of *Croton cajucara* extract on serum lipids of rats fed with high fat diet, *Phytother Res* **10**(8), 697-99 (1996)].

Administration of *trans* dehydrocrotonin, a constituent of *C. cajucara,* to triton (WR-1339)- induced hyperlipidemic mice (at doses of 25 and 50 mg/kg) caused significant reduction of serum cholesterol and triglyceride levels. The results were comparable to gemifibrozil (100mg/kg), a known antihyperlipidemic agent. The use of *trans* dehydrocrotonin to combat the problems associated with hyperlipidemia is suggested. [Silva RM, Santos FA, Maciel MAM, Pinto AC, Rao VSN; Effect of trans dehydrocrotonin, a 19-nor-clerodane diterpene from *Croton cajucara* on experimental hypertriglyceridemia and hypercholesterolemia induced by triton WR -1339 (tylaxopal) in mice, *Planta Med* **67**(8), 763-65 (2001)].

Cucumis sativus (H. Khira, S. Sukasa): See Pectin in Appendix: [Prasanna Kumar et al.; *J Food Sci Technol* **34**(2), 103-07 (1997)].

The oral administration of the pectin extracted from the fruit of *C. sativus* at a dose of 5g/kg body weight/day showed significant hypolipidemic action in normal as well as cholesterol-fed experimental animals. Concentrations of cholesterol, triglycerides, phospholipids and free fatty acids in the serum and tissues of experimental animals were significantly reduced by *Cucumis* pectin. Pectin administration enhanced the activity of HMG CoA reductase, decreased the activities of glucose-6-phosphate dehydrogenase and malate dehydrogenase and increased the activities of lipoprotein lipase and plasma LCAT. Incorporation of labelled 14C acetate into free cholesterol was significantly higher in the liver of pectin-treated rats. Concentrations of bile acids (hepatic and faecal) and faecal neutral sterols showed significant increases in the pectin administered groups. [Sudheesh S, Vijayalakshmi NR; Lipid-lowering action of pectin from *Cucumis sativus*, *Food Chem* **67**(3), 281-86 (1999)].

Cuminum cyminum (Cumin, H. Jira, S. Jiraka): Ethereal extract of both cumin and turmeric inhibited arachidonate-induced platelet aggregation. Extracts from these spices inhibited thromboxane B2 production from exogenous 14C arachidonic acid in washed platelets; a simultaneous increase in the formation of lipoxygenase-derived products was observed. Turmeric extract inhibited incorporation of ^{14}C arachidonic acid into platelet phospholipids and deacylation of arachidonic acid -labelled phospholipids on stimulation with calcium ionophore A23187. Cumin extract was devoid of such effects. [Srivastava KC; Extracts from two frequently consumed spices— cumin (*Cuminum cyminum*) and turmeric (*Curcuma longa*)— inhibit platelet aggregation and alter eicosanoid biosynthesis in human blood platelets. *Prostaglandins Leukot Essent Fatty Acids* **37**(1), 57-64 (1989).].

Oral administration of of *C. cyminum* (0.25 g / kg bw) to diabetic rats for 6 weeks resulted in a significant reduction in plasma and tissue cholesterol, phospholipids, free fatty acids and triglycerides. [Dhandapani S, Subramanian VR, Rajagopal S, Namasivayam N; Hypolipidemic effect of *Cuminum cyminum* L. on alloxan-induced diabetic rats, *Pharmacol Res* **46**(3), 251-55 (2002)].

Curcuma amada (H. Amhaldi, S. Karpura haridra, Amragandhi): See *Curcuma longa*

[Pachauri & Mukherjee; *J Res Indian Med* **5**(1), 27-30 (1970)].

Curcuma comosa: Intraduodenal administration of butanol and ethyl acetate extracts of *C. comosa* induced a dose-dependent stimulation of bile secretion. High dose of extract increased bile flow rate with lower bile salt concentration, whereas low doses of the drug enhanced bile flow rate without affecting the bile salt contents alongwith reducetion of plasma cholesterol levels. [Piyachaturawat P, Gansar R, Suksamrarn A; Choleretic effect of *Curcuma comosa* rhizome extracts in rats, *Int J Pharmacogn* **34**(3), 174-78 (1996)].

The hypolipidemic effect of an ethyl acetate extract of the rhizome of *C. comosa* Roxb was investigated in mice. Intragastric administration of the extract significantly decreased plasma lipid levels of both triglyceride and cholesterol but increased liver triglyceride content. The lower plasma cholesterol activity of *C. comose* extract was found to be essentially associated with elevation of plasma HDL-cholesterol level, increased excretion of faecal cholesterol and bile salt. The results suggest that *C. comosa* exerts hypocholesterolemic activity by accelerating mobilization of cholesterol from peripheral tissues into liver and enhancing excretion of cholesterol and bile salt into faeces. [Piyachaturawat P, Teeratagolpisal N, Toskulkao C, Suksamrarn A; Hypolipidemic effect of *Curcuma comosa* in mice, *Artery* **22**(5), 233-41 (1997)].

Oral adminstration of ethyl acetate extract of *C. comosa* to hypercholesterolemic hamsters for 7 days caused lowering of serum cholesterol and triglycerides in a dose dependant manner. A significant increase in the hepatic cholesterol contents without much change in the hepatic triglyceride contents was noted in these treated animals. Extract of *C. comosa* also enhanced serum high density lipoprotein cholesterol along with a decrease in the low density lipoprotein cholesterol. *Curcuma comosa* was considered to reduce lipids by accelerating mobilisation of lipid from extra hepatic tissue to liver and thus facilitating cholesterol excretion. [Piyachaturawat P, Charoenpiboonsin J, Toskulkao C, Suksamrarn A; Reduction of plasma cholesterol by *Curcuma comosa* extract in hypercholesterolemic hamsters, *J Ethnopharmacol* **66**(2), 199-204 (1999)].

Curcuma longa (Turmeric, H. Haldi, S. Haridra): Simultaneous feeding of curcumin, extracted from *C. longa* with cholesterol to rats significantly reduced the serum and liver cholesterol levels compared to group of rats fed cholesterol without curcumin. Cholesterol deposition in liver was also comparatively less in curcumin treated rats. Curcumin also enhanced the faecal bile acids and cholesterol excretion in hypercholesterolemic rats. [Subbarao D, Chandrashekhara N, Satyanarayana MN, Srinivasan M; Effect of curcumin on serum and liver cholesterol levels in the rats, *J Nutr* **100**(July-Dec), 1307-16(1970)].

Effect of ether and alcholic extracts of *Curcuma longa* and *C. amada* on the lipid metabolism was evaluated in cholesterol induced-hypercholesterolemic rabbits.

Administration of ether extract of *C. amada* significantly reduced the serum cholesterol levels. The cholesterol / phospholipid ratio was also decreased in *C. amada* extract treated hypercholesterolemic animals. However, the cholesterol lowering effect of alcoholic extract of C. amada or alcoholic or ether extract of *C. longa* was comparable. [Pachauri SP, Muckerjee SK; Effect of *Curcuma longa* (Haridra) and *Curcuma amada* (Amragandhi) on the cholesterol levels in experimental hypercholesterolemia of rabbits, *J Res Indian Med* **5**(1), 27-30 (1970)].

Administration of curcumin, isolated from turmeric, to cholesterol-fed (1% in diet) albino rats for 4 weeks at 0.2, 0.1 and 0.05% levels elicited marked hypocholesterolemic activity. [Patil TN, Srinivasan M; Hypocholesterolemic effect of curcumin in induced hypercholesterolemic rats, *Indian J Exp Biol* **9**(April), 167-69 (1971)].

In high fat diet (30% saturated fat)-fed rats, hypolipidemic effect of curcumin, ferulic acid (25 mg%) and capsaicin (0.2mg%) was investigated. Capsaicin feeding to female rats with high fat diet decreased the rate of weight gain, liver and serum triglycerides and adipose tissue lipoprotein lipase activity alongwith enhancement of hormone sensitive lipase and free fatty acids. Curcumin and ferulic acids given with high fat diet also lowered the rate of weight gain, liver total lipid and serum triglyceides. [Srinivasan MR, Satyanarayana MN; Influence of capsaicin, curcumin and ferulic acid in rats fed high fat diet, *J Biosci* **12**(2), 143-52 (1987)].

See *Allium sativum* (Garlic): [Arora *et al.*; *Hamdard Medicus* **30** (1-2) 163-74 (1987)].

Feeding of ethanolic (50%) extract of *Curcuma longa* (tuber) and *Nardostachys jatamansi* (whole plant) to rats was found to elevate HDL-cholesterol/total cholesterol ratio. The extracts also caused a significant reduction in the ratio of total cholesterol/ phospholipids. *Curcuma longa* exhibited better cholesterol and triglyceride lowering activity as compared to *N. jatamansi* in triton-induced hyperlipidaemic rats. [Dixit VP, Jain P, Joshi SC; Hypolipidemic effects of *Curcuma longa* L and *Nardostachys jatamansi* DC in Triton-induced hyperlipidemic rats, *Indian J Physiol Pharmacol* **32**(4), 299-304 (1988)].

See *Cuminum cyminum:* [Srivastava KC; *Prostaglandins Leukot Essent Fatty Acids.* **37**(1), 57-64 (1989).].

See *Saccharum officinarum:* [Tarvady & Dhar; *Biomedicine* **9** (1) 39-42 (1989); *Indian J Exp Biol* **28**(7), 657-60 (1990)].

Several pharmacological and clinical studies revealed hypocholesterolemic, antiplatelet, antioxidant, anti-inflammatory, antimicrobial and anticancer activities of *Curcuma longa*. Therapeutic indications and contraindications of *C. longa* and its active principle curcumin were discussed. [Bone K; Turmeric-The spice of life ? *Brit J Phytother* **2**(2), 51-60 (1991)].

The activity of hepatic cholesterol-7 α-hydroxylase, the rate-limiting enzyme of bile acid biosynthesis, was significantly elevated in curcumin, capsaicin (red pepper), ginger and mustard treated animals. Serum and liver microsomal cholesterol contents were significantly higher in the curcumin and capsaicin treated animals. The study suggested that the spices tumeric, red pepper, ginger and mustard can stimulate the conversion of cholesterol to bile acids, an important pathway of elimination of cholesterol from the body. However, simultaneous stimulation of cholesterol synthesis by the spice principles - curcumin and capsaicin-suggests that there may not be any significant contribution of stimulation of bile acid biosynthesis to the hypocholesterolemic action of these spices, and the latter action may solely be due to interference with exogenous cholesterol absorption. [Srinivasan K, Sambaiah K; The effect of spices on cholesterol–7 α-hydroxylase activity and on serum and hepatic cholesterol levels in the rat, *Int J Vitamin Nutr Res* **61**(4), 364-69 (1991)].

Hypolipidemic, antithrombotic, antibacterial, antifungal, hepatoprotective, antitumor and anti-inflammatory activities of *C. longa* have been discussed. [Srimal RC, Curcumin: A modern drug, *Indian Spices* **30**(2-3), 21-25 (1993)].

See *Glycine max* (Soya bean, soybean): [Lanksy PS; *Acta Horticulturae* (332), 131-36 (1993)].

See *Oryza sativa:* [Seetharamaiah & Chandrashekhara; *J Food Sci Technol* **30**(4), 249-52 (1993)].

Effect of feeding 0.5% curcumin diet or 1% cholesterol diet was examined in albino rats rendered diabetic with streptozotocin injection. Diabetic rats fed a curcumin diet showed lowered lipid peroxidation in plasma and urine when compared to other diabetic groups. The study reveals that curcumin feeding improves the metabolic status in diabetic condition, despite no effect on hyperglycemic status or the body weights. The mechanism by which curcumin improves this situation is probably by virtue of its hypocholesterolemic influence, antioxidant nature and free radical scavenging property. [Babu PS, Srinivasan K; Influence of dietary curcumin and cholesterol on the progression of experimentally induced diabetes in albino rat, *Mol Cell Biochem* **152**(1), 13-21 (1995)].

Treatment of 5% turmeric extract mixed with standard diet to hypercholesterolemic mice significantly decreased serum and hepatic cholesterol, triglycerides and total lipids levels. Feeding with 10% turmeric extract diet brought the levels comparable to those in normal untreated mice. [Godkar PB, Narayanan P, Bhide SV; Hypocholesterolemic effect of turmeric extract on Swiss mice, *Indian J Pharmacol* **28**(3), 171-74 (1996)].

In normal and hyperlipidemic subjects, the effect of turmeric extract on lipid profile was studied. Administration of turmeric extract (1g twice daily) for 15 days significantly reduced the serum total cholesterol, triglycerides and LDL-cholesterol levels. Hyperlipidemic subjects showed more pronounced fall in cholesterol and triglyceride levels as compared to those who had normal levels of cholesterol and triglycerides prior to administration of turmeric extract. It was suggested that possibly the hypolipidemic activity could be attributed to its antioxidant action. [Deshpande UR, Joseph LJ, Manjure SS, Bhide SV, Samuel AM; Effect of turmeric extract on lipid profile, *International Seminar on Free Radical Mediated Diseases and Ayurveda,* Faculty of Ayurveda, IMS, BHU Varanasi, India, (A-22), September 2-4, 1996].

See *Allium sativum* (Garlic): [Dwivedi S; *Ann Natl Acad Med Scs* (India) 32(3&4) 159- 175(1996)].

Blood cholesterol was lowered significantly by dietary curcumin in streptozotocin-induced diabetic animals. Cholesterol decrease was exclusively from LDL-VLDL fraction. Significant decrease in blood triglyceride and phospholipids was also brought about by dietary curcumin in diabetic rats. Curcumin also exhibited lowering of cholesterol and phospholipid in diabetic animals maintained on a high cholesterol diet. Dietary curcumin showed a distinct tendency to counter the changes in lipid fractions of liver under diabetic conditions. Hepatic cholesterol-7α- hydroxylase activity was markedly higher in curcumin-fed diabetic animals suggesting a higher rate of cholesterol catabolism. [Babu PS, Srinivasan K; Hypolipidemic action of curcumin, the active principal of turmeric (*Curcuma longa*) in streptozotocin induced diabetic rats, *Mol Cell Biochem* **166**(1-2), 169-75 (1997)].

See *Allium sativum:* [Sharma & Dwivedi; *Indian Drugs* **34**(5), 242-51 (1997)].

The antioxidant and hypocholesterolaemic effects of curcumin against alcohol-induced lipid peroxidation and hyperlipidaemia were investigated. Ethanol-induced liver injury was assessed by the activities of serum aspartate transaminase and alkaline phosphatase, which were elevated in ethanol-treated rats. The liver injury was associated with lipid peroxidation and a disruption in the antioxidant defence mechanism, as evidenced by raised levels of thiobarbituric acid reactive substances (TBARS), lowered levels of glutathione and decreased activities of superoxide dismutase and catalase. Curcumin administration resulted in returning alkaline phosphatase and aspartate transaminase activities to near normal state. Curcumin's antioxidant properties were clearly indicated by diminished TBARS levels and raised superoxide dismutase and catalase activities. The levels of cholesterol and free fatty acids declined after curcumin treatment in alcohol-fed rats, showing its hypolipidaemic property. Histopathological studies also indicated the protective role of curcumin against the adverse effect of alcohol. [Rajakrishnan V, Viswanathan P, Rajasekaran KN, Gunashekaran G, Menon VP; Role of curcumin in alcoholic hepatotoxicity, *Medical Sci Res* **26**(10), 715-19 (1998)].

The oxidation of low density lipoproteins (LDL) plays an important role in the development of atherosclerosis. Administration of an ethanol-aqueous extract obtained from rhizomes of *C. longa* (at a dose of 1.66 mg/kg body weight) to diet-induced atherosclerotic rabbits decreased the susceptibility of LDL to lipid peroxidation and proved useful in the management of cardiovascular disease in which atherosclerosis is important. [Ramirez-Tortosa MC, Mesa MD, Aguilera MC, Quiles JL, Baro L, Ramirez-Tortosa CL, Martinez-Victoria E, Gil A; Oral administration of a turmeric extract inhibits LDL oxidation and has hypocholesterolemic effects in rabbits with experimental atherosclerosis, *Atherosclerosis* **147**(2), 371-78 (1999)].

Curcumin, the yellow pigment in turmeric, was found to lower serum cholesterol concentration, hepatic cholesterol and triglyceride contents, and accumulation of cholesterol in the artery. The cholesterol-lowering effects of curcumin, together with its anti-oxidative and anti-inflammatory activities, may play some important roles in preventing atherosclerosis. [Kim TG, Kim SH, Kang SY, Jung KK, Park YB, Choi MS, Lee HS, Han HM; Anti-atherogenic effects of curcumin in hypercholesterolemic rabbits, *Yakhak Hoeji* **44**(1), 71-79 (2000) Article in Korean].

Curcumin, curcuminoids (compounds, structurally related to curcumin) and the yellowish phenolic pigments of turmeric are known to display antioxidative and hypocholesterolemic activities. The effects of dietary supplemented curcuminoids (commercial grade curcumin: a mixture of curcumin (73.4%), demethoxycurcumin and bisdemethoxycurcumin) on lipid metabolism were studied in male Sprague-Dawley rats. The results of the investigation indicate that dietary curcuminoids have lipid-lowering potency *in vivo*, probably due to alterations in fatty acid metabolism. [Asai A, Miyazawa T; Dietary curcuminoids prevent high fat diet-induced lipid accumulation in rat liver and epididymal adipose tissue, *J Nutr* **131**(11), 2932-35 (2001)].

In rats rendered hypercholesterolemic by maintaining them on a cholesterol-enriched diet (0.5%) for 8 weeks, inclusion of curcumin (0.2%), a constituent of *C. longa*, produced the expected hypolipidemic effect. Erythrocyte membranes of hypercholesterolemic rats were relatively enriched in cholesterol, which was about 120% of basal control, while membrane phospholipid was unaffected. This resulted in a significant alteration in cholesterol to phospholipid ratio of RBC membranes. Dietary curcumin was observed to counter this altered lipid profile of erythrocyte membranes in hypercholesterolemic situation by producing a significant (10-14%) decrease in membrane cholesterol content. Increased fragility of erythrocytes in hypercholesterolemic rats was also corrected by dietary curcumin. [Kempaiah RK, Srinivasan K; Integrity of erythrocytes of hypercholesterolemic rats during spices treatment, *Mol Cell Biochem* **236**(1-2), 155-61 (2002)].

See *Zingibar officinale:* [Singh VK, Singh S, Singh DK; Pharmacological effects of spices: Recent progress in medicinal plants: Phytochemistry and pharmacology, JN Govil, VK Singh (eds.) Studium press, LLC, Houston, Texas, USA, 2, p 321-353 (2003)].

See *Typha angustifolia*: [Park *et al.*; *Phytother Res* **18**(3), 224-29 (2004)].

Inclusion of spice principles {curcumin (0.2%) or capsaicin (0.015%) or garlic (2.0%)} in the diet of rats, rendered hyperlipidemic by maintaining them on a high fat diet, produced hypotriglyceridemic effect. The spice principles were also effective in reducing oxidant stress. [Kempaiah RK, Srinivasan K; Influence of dietary curcumin, capsaicin and garlic on the antioxidant status of red blood cells and the liver in high fat-fed rats, *Ann Nutr Metab* **48**(5), 314-20 (2004)].

***Curcuma xanthorrhiza*:** Two new phenolic diarylheptanoids, 5-hydroxy-7-(4-hydroxyphenyl)-1-phenyl-(1*E*)-1-heptene and 7-(3,4-dihydroxyphenyl)-5-hydroxy-1-phenyl- (1*E*)-1-heptene, isolated from rhizomes of *C. xanthorrihiza* elicited significant hypolipidemic activity by inhibiting liver triglyceride secretion .[Suksamrarn A, Eiamong S, Piachaturawat P, Charoenpiboonsin J; Phenolic diaryl heptanoids from *Curcuma xanthorrhiza, Phytochem* **36**(6), 1505-08 (1994)].

Curcuma zedoaria (H. Kachura, S. Sati)**:** Epidemiological studies have shown that hypercholesterolemia is a major risk factor for coronary artery disease. Clinical trials of lipid lowering therapy, using 3-hydroxy-3-methylglutaryl coenzyme A (HMG Co-A) reductase inhibitors, have been shown to decrease coronary events and mortality. Among 100 traditional Chinese herbs used for the study, only two herbs: *Curcuma zedoaria* Roscoe and *Poncirus trifoliata* Raf showed significant HMG Co-A reductase inhibitor activity. [Liu JC, Chan P, Hsu FL, Chen YJ, Hsieh MH, Lo MY, Lin JY; The *in vitro* inhibitory effects of crude extracts of traditional Chinese herbs on 3-hydroxy-3-methylglutaryl-coenzyme A reductase on Vero cells, *Am J Chin Med* **30**(4), 629-36 (2002)].

Cyamopsis. tetragonoloba (Cluster bean, Guar, H. Gowar, S. Bakuchi): See Polysaccharides in Appendix: [Tsuji *et al.*; *Annual Report National Inst Nutr* (24), 83-91 (1975)].

Guar gum, a form of dietary fibre obtained from the plant, was administered to 10 patients with type IIa or IIb hyperlipidemia for 2 weeks. Serum cholesterol levels of all patients fell by about 10.6% after 2 weeks of guar gum (5g, thrice daily) administration. Serum triglyceride was not changed significantly. Guar gum, which can be incorporated into foods, merits further study as a potential hypocholesterolemic agent. [Jenkins DJA, Leeds AR, Slavin B, Mann J, Jepson EM; Dietary fibre and blood lipids reduction of serum cholesterol in type II hyperlipidemia by guar gum, *Am J Clin Nutr* **32**(1), 16-18 (1979)].

Total serum cholesterol level fell by 13% when both guar gum and pectin were fed to twenty-two healthy volunteers respectively, at a dose of 20g/d and 31g/d alongwith controlled diets for a period of 3 weeks. No significant change in high density lipoprotein cholesterol was observed. [Jenkins DJA, Reynolds D, Leeds AR, Waller AL, Cummings JH; Hypocholesterolemic action of dietary fibre unrelated to faecal bulking effect, *Am J Clin Nutr* **32**(12), 2430-35 (1979)].

Consumption of 13 g guar gum in crisp bread by 11 hyperlipidemic patients for 2-8 weeks duration reduced total serum cholesterol (13%) without any change in HDL cholesterol at the end of 8 weeks. [Jenkins DJA, Reynolds D, Slavin E, Leeds AR, Jenkins AL, Jepson EM; Dietary fibres and blood lipids; Treatment of hypercholesterolemia with guar crisp bread, *Am J Clin Nutr,* **33**(3), 575-81 (1980)].

Oral administration of guar flour (10g/d) to 50 normal male subjects for 2 weeks significantly reduced serum cholesterol, total lipids and uric acid levels alongwith progressive and significant increase in serum total protein levels [Khalsa N, Sharma PK; Effect of guar (*Cyamopsis tetragonoloba*) on serum lipids, uric acid and proteins, *Indian J Nutr Dietet* **17**(8), 297-301 (1980)].

See Pectin in Appendix: [Sharma *et al.*; *Indian J Physiol Pharmacol* **24**(2), 136-38 (1980)].

Hypocholesterolemic and hypoglycemic effects of guar gum in rats have been reported. [Joshi LD, Singhal PC, Gupta RK; Variation effects of guar gum on blood sugar and serum cholesterol levels in experimental rats, *Indian J Pharm Sci* **43**(5), 166-68 (1981)].

Modification of diet of 10 insulin-dependent diabetics, by addition of guar gum to butter milk rusks significantly lowered the serum cholesterol levels without controlling diabetes. [Botha APJ, Steyn AF, Esterhuysen AJ, Slabbert M; Glycosylated haemoglobin, blood glucose and serum cholesterol levels in diabetics treated with guar gum, *South Afr Med J* **59**(10), 333- 34 (1981)].

Particulate fibres, such as wheat bran, do not appear to significantly alter plasma lipids or lipoprotein distributions in humans, or the atherogenicity of diets in experimental animals. Dietary fibres found in fruits, legumes, and vegetables, in contrast, show more definitive responses. Among the fibre isolates, the gelling and mucilaginous fibres, such as pectins and guar gum, predictably decrease circulating lipids in humans and animals and increase excretion of faecal metabolites of cholesterol, the bile acids. These fibres and fibre components can be shown to influence luminal solubility of lipids and the extent of lymphatic absorption of both cholesterol and triglyceride. [Vahouny GV; Dietary fibre, lipid metabolism, and atherosclerosis, *Fed Proc* **41**(11), 2801-6 (1982)].

In hypercholesterolemic rats, administration of decoction of green guar pods, progressively lowered serum, liver and aortic total cholesterol levels. Feeding of guar decoction to hypercholesterolemic rabbits also significantly reduced the serum, liver and aortic total cholesterol and triglyceride contents. The decoction enhanced faecal sterols and bile acid excretion. Hypolipidemic activity of this drug was attributed to its high fibre contents. [Santhakumari G, Nair RB, Varma RR; Effect of guar feeding on the lipid profiles of hypercholesterolemic rats and rabbits, *Planta Med* **44**(1), 57-60 (1982)].

Hypocholesterolemic effects of *Cyamopsis tetragonoloba* whole seed, its solvent extracts and residual seed meal were investigated. Feeding of whole seed of *C. tetragonoloba* to hypercholesterolemic rats for 2 weeks caused significant lowering of serum cholesterol and blood sugar levels. Petroleum ether extract also showed hypocholesterolemic activity but it enhanced blood sugar levels. However, the residual seed meal of the plant elicited both hypocholesterolemic and hypoglycemic effect. [Joshi LD, Singhal PC, Gupta RK; Changes in serum cholesterol and blood sugar levels on feeding with *Cyamopsis tetragonoloba* (Guar) and its solvent extracts, *Curr Sci* **51**(21), 1037-39 (1982)].

Feeding of *Cyamopsis. tetragonoloba* (15.6g/d) with benzafibrate (600mg/d) to 12 patients of familial hypercholesterolemia for three months lowered the plasma cholesterol and LDL-cholesterol without affecting the HDL and VLDL-cholesterol levels. However, plasma glucose levels and body weight did not change following administration of *C. tetragonoloba*. [Wirth A, Middelhoff G, Braeuning Ch, Schlierf G; Treatment of familial hypercholesterolemia with combination of benzafibrate and guar, *Atherosclerosis* **45**(3), 291-97 (1982)].

Tender cluster bean pod (*Cyamopsis tetragonoloba*) is a vegetable commonly consumed in South India and contains 20% of guar gum on dry weight basis. Effects of incorporating this vegetable into a hypercholesterolemic diet of rats were studied. Cluster bean at 0.5 and 2.5% levels, commercial guar gum (0.5%),. cluster bean partially free from guar gum (1.6%) and neutral detergent fibre of cluster bean (0.6%)-exerted a hypocholesterolemic effect and also lowered liver cholesterol concentration, but did not alter liver weights. [Sarathy R, Saraswathi G; Effect of tender cluster bean pods (*Cyamopsis tetragonoloba*) on cholesterol levels in rats, *Am J Clin Nutr* **38**(2), 295-9 (1983)].

Guar gum has been shown to be a potent hypocholesterolemic agent. Guar gum reduces not only cholesterol but also triglyceride levels in patients affected by familial combined hyperlipoproteinemia. Further studies are needed to confirm the suggestion that the different distribution of very low density lipoprotein apoC-III isoforms induced by guar gum supplementation may influence the behaviour of plasma triglycerides. [Bosello O, Cominacini L, Zocca I, Garbin U, Ferrari F, Davoli A; Effects of guar gum on plasma lipoproteins and apolipoproteins CII and CIII in patients affected by familial combined hyperlipoproteinemia, *Am J Clin Nutr* **40**(6), 1165-74 (1984)].

The effect of guar-enriched pasta with a 20% (w/w) content of guar gum was tested in normal volunteers, diabetic hyperlipidemic patients in different out and in-patient protocols. Plasma glucose and triglyceride rises were almost completely prevented by the pasta in normal volunteers; plasma insulin levels were modified to a lesser extent. In hyperlipidemics, a reduction of triglyceride levels was particularly evident. In mixed types of hyperlipidemias, a significant hypocholesterolemic effect was also demonstrated. Guar gum pasta may provide a simple dietary addition for the management of common metabolic disorders. [Gatti E, Catenazzo G, Camisasca E, Torri A, Denegri E, Sirtori CR; Effects of guar enriched pasta in the treatment of diabetes and hyperlipidemia, *Ann Nutr Metab* **28**(1), 1-10 (1984)].

The failure of guar gum and lignin to significantly decrease the amount of solubilised lipid suggests that the hypocholesterolemic effect of these fibres is due more to their bile acid binding capacity than to an effect on lipid solubilisation. [Gallaher D, Schneeman BO; Intestinal interaction of bile acids, phospholipids, dietary fibres, and cholestyramine, *Am J Physiol* **250**(4 Pt 1), G420-26 (1986)].

Feeding of guar whole seed to normal and alloxan diabetic guinea pigs for 4 weeks significantly reduced total lipids and sugar levels. In normal guinea pigs both free and esterified cholesterol contents were decreased whereas in diabetic animals only esterified cholesterol was lowered following guar feeding. Levels of triglycerides, phospholipid and total lipids were also decreased in these animals. [Srivastawa A, Longia GS, Singh SP, Joshi LD; Hypoglycemic and hypolipemic effect of *Cyamopsis tetragonoloba* (guar) in normal and diabetic guinea pigs, *Indian J Physiol Pharmacol* **31**(2), 77-83 (1987)].

Serum cholesterol and triglycerides were significantly reduced following administration of guar gum to rats. However, guar seeds and splits failed to show such hypolipidemic activity. In cholesterol-induced hyperlipidemic rabbits, guar gum (*C. tetragonoloba* 50mg/kg) significantly lowered serum and liver lipids at 60 and 90 days. The hypolipidemic activity of guar gum is attributed to increased faecal bile acids excretion and inhibition of cholesterol biosynthesis in liver. [Singh L, Nityananda S; Hypolipidemic effect of guar gum in rats and rabbits, *Indian J Med Res* **88**(Dec), 550-57 (1989)].

Guar gum from endosperm of *C. tetragonoloba* elicited hypocholesterolemic and hypoglycemic activity. A monograph containing botany, chemistry, pharmacology and toxicology of guar gum has been published. [Guar gum: A monograph, *Lawrence Review of Natural Products* No 1-2, (1990)].

The hypolipidemic effect of guar gum (30 g/day) was examined in a double blind placebo controlled crossover study in 9 patients with primary hyperlipidemia, the treatment period being of six weeks duration. Cholesterol levels in low density lipoprotein and in intermediate density lipoprotein were decreased. Plasma cholesterol levels were also reduced. [Turner PR; Tuomilehto J, Happonen P, La-Ville AE, Shaikh M, Lewis B; Metabolic studies on the hypolipidemic effect of guar gum, *Atherosclerosis* **81**(2), 145-50 (1990)].

The hypolipidemic effect of guar gum (15g/d) was compared with that of an oat (*Avena sativa*) fibre source (77g/d). Both treatments supplied the same amount of total dietary fibre (11 g/d) and were taken with water three times a day for 3 weeks at mealtime. Both treatments were effective in reducing elevated total cholesterol, guar gum at the level fed was significantly more effective in reducing total cholesterol. Neither treatment induced significant changes in high density lipoprotein cholesterol or very low density lipoprotein cholesterol. [Spiller GA, Farquhar JW, Gates JE, Nichols SF; Guar gum and plasma cholesterol: Effect of guar gum and an oat fibre source on plasma lipoproteins and cholesterol in hypercholesterolemic adults, *Arterioscler*

Thromb **11**(5), 1204-08 (1991)].

Consumption of 15 g guar gum (a mucilage type dietary fibre from endosperm layer of seeds of *C. tetragonoloba*) with normal diet for 6 weeks by overweight adults, significantly decreased plasma cholesterol, LDL-c and cholesterol /HDL- c ratio. However, HDL-c levels did not change in these subjects. [Kawatra A, Kapoor AC, Sehgal S; Hypocholesterolemic effect of guar gum in overweight adults, *Plant Foods Hum Nutr* **41**(3), 241-45 (1991)].

Guar gum was fed together with either 50.3% starch or 50.3% sucrose in a balanced diet to pigs and its effect on serum lipids was examined. With the cornstarch-based diet neither 15 g nor 30 g guar gum had an influence on serum total cholesterol or triglyceride levels. In the presence of sucrose the supplementation of 30 g guar led to a significant decrease of the cholesterol concentrations in the very low density lipoproteins (VLDL) and high density lipoproteins (HDL). There was also a tendency for decreased cholesterol levels in the low density lipoproteins (LDL) after adding 30 g guar to the sucrose diet. The study demonstrates that guar gum exerts a hypocholesterolemic effect in the presence of sucrose in the diet, but not in the case of starch consumption. [Ahrens F, Pfeuffer M, Hagemeister H, Barth CA; The hypocholesterolemic effect of guar gum depends on dietary sucrose: Studies in minipigs, *Zeitschrift fuer Ernaehrungswissenschaft* **30**(2), 109-17 (1991)].

Guar gum at 6% and 12% in the diet reduces total serum cholesterol by 31% and 51%, respectively, in male sea quails, fed with a diet containing 0.5% cholesterol for a period of one week. The potency of hypocholesterolemic action of guar gum in cholesterol-fed sea quails is much less than that in cholesterol-fed chickens. [Day CE; Guar gum reduces serum cholesterol in sea quails fed a cholesterol diet, *Artery* **18**(3), 107-14 (1991)].

The effects of guar gum and its enzyme hydrolysate as well as of fructo-oligosaccharide on lipid metabolism were compared in rats fed high fat diets employing lard or palm oil as dietary fat. Not only guar gum but also the hydrolysate and the oligosaccharide reduced serum cholesterol levels irrespective of dietary fat sources. The triglyceride-lowering effects of the hydrolysate and the oligosaccharide were comparable to that of guar gum. Guar gum and its hydrolysate suppressed HMG-CoA reductase activities in the ileum where dietary fat was lard. [Ide T, Moriuchi H, Nihimoto K; Hypolipidemic effects of guar gum and its enzyme hydrolysate in rats fed highly saturated fat diets, *Ann Nut Metab* **35**(1), 34-44 (1991)].

See *Avena sativa* (Oat): [Jonnalagadda *et al*,; *J Nutr* **123**(8), 1377-82 (1993)].

The effect of viscosity and fermentability of soluble dietary fibres on plasma and liver cholesterol concentration was assessed on hamsters. Plasma cholesterol concentrations at 3, 6 and 11 weeks and liver cholesterol concentrations at 6 and 11 weeks were significantly lower in hamsters, fed diets containing 0.12% cholesterol and 5% fibre as high viscosity hydroxypropyl methylcellulose, compared to those receiving low viscosity hydroxypropyl methylcellulose. Again plasma and liver cholesterol were significantly lower in hamsters, fed diets containing 0.12% cholesterol and high viscosity guar gum compared to those receiving low viscosity guar gum at 6 weeks, but not at 3 or 11 weeks. Hepatic sterol synthesis rates were not affected by any of the diets. This study shows that greater viscosity of intestinal contents is strongly associated with cholesterol reduction, but that the contribution of fibre fermentation remains uncertain. [Gallaher DD, Hassel CA, Lee KJ, Gallaher CM; Viscosity and fermentability as attributes of dietary fibre responsible for the hypocholesterolemic effect in hamsters, *J Nutr* **123**(2), 244-52 (1993)].

Hypolipidemic effect of a powder containing *C. tetragonoloba*, *Trigonella foenum-graecum*, *Cephalandra indica* and *Gymnema sylvestre* was investigated in 30 control and 30 diabetic patients (NIDDM) and a significant reduction of total cholesterol and LDL- cholesterol was observed. However, HDL-c, VLDL-c and triglyceride levels remained unaltered after the therapy. [Bharadwaj PK, Dasgupta DJ, Parashar BS, Kaushal SS; Effective reduction of LDL-cholesterol by indigenous plant product, *J Indian Med Assoc* **92**(3), 80-81 (1994)].

γ-Irradiation abolished the cholesterol-lowering effect of guar gum, whereas sterilisation by heat preserved this effect. [Alvarez-Leite JI, Andrieux C, Ferezou J, Riottot M, Vieira EC; Heat or γ-irradiation sterilisation affects the hypocholesterolemic effect of guar gum in axenic and heteroxenic rats, *Brazilian J Med Biol Res* **27**(3), 677-89 (1994).

[Germ-free and heteroxenic rats were given a hypercholesterolemic diet with or without 5% guar gum for 4 weeks. Rats fed guar gum diets showed a lower hepatic and plasmatic cholesterol level when compared with rats fed hypercholesterolemic diet. This reduction of cholesterolemia was due to a decrease in the chylomicron and very low density lipoprotein fraction. The caecal and portal concentrations of propionate were 30% higher in rats fed with guar gum diet than in those fed the hypocholesterolemic diet. These results exclude the participation of the intestinal microflora in the hypocholesterolemic effect of guar gum. [Alvarez-Leite JI, Andrieux C, Ferezou J, Riottot M, Vieira EC; Evidence for the absence of participation of the microbial flora in the hypocholesterolemic effect of guar gum in gnotobiotic rats, *Comparative Biochem Physiol* (A) *Comparative Physiol* **109**(2), 503-10 (1994)].

In cholesterol-induced hyperlipidemic rabbits, petroleum ether extract of guar gum and ethanolic extract of ginger (200mg/kg) significantly decreased the serum total cholesterol, triglycerides and phospholipids and increased the HDL-cholesterol levels compared to hypercholesterolemic untreated rabbits. These drugs also lowered the streptozotocin-induced increased blood sugar levels. [Bhandari U, Sharma JN; Comparision of hypolipidemic and hypoglycemic activity of *Cyamopsis tetragonoloba* and *Zingiber officinale* (ginger) in experimental animals, *Int Conf Curr Prog Med Aromat Plant Res*, Calcutta (India), p. 133, Dec 30, 1994-Jan 1, 1995].

See Plant Fibres in Appendix: [Fernandez *et al.*; *J Lipid Res* **36**(10), 2191-202 (1995)].

The lipid-lowering capacity of two different polysaccharides; a high viscosity and a low viscosity guar gum were investigated in male Wistar rats. The high viscosity guar gum (HVGG) diet was more potent in enhancing bile acid excretion and producing a potent cholesterol-lowering effect than the low viscosity guar gum (LV-GG) diet. HV-GG also showed a marked effect of on sterol excretion, whereas LV-GG had a marginal effect on this process. Both LVGG and HV-GG depressed plasma triglycerides, and lowered high density lipoprotein-2 (HDL- 2) cholesterol, whereas only the HV-GG diet depressed low density lipoprotein (LDL) and (HDL-1)-cholesterol. The decreased efficiency of the LV-GG diet to produce a hypocholesterolemic response resulted in a decreased stimulation of hydroxymethyl glutaryl coenzyme A (HMG CoA) reductase, and this could explain the lesser efficiency of LV-GG diet to develop a cholesterol-lowering effect. [Favier ML, Bost PE, Guittard C, Demigne C, Remesy C; Reciprocal influence of fermentations and bile acid excretion on cholesterol-lowering effect of fermentable carbohydrate, *J Nutr Biochem* **8**(3), 127-32 (1997)].

The rats fed with guar gum for 60 days elicited significant lowering of serum cholesterol, triglycerides and body weight. These animals also exhibited an increase in high density lipoprotein cholesterol (HDL-c) along with elevation of HDL/LDL-cholesterol ratio. Guar gum increased the length of the small intestine (10 %) with 25 % retardation in the intestinal transit. [Frias ACD, Sgarbieri VC; Guar gum effects on food intake, blood serum lipids and glucose levels of Wistar rats, *Plant Foods Hum Nutr* **53(1),** 15-28 (1998)].

After 8 days of adaptation, rats were fed with diets containing either sucrose (controls) or experimental fibres (guar gum and a low molecular weight pectin) for three weeks. Compared with controls, rats fed soluble fibres showed a significant decrease of triacylglycerol, total cholesterol and insulin concentrations without changes in postprandial blood glucose levels. Glucagon was upregulated. Compared to rats fed with low molecular weight pectin, a significant decrease of postprandial corticosterone was observed in rats fed guar gum. It is suggested that the decrease of corticosterone and insulin levels may partly explain the more important hypolipidemic effect observed in this group. [Grizard D, Dalle M, Barthomeuf C; Changes in insulin and corticosterone levels may partly mediate the hypolipidemic effect of guar gum and low-molecular weight pectin in rats, *Nutr Res* **21**(8), 1185-90 (2001)].

The hypocholesterolemic effect of the ingestion of three different hydrocolloids (guar gum, xanthan gum and pre-gelatinised cornstarch) at 1.5% concentration was assessed on rats, cellulose being used as control. In the first stage of the experiment, all animals were fed with a hypercholesterolemic diet that produced a significant increase in the mean concentration of total cholesterol. In the subsequent stage, 1.5% of the starch was replaced with each of the three hydrocolloids in the experimental ration. Under the conditions of the present study, the hypocholesterolemic effect of hydrocolloid ingestion at a dose of 1.5% of the ration was not significant in comparison to the effect produced by the reduction and change of lipids in the diet. [Castro IA, Tirapegui J, Benedicto ML; Effects of diet supplementation with three soluble polysaccharides on serum lipid levels of hypercholesterolemic rats, *Food Chem* **80**(3), 323-30 (2003)].

See *Trigonella foenum-graecum:* [Venkatesan et *al.*; *Eur J Nutr* **42**(5), 262-71 (2003)].

Cyanodon dactylon (H. Dhub, S. Dhurva): See *Hibiscus rosa-sinensis* [Shanmugasundaram *et al.*; *J Ethnopharmacol* **31**, 85-89 (1991)].

Cyclocarya paliurus (Batal): A single oral administration of *C. paliurus* extract (250 mg/kg) suppressed an increase in plasma triacylglycerol (TG) levels when fed with 5 ml/kg of lard or olive oil. The inhibition rates were 28.6% and 24.1%, respectively, but free fatty acid levels in plasma were not significantly affected as compared with control group mice. In addition, *C. paliurus* extract showed inhibitory activity toward pancreatic lipase, a key enzyme of dietary TG absorption, with an IC_{50} of 9.1 μg/ml *in vitro*. The results of investigation suggested that the hypolipemic action of *C. paliurus* extract was probably interrelated with suppression of the activity of digestive lipase. [Kurihara H, Asami S, Shibata H, Fukami H, Tanaka T; Hypolipemic effect of *Cyclocarya paliurus* (Batal) Iljinskaja in lipid-loaded mice, *Biol Pharm Bull* **26**(3), 383-85 (2003)].

Cymbopogon proximus (Halfa-barr): See *Zygophyllum coccineum:* [Newairy *et al.*; *J Environ Sci Health* **B. 37**(5), 475-84 (2002)].

Cynanchum viminale: See *Saccharum officinarum:* [Tarvady & Dhar; *Biomedicine* **9** (1) 39-42 (1989); *Indian J Exp Biol* **28**(7), 657-60 (1990)].

Cynara scolymus (Artichoke, H. Hatichoke): Artichoke leaf extract was considered a safe and effective hypolipidemic agent because of its known inhibitory action on cholesterol biosynthesis and LDL oxidation and enhancement of biliary cholesterol excretion. In view of these actions, artichoke was also suggested to be effective in preventing atherosclerosis. [Fintelmann V; Therapeutic profile and mechanism of action of Artichoke leaf extract: hypolipemic, antioxidant, hepatoprotective and choleretic properties, *Phytomedicine* **3**(Suppl 1), 50 (1996/97)].

High dose of aqueous extracts from artichoke leaves were found to inhibit cholesterol biosynthesis from 14C-acetate in primary cultured rat hepatocytes in a concentration-dependent biphasic manner with moderate inhibition between 0.007 and 0.1 mg/ml and more strong inhibition at 1 mg/ml. Replacement of 14C-acetate by 14C-mevalonate largely omitted the inhibiting effect of artichoke extracts indicating an inhibition at the level of hydroxymethyl glutaryl-CoA-reductase. However, no direct inhibition of this enzyme could be detected and no other enzymic steps later in the biosynthetic pathway for cholesterol seemed to be affected. Instead, inhibition was found to occur in a time-dependent manner, to last for several hours even after washing out the extracts by fresh medium and to be fully reversible within 20 hr after removal of the extracts. In addition, the stimulation of HMGCoA-reductase activity by insulin was efficiently blocked by the extracts, although other insulin-dependent phenomena were not influenced. Screening of several known constituents of artichoke extracts revealed that cynaroside and particularly its aglycone luteolin were mainly responsible for inhibition. The results demonstrated that artichoke extracts inhibited hepatic cholesterol biosynthesis in an indirect but efficient manner and, thus, contributed *via* this action to the recently confirmed hypolipidemic influence of this phytopharmacon in man. [Gebhardt R; Inhibition of cholesterol biosynthesis in primary cultured rat hepatocytes by artichoke (*Cynara scolymus* L.) extracts, *J Pharmacol Exp Ther* **286**(3), 1122-28 (1998)].

It is currently believed that oxidative stress and inflammation play a significant role in atherogenesis. Artichoke extract exhibits hypolipemic properties and contains numerous active substances with antioxidant properties *in vitro*. Aqueous and ethanolic extracts from artichoke were found to inhibit basal and stimulated reactive oxygen species (ROS) production in endothelial cells and monocytes in a dose dependent manner. In endothelial cells, the ethanolic and aqueous extracts (50 μg/ml) reduced oxidized LDL (ox-LDL)-induced intracellular ROS production by 60% and 43%, respectively. The ethanolic extract (50 μg/ml) reduced ox-LDL-induced intracellular ROS production in monocytes by 76%. Effective concentrations (25-100 μg/ml) were well below the cytotoxic levels of the extracts. [Zapolska-Downar D, Zapolski- Downar A, Naruszewicz M, Siennicka A, Krasnodebska B, Koldziej B; Protective properties of artichoke (*Cynara scolymus*) against oxidative stress induced in cultured endothelial cells and monocytes, *Life Sci* **71**(24), 2897-908 (2002)].

In olive oil-fed mice, methanolic extract of *C. scolymus* prevented increase of serum triglyceride levels. Sesquiterpenes and sesquiterpene glycosides, isolated from this plant, were the active components. The antihyperlipidemic activity of this plant was partially attributed to its gastric emptying inhibitory effect. [Shimoda H, Ninomiya K, Nishida N, Yoshino T, Morikawa T, Matsuda H, Yoshikawa M; Antihyperlipidemic sesquiterpenes and new sesquiterpene glycosides from the leaves of artichoke (*Cynara scolymus* L.): Structure requirement and mode of action, *Bioorg Med Chem Lett* **13**(2), 223-28 (2003)].

D

***Dalbergia odorifera*:** Detailed phytochemical analysis of *Dalbergia odorifera*, a known antihypercholesterolemic drug, was made and thirteen compounds were isolated and fully characterized. [Yahara S, Ogata T, Nohara T; Studies on the constituents of the crude drug effective for antihypercholesterolemia-*Dalbergia odorifera*, *J Pharm Sci* **76**(11), S210 (1987)].

***Daphne koreana*:** Oral administration of daphnetin, isolated from *D. koreana*, elevated serum levels of high density lipoprotein cholesterol (HDL-c) and ratio of HDL-c/total cholesterol in normal rats without much change in the lipid levels in normal mice. Daphnetin (800mg/kg/d) significantly decreased serum total cholesterol in yolk (0.5ml)-treated mice. In hyperlipidemic rats also, serum HDL-c and its ratio to total cholesterol were significantly increased following treatment with daphnetin. [Jiang XI, Qu SY, Li W, Pan G, Chen XL; Effect of daphnetin on lipoprotein cholesterol contents in serum, *Acta Pharm Sin* **22**(1), 53-55 (1987)].

Daucus carota (Carrot, H. Gajar, S. Sikha-mulam)**:** Administration of carrot fibre (10g twice daily) for twelve weeks to ten patients produced significant lowering of serum cholesterol and LDL-cholesterol levels. The treated patients also exhibited increase in the HDL-cholesterol contents. [Shahni SR, Banavalikar MM, Chotalia CS, Kulkarni VS, Biyani MK; The effect of rufage (carrot fibre) on hypercholesterolemic patients, *The Indian Practioner* **55**(9), 585-88 (2002)].

***Dioscorea panthaica*:** The anti-hypercholesterolemic and cholesterol absorption inhibitory activities between total saponin of *D. panthaica* and diosgenin were compared. The preventive and therapeutic activity of diosgenin against hypercholesterolemia, induced by cholesterol in mice or rats, was found to be stronger than that of the total saponin of *D. panthaica*. The mechanism of anti-hypercholesterolemic activity of diosgenin is probably related with its cholesterol absorption inhibitory activity. [Ma Hai ying, Zhao Zhi tao, Wang LJ, Wang Y, Zhou QL, Wang BX; Comparative study on anti-hypercholesterolemie activity of diosgenin and total saponin of *Dioscorea panthaica, Zhongguo Zhongyao Zazhi* **27**(7), 528-31 (2002) Article in Chinese].

Dioscorea species: See *Glycine max*: [Lanksy PS; *Acta Horticulturae*, (332), 131-36 (1993)].

Diospyros kaki (Japanese Persimmon, H. Halwa tendu): The effect of dietary persimmon on lipid metabolism and antioxidant activity was investigated in male Wistar rats adapted to cholesterol-free or 1% cholesterol diets. The results of the investigation demonstrated hypolipidemic and antioxidant properties of persimmon. These properties are attributed to its water-soluble dietary fibre, carotenoids and polyphenols. [Gorinstein S, Bartnikowska E, Kulasek G, Zemser M, Trakhtenberg S; Dietary persimmon improves lipid metabolism in rats fed diets containing cholesterol, *J Nutr* **128**(11), 2023-27 (1998)].

The hypocholesterolemic and antioxidant effects of dry persimmon peel and dry persimmon pulp were studied in rats. The results demonstrate that persimmon fruit exerts hypocholesterolemic and antioxidant effects and, therefore, is considered for an antiatherosclerotic diet. A diet fortified with dry persimmon peel is more efficient than the same diet fortified with dry persimmon pulp. [Gorinstein S, Kulasek GW, Bartnikowska E, Leontowicz M, Zemser M, Morawiec M, Trakhtenberg S; The influence of persimmon peel and persimmon pulp on the lipid metabolism and antioxidant activity of rats fed cholesterol, *J Nutr Biochem* **9**(4), 223-27 (1998)].

Diospyros virginiana (Common Persimmon): Dietary fibres, major phenolics, main minerals, and trace elements in persimmons and apples (*Malus domestica*) were analyzed and compared in order to choose a preferable fruit for an antiatherosclerotic diet. Total, soluble, and insoluble dietary fibres, total phenols, epicatechin, gallic and *p*-coumaric acids, and concentrations of Na, K, Mg, Ca, Fe, and Mn in whole persimmons, their pulps, and peels were significantly higher than in whole apples, pulps, and peels. The relatively high contents of dietary fibres, total and major phenolics, main minerals, and trace elements make persimmon preferable for an antiatherosclerotic diet. [Gorinstein S, Zachwieja Z, Folta M, Barton H, Piotrowicz J, Zemser M, Weisz M, Trakhtenberg S, Martin-Belloso O; Comparative contents of dietary fibre, total phenolics, and minerals in persimmons and apples, *J Agric Food Chem* **49**(2), 952-7 (2001)].

Dolichos lablab (H. Sem, S. Shimbi): See *Phaseolus anguris:* [Chan *et al*,; *J Agric Food Chem* **46**(9), 3698-3701(1998)].

Dracocephalum kotschyi: Administration of aqueous alcoholic extract of *D. kotschyi* leaves as well as of its polyphenolic fraction to high fat diet-induced hyperlipidemic rats produced a significant decrease of blood triglyceride, total cholesterol and LDL-cholesterol levels and an increase of HDL-cholesterol level. [Ebrahim Sajjadi S, Movahedian Atar AM, Yektaian A; Antihyperlipidemic effect of hydroalcoholic extract, and polyphenolic fraction from *Dracocephalum kotschyi* Boiss, *Pharm Acta Helv* **73**(3), 167-70 (1998)].

E

***Echium plantagineum*:** Concentrations of long-chain (n-3) polyunsaturated fatty acids, including eicosapentaenoic acid, increased in plasma and neutrophils when subjects consumed Echium oil (oil obtained from *E. plantagineum* seeds). Dietary plant oils rich in stearidonic acid are metabolized to longer-chain, more unsaturated (n-3) polyunsaturated fatty acids. These oils appear to possess hypotriglyceridemic properties typically associated with fish oils. [Surette ME, Edens M, Chilton FH, Tramposch KM; Dietary echium oil increases plasma and neutrophil long-chain (n-3) fatty acids and lowers serum triacylglycerols in hypertriglyceridemic humans, *J Nutr* **134**(6), 1406-11 (2004)].

Eleusine coracana (Ragi, H. Mandua, S. Rajika): See Plant Fibres in Appendix: [Thomas *et al.*; *J Food Sci Technol* **27**(5), 290-93 (1990)].

The effect of carbohydrate-rich diets i.e., *Eleusine coracana* (ragi), *Oryza sativa* (rice) and *Manihot utilisima* (tapioca) on lipids and glycemic response was investigated on individuals of both sexes. Ragi reduced total serum cholesterol, low density lipoprotein cholesterol and triglycerides alongwith enhancement of high density lipoprotein cholesterol levels. However, glycemic response did not alter following consumption of above mentioned carbohydrate diets as compared to isocaloric wheat supplemented basal diet. [Kurup PG, Krishnamurthy S; Glycemic response and lipemic index of rice, ragi and tapioca as compared to wheat diet in humans, *Indian J Exp Biol* **31**(3), 291-93 (1993)].

***Elsholtzia splendens*:** See *Acanthopanax senticocus:* [Zhizhen & Chenglin; *Chinese Journal of Integrated Traditional and Western Medicine* **10**(3), 155-56 (1990)].

Emblica officinalis (H. Amla, S. Amalki): Administration of fresh *E. officinalis* fruits (1g/d) to cholesterol (0.5g/d) and clarified butter (1g/d)-fed rabbits significantly lowered the serum cholesterol. [Mishra M, Pathak UN, Khan AB; *Emblica officinalis* Gartin. And serum cholesterol levels in experimental rabbits, *Brit J Exp Pathol* **62**(5), 526-28 (1981)].

Oral administration of *E. officinalis* and *Terminalia chebula* for 60 days significantly reduced the blood sugar levels in diabetic patients. However, these drugs did not show any effect on serum cholesterol levels. [Mishra SK, Pandey SK, Sharma SH, Singh GD; Effect of Amalki-Haritaki on Madhumeha, *Nagarjun* **26**(5), 105-07 (1983)].

In cholesterol-induced hyercholesterolemic and atherosclerotic rabbits, the effects of *E. officinalis* and vitamin C on the cholesterol levels and atherosclerosis were studied. Administration of *E. officinalis* and vitamin C for 16 weeks significantly lowered serum cholesterol levels in hypercholesterolemic rabbits. However, the serum cholesterol levels were higher in *E. officinalis* treated group of rabbits as compared to vitamin C treated ones. The study showed that though both *E. officinalis* and vitamin C were capable of reducing cholesterol levels, *E. officinalis* also exerted antiatherogenic effect. It was suggested that vitamin C alone might not be related to antiatherogenic properties of *Emblica officinalis*. [Thakur CP, Mandal K; Effect of *Emblica officinalis* on cholesterol induced atherosclerosis in rabbits, *Indian J Med Res* **79**(Jan), 142-46 (1984)].

Serum, aortic and hepatic cholesterol levels were significantly lowered following administration of *E. officinalis* to rabbits. However, it did not affect euglobulin clot lysis time, platelet adhesiveness or serum triglyceride levels. [Thakur CP, *Emblica officinalis* reduces serum, aorotic and hepatic cholesterol in rabbits, *Experientia* **41**(3), 423-24 (1985)].

In cholesterol-fed rats, effect of amla juice, pulp and vitamin C on the atheroma formation was investigated. The dose of amla was calculated so as to provide approximately 35mg/kg ascorbic acid per day. Amla juice, pulp and vitamin C prevented the rise in serum cholesterol and triglyceride in cholesterol fed rats. The platelet aggregation was also inhibited in the treated animals. Amla and vitamin C significantly prevented the atheroma formation in these animals. Amla juice and pulp was found to be relatively more effective than vitamin C in lowering lipids and preventing the atheroma. [Bordia A, Verma SK, Mehta LK, Andreais AMR; Comparative effect of amla juice, pulp and vitamin C on atheroma in cholesterol fed rats, *Indian Heart J* **37**(3), 179-82 (1985)].

In normal and hypercholesterolemic men (35-55 years), the effect of supplementation of diet with *E. officinalis* in raw form on total serum cholesterol and its lipoprotein fractions was investigated. Following consumption of *E. officinalis,* both normal and hypercholesterolemic volunteers exhibited a significant decrease in cholesterol levels. However, after two weeks of withdrawl of *E. officinalis*, a significant increase in the serum cholesterol levels was noted in hypercholesterolemic subjects. [Jacob A, Pandey

M, Kapoor S, Saroja R; Effect of Indian goose berry (amla) on serum cholesterol levels in men aged 35-55 years, *Euro J Clin Nutr* **42**(1), 939-44 (1988)].

See *Terminalia chebula* ((Bala Haritaki): [Thakur *et al.*; *Int J Cardiol* **21**(2), 167-75 (1988)].

Feeding of *E. officinalis* to hypercholesterolemic rabbits initially raised plasma cholesterol and lipid levels, which was followed by a significant fall in these levels at the end of 12 weeks. Hepatic lipid levels were also reduced in these animals. Aortic lipid content was much less in treated rabbits compared to hyperlipidemic animals. [Mand JK, Soni JL, Gupta PP, Rattan Singh; Effect of Amla (*Emblica officinalis*) on the development of atherosclerosis in hypercholesterolemic rabbits, *J Res Edu Indian Med* **10**(2), 1-7 (1991)].

Administration of *E. officinalis* juice (0.5ml/kg bw) to cholesterol-fed rabbits for 60 days significantly decreased serum cholesterol (82%), triglycerides (66%), phospolipid (77%) and LDL–cholesterol (90%). The juice elicited regression of aortic plaques alongwith lowering of tissue lipids. Cholesterol and phospolipid excretion was also enhanced in treated rabbits. [Mathur R, Sharma A, Dixit VP, Varma M; Hypolipidemic effect of fruit juice of *Emblica officinalis* in cholesterol-fed rabbits, *J Ethnopharmacol* **50**(2), 61-68 (1996)].

See *Allium sativum* (Garlic): [Dwivedi S; *Ann Natl Acad Med Sci* (India) 32(3&4) 159- 175(1996)].

See *Allium sativum:* [Sharma & Dwivedi; *Indian Drugs* **34**(5), 242-51 (1997)].

See *Terminalia chebula:* [Nalini et *al.*; *Plant Foods Human Nutr* **53**(4), 343-49 (1999)].

Flavonoids isolated from *E. officinalis, Sesamum indicum* and *Momordica charantia* were examined for their hypolipidemic and hypoglycemic activities. Of the three sources, flavonoids isolated from *E. officinalis* showed maximum hypolipidemic and hypoglycemic activities. Besides, these flavonoids also improved the haemoglobin levels in rats. [Anila L, Vijayalakshmi NR; Beneficial effects of flavonoids from *Sesamum indicum, Emblica officinalis* and *Momordica charantia, Phytother Res* **14**(8), 592-95 (2000)].

See *Allium sativum* (Garlic): [Augusti *et al.*; *Indian J Exp Biol.* **39**(8), 760-66 (2001)].

Flavonoids from *E. officinalis* and *Mangifera indica* were found to reduce effectively lipid levels in serum and tissues of hyperlipidemic rats. While hepatic HMG CoA reductase activity was significantly inhibited in rats fed *E. officinalis* flavonoids, an increase of this enzyme was observed in rats administered *M. indica* flavonoids. The degradation and elimination of cholesterol was highly enhanced by flavonoids of both the plants. The mechanism of hypolipidemic action of *E. officinalis* was due to the concerted action of inhibition of synthesis and enhancement of degradation of cholesterol. *M. indica* flavonoids did not inhibit cholesterogenesis but enhanced degradation of cholesterol significantly. [Anila L, Vijayalakshmi NR; Flavonoids from

Emblica officinalis and *Mangifera indica*-effectiveness for dyslipidemia, *J Ethnopharmacol* **79**(1), 81-87 (2002)].

***Engelhardtia chrysolepis*:** Astilbin, in kohki tea from the leaves of *E. chrysolepis* (Chinese name huang -qui), and its aglycone taxifolin significantly decreased total hepatic cholesterol and phospholipid contents in rats, fed with cholesterol-free diet. Besides this, astilbin and taxifolin also lowered serum and liver TBARS (Thiobarbituric acid reactive substances) without affecting the antioxidative enzyme activity [Igarashi K, Uchida Y, Murakami N, Mizutani K , Masuda H; Effect of astilbin in tea processed from leaves of *Engelhardtia chrysolepis* on the serum and liver lipid concentration and the erythrocyte and liver antioxidative enzyme activities in rats, *Biosci Biotechnol Biochem* **60**(3), 513-15 (1996)].

***Ephedra equisetina*:** See Proanthocyanidin polymer in Appendix: [Khushbaktova *et al.; Khim Farma Zh* **23**(9), 1111-15 (1989)].

***Eremurus regelii*:** See Polysaccharides in Appendix: [Zhushbaktova *et al.*; *Khim Farm Zh* **21**(11), 1348-52 (1987)].

Eucommia ulmoides (*Eucommiae cortex*): See *Acanthopanax senticosus* [Whang et *al.*; *Korean J Pharmacogn* **27**(1), 65-74 (1996)].

Eugenia aromatica (Syn. *Syzygium aromaticum,* H. Laung, S. Lavanga)**:** See *Zingibar officinale:* [Singh VK, Singh S, Singh DK; Pharmacological effects of spices. Recent progress in medicinal plants: Phytochemistry and pharmacology, JN Govil, VK Singh (eds.) Studium press, LLC, Houston, Texas, USA, 2, p 321-353(2003)].

Eugenia jambolana (Syn. *Syzygium cumini,* H. Jamun, S. Jambu): In addition to hypoglycemic activity, ethanolic extract of seeds *E. jambolana* exhibited significant hypolipidemic effect as evident from fall in total serum cholesterol (TC)/high density lipoprotein cholesterol (HDL-c) ratio, serum low density lipoprotein cholesterol (LDL-c) levels and decreased activity of HMG-CoA reductase. [Sharma SB, Nasir A, Prabhu KM, Murthy PS, Dev G; Hypoglycaemic and hypolipidemic effect of ethanolic extract of seeds of *Eugenia jambolana* in alloxan-induced diabetic rabbits, *J Ethnopharmacol.* **85**(2-3), 201-06 (2003)].

Administration of an active compound isolated from *E. jambolana* (7mg/kg) to streptozotocin and alloxan-induced diabetic rabbits significantly decreased hyperlipidemia. This compound also elicited antihyperglycemic activity in both the models of experimental diabetes. Plasma insulin levels were increased in treated diabetic animals. [Sharma SB, Nasir A, Murthy PS, Prabhu KM; Novel herbal antidiabetic drugs from *Eugenia jambolana* IUPAC *International Conference on Biodiversity and Natural Products Chemistry and Medicinal Applications,* New Delhi, p. 27, 26-31 January, 2004].

***Eupatorium hyssopifolium*:** See *Balduina angustifolia*: [Hall *et al.*; *J Pharm Sci* **69**(6), 694- 97 (1980)].

F

Fagopyrum esculentum (Buckwheat, H. Kotu): Administration of buckwheat leaf extracts to high fat diet-fed rabbits for 12 weeks, significantly lowered the hepatic tissue total cholesterol, triglycerides and malondialdehyde. The leaf extract also increased serum testosterone levels along with lowering of serum insulin levels. [Wojeicki J, Samochowiec L, Gonet B, Juzwiak S, Dabrowska Zamojcin E, Katdonska M, Tustanowski S; Effect of buckwheat extract on free radical generation in rabbits administered high fat diet, *Phytother Res* **9**(5), 323-26 (1995)].

The effects of buckwheat protein on cholesterol metabolism were compared with those of soybean protein and casein. The rats were fed a cholesterol-rich semipurified diet containing the buckwheat protein extract, soybean protein or casein as protein source for 3 weeks. Plasma cholesterol levels were decreased in the rats, fed the buckwheat protein extract diet compared to the rats fed the soybean protein or casein diet. Concentrations of hepatic cholesterol were also significantly decreased in the rats fed with the buckwheat protein extract diet as compared to the rats fed other protein diets. [Kayashita J, Shimaoka I, Nakajyoh M; Hypocholesterolemic effect of buckwheat protein extract in rats fed cholesterol enriched diets, *Nutr Res* **15**(5), 691-98 (1995)].

Consumption of buckwheat protein lowers plasma cholesterol and its cholesterol-lowering effect is mediated by higher faecal excretion of neutral sterols. Lower digestibility of buckwheat protein is at least partially responsible for the effect. [Kayashita J, Shimaoka I, Nakajoh M, Yamazaki M, Kato N; Consumption of buckwheat protein lowers plasma cholesterol and raises faecal neutral sterols in cholesterol-fed rats because of its low digestibility, *J Nutr* **127**(7), 1395-400 (1997)].

Ferula asafoetida (Asafoetida, H. Hing, S. Hingu): See *Adenocalymma alliaceum:* [Srinivasan and Srinivasan; *Indian J Exp Biol* **33**(1), 64-66 (1995)].

Ferula varia: See Flavonoids in Appendix: [Khushbaktova *et al.; Khim Farma Zh* **25**(4), 53- 57 (1991)].

Ficus bengalensis (Banyan tree, H. Bargad): See *Capparis deciduas:* [Agarwal and Chauhan; *Plant Foods Hum Nutr* **38**(2), 189-97 (1988)].

Leucopelargonidin glycoside, isolated from the bark of the plant, demonstrated significant hypoglycemic, hypolipidemic and serum insulin raising effects in moderately diabetic rats with close similarities to the effects of a minimal dose of glibenclamide. However, unlike glibenclamide, the glycoside significantly enhanced the faecal excretion of sterols and bile acids. [Cherian S, Augusti KT; Antidiabetic effects of a glycoside of leucopelargonidin isolated from *Ficus bengalensis* Linn. *Indian J Exp Biol.* **31**(1), 26-29 (1993)].

Administration of aqueous extract of bark of *F. bengalensis* to cholesterol-fed rabbits, led to the lowering of serum cholesterol, LDL, VLDL-cholesterol and triglyceride levels. HDL-cholesterol levels were enhanced in treated hypercholesterolemic rabbits [Shukla R, Anand K, Prabhu KM, Murthy S; Hypocholesterolemic effect of water extract of the bark of banyan tree, *Ficus bengalensis, Indian J Clin Biochem* **10**(1), 14-18(1995)].

Feeding of aqueous extract of *F. bengalensis* (50mg/kg/d) for 30 days to subdiabetic and diabetic rabbits significantly reduced the serum total cholesterol, LDL-cholesterol and VLDL-cholesterol levels. This extract also brought down the levels of triglycerides and glycosylated haemoglobin in diabetic rabbits. [Shukla R, Anand K, Prabhu KM, Murthy PS; Hypolipidemic effect of water extract of *Ficus bengalensis* in alloxan induced diabetes mellitus rabbits, *Indian J Clin Biochem* **10**(2), 119-121(1995)].

Leucopelargonidin-3-O- α-L-rhamnoside and leucocyanidin-3-O- α-D-galactosyl cellobioside, isolated from the bark of *F. bengalensis* were methylated respectively, to their 5,7- and 5,3'-dimethyl ethers. The antioxidant action of these flavonoid derivatives was evaluated in hyperlipidemic rats and compared with that of quercetin. The *Ficus* compounds showed significant antioxidant effects, which might be attributed to their polyphenolic nature. The methylation of two hydroxyl groups in the *Ficus* flavonoids might have slowed down their antioxidant action as compared to quercetin. [Daniel RS, Mathew BC, Devi KS, Augusti KT; Antioxidant effect of two flavonoids from the bark of *Ficus bengalensis* Linn in hyperlipidemic rats, *Indian J Exp Biol* **36**(9), 902-06 (1998)].

Administration of two *Ficus* flavonoids (leucopelargonin and leucocyanin derivatives) as well as quercetin to cholesterol-fed rats at a dose of 100mg/kg caused lowering of atherogenic index and increased hepatic HMG CoA reductase. These compounds also significantly increased the incorporation of labeled acetate into free and ester cholesterol in liver tissue of hyperlipidemic rats. However, the hepatic bile acids, sterols and lipogenic enzyme activity did not change much following treatment with these drugs. [Daniel RS, Devi KS, Augusti KT; Mechanism of action of antiatherogenic and related effects of *Ficus bengalensis* Linn. Flavonoids in experimental animals, *Indian J Exp Biol* 41(4), 296-303 (2003)].

The antioxidant effect of aqueous extract of the bark of *F. bengalensis* was evaluated in hypercholesterolemic rabbits. Treatment with water extract decreased the levels of serum cholesterol, triacylglycerol and LDL + VLDL-cholesterol. It also led to a decrease in lipid peroxidation, as evidenced by fall in thiobarbituric acid reactive substances with a corresponding increase in blood glutathione content. A significant increase in the activities of antioxidant enzymes; superoxide dismutase, catalase, glutathione peroxidase and glutathione reductase was also noticed. The water extract of the bark of *F. bengalensis* was thus found to show significant antioxidant effect, in addition to hypolipidemic effect. [Shukla R, Gupta S, Gambhir JK, Prabhu KM, Murthy PS; Antioxidant effect of aqueous extract of the bark of *Ficus bengalensis* in hypercholesterolaemic rabbits, *J Ethnopharmacol* **92**(1), 47-51 (2004)].

Ficus carica (H. Anjir, S. Anjira)**:** Oral administration of a decoction of *F. carica* leaves significantly reduced the blood triglyceride levels in streptozotocin-induced diabetic rats. Intraperitoneal administration of *F. carica* extract also lowered the plasma triglyceride levels in diabetic rats. However, this extract did not affect the cholesterolemia. [Dominguez E, Canal JR, Torres MD, Camillo JE, Perez C; Hypolipidemic activity of *Ficus carica* leaf extracts in streptozotocin diabetic rats, *Phytother Res* **10**(6), 526-28 (1996)].

Intraperitoneal administration of *F. carica* leaf decoction (50g dry wt/kg bw) to experimentally induced hyperetriglyceridemic rats, dcreased the plasma triglyceride levels. However, plasma cholesterol levels did not change significantly in treated rats. [Perez C, Canal JR, Canopillo JE, Romero A, Torres DM; Hypotriglyceridemic activity of *Ficus carica* leaves in experimental hypertriglyceridemic rats, *Phytother Res* **13**(3), 188-91 (1999)].

Experiments confirm that antioxidant status is affected in the diabetes syndrome, and that *Ficus carica* extracts tend to normalise it. [Perez C, Canal JR, Torres MD; Experimental diabetes treated with *Ficus carica* extract: Effect on oxidative stress parameters, *Acta Diabetologica* **40**(1), 3-8 (2003)].

Ficus glomerata (H. Gular, S. Udumbara)**:** See *Capparis deciduas:* [Agarwal and Chauhan; *Plant Foods Hum Nutr* **38**(2), 189-97 (1988)].

Ficus religiosa (H. Pipal, S. Asvattha)**:** See *Capparis deciduas:* [Agarwal and Chauhan *Plant Foods Hum Nutr* **38**(2), 189-97 (1988)].

Ficus robusta (*F. elastica*, Rubber plant)**:** Rubber seed oil, rich in polyunsaturated fats shows hypolipidemic effect both in experimental hyperlipidemic animals as well as in hyperlipoproteinemic patients. It was also able to depress the induced aortic atherosclerotic lesion in rabbits, fed with cholesterol-rich diet for 2.5 months. Rubber seed oil could facilitate regression of aortic atherosclerosis to some extent. The possible mechanism of this effect of rubber seed oil has been discussed. [Liu C, Tang C, Yang L et al.; Effect of rubber seed oil on the development and regression of experimental atherosclerosis of the aorta in rabbits, *Zhonghua Xinxueguanbing Zazhi* **9**(1), 54-57 (1981)].

Flueggea microcarpa (H. Dalme, S. Nilishila)**:** Oral administration of bergenin, isolated from the leaves of *F. microcarpa,* to hyperlipidemic rats for 14 days significantly decreased serum total lipid without much changes in serum cholesterol and triglycerides. However, after 21 days of administration the serum cholesterol, triglycerides, low density lipoprotein cholesterol (LDL-c) and very low density lipoprotein cholesterol (VLDL-c) levels were significantly reduced, while the serum high density lipoprotein cholesterol (HDL-c) level was elevated . Atherogenic index was also significantly decreased in bergenin-treated rats [Farboodniay Jahromi MA, Chansouria J.P.N., Ray AB; Hypolipidemic activity in rats of bergenin, the major constituent of *Flueggea microcarpa, Phytother Res* **6**(4), 180-83 (1992)].

***Fructus corni*:** In normal mice, oral administration of alcoholic extract of *F. corni* (10- 20g/kg) for 7 days decreased blood lipid and glucose levels. Similarly in alloxan-diabetic mice also this drug (10-20g/kg for 3 days) significantly reduced blood sugar levels. Inhibition of platelet aggregation and a decrease in the viscosity of blood was also noted following treatment with *F. corni* in rabbits. [Lill Baoling, Zhu Danni, Yu Zhiling, Yan Yongqing; Effect of alcoholic extract of *Fructus corni* on blood glucose. lipid levels and platelet aggregation in experimental animals, *J China Pharm Univ* **23**(1), 19-21 (1992)].

G

Garcinia cambogia: Administration of dexamethasone (10 mg/kg bw/d sc.) in rats resulted in marked increase in the levels of triglycerides and cholesterol and free fatty acids in both plasma and liver. The level of phospholipids also increased in the plasma but decreased significantly in liver tissue as compared to those in normal rats. The lipid levels were maintained at near normalcy when co-treated with *Garcinia cambogia* fruit extract (1 g/kg bw/d, p o.) in dexamethasone administered rats. [Mahendran P, Devi CS; Effect of *Garcinia cambogia* extract on lipids and lipoprotein composition in dexamethasone administered rats, *Indian J Physiol Pharmacol* **45**(3), 345-50 (2001)].

The modulating effect of *G. cambogia* fruit extract on ethanol-induced peroxidative damage in rats was determined. Ethanol administered rats were treated concomitantly with *G. cambogia* fruit extract (1g/kg bw/d) orally for 45 days. Co-treatment of the rats with *G. cambogia* significantly inhibited the rise in lipid levels and also the peroxidative damage caused by ethanol. The imbalance in lipid metabolism is considered to be the reason for increase in lipid peroxidation and the hypolipidemic property of *G. cambogia* reduces the peroxidative damage, enhanced by ethanol. [Mahendran P; Devi CS; The modulating effect of *Garcinia cambogia* extract on ethanol induced peroxidative damage in rats, *Indian J Pharmacol* **33**(2), 87-91 (2001)].

Administration of flavonoids from *G. cambogia*, at a dose of 1 mg/100g bw/d, significantly lowered lipid levels in rats fed with normal and cholesterol-containing diets. The HMG-CoA reductase showed significant reduction in normocholesterolemic rats. Activities of glucose-6- phosphate dehydrogenase and isocitrate dehydrogenase were reduced significantly. Highly stimulated activities of the enzymes lipoprotein lipase and plasma lecithin cholesterol acyl transferase were noted in flavonoid-administered animals. Hepatic and faecal bile acids and faecal neutral sterol levels were elevated substantially, indicating a higher rate of degradation of cholesterol. Thus hypolipidemic activity of these flavonoids may be due to a lower rate of lipogenesis and higher rate of degradation. [Koshy AS, Anila L, Vijayalakshmi NR; Flavonoids from *Garcinia cambogia* lower lipid levels in hypercholesterolemic rats, *Food Chem* **72**(3), 289-94 (2001)].

Gardenia jesminoides (S. Gandharaj): See *Artemisia* species: [Jing *et al.*; *Chinese Journal of Integrated Traditional and Western Medicine* **6**(1), 21-23 (1986)].

Geranium thunbergii: Administration of geraniin, a tannin isolated from *G. thunbergii*, to puromycin aminonucleoside-induced nephrotic animals, lowered serum cholesterol and lipid peroxide levels. [Nakanishi Y, Kubo M, Okuda T, Abe H; Effect of geraniin on aminonucleoside nephrosis in rats, *Natural Medicine* **53**(2), 94-100 (1999)].

Glycine max (Soya bean, soybean, H. Bhat): Effect of wheat, rice, or soya bran on plasma lipids was studied on monkeys (*Macaca fascicularis*) for 9 months. None of the brans reduced plasma levels of cholesterol, whereas cholestyramine produced marked hypocholesterolemic effects. [Malinow MR, McLaughlin P, Papworth L, Naito HK, Lewis LA; Effect of bran and cholestyramine on plasma lipids in monkeys, *Am J Clin Nutr* **29**(8), 905-11 (1976)].

Substitution of animal proteins in a group of 20 patients with type-II hyperlipoproteinemia by soybean textured protein induced a 14% decrease of plasma-cholesterol levels after 2 weeks and 21% after 3 weeks. The addition of cholesterol (500mg/d) to soy protein did not modify the hypocholesterolemic response and this observation supported the hypothesis that a soy protein has a hypocholesterolemic action *per se*. [Sirtori CR, Agradi E, Conti F, Mantero O, Gatti E; Soybean protein diet in the treatment of type II hyperlipoproteinemia, *Lancet* **1**(8006), 275-77 (1977)].

The effect of dietary protein on the level of plasma cholesterol in young, healthy, normolipidemic women was investigated. In this study, the mean plasma cholesterol level was found to be significantly lower in women who were given soybean protein in their diet. [Carroll KK, Giovannetti PM, Huff MW, Moase O, Roberts DC, Wolfe BM; Hypocholesterolemic effect of substituting soybean protein for animal protein in the diet of healthy young women, *Am J Clin Nutr* **31**(8), 1312-21 (1978)].

The hypocholesterolemic action of soy protein was clearly demonstrated in swine, fed a high fat, high cholesterol diet. [Kim DN, Lee KT, Reiner JM, Thomas WA; Effects of a soy protein product on serum and tissue cholesterol concentrations in swine-fed high fat, high-cholesterol diets, *Exp Mol Pathol* **29**(3), 385-99 (1978)].

A group of rabbits were given in sequence a laboratory stock diet (I), a semi-purified diet containing 25% casein (II) and a similar diet in which soybean meal replaced casein (III). On changing from diet I to II, plasma cholesterol rose 4-fold after 16 weeks, but fell 50% after 12 weeks on changing from diet II to III. Replacement of casein with soybean meal in the semi-purified diet caused an increased faecal excretion of sterols but not of bile acids. The hypocholesterolemic effect of soybean meal is probably due to its action in increasing the excretion of faecal neutral sterols. [Fumagalli R, Paoletti R, Howard AN; Hypocholesterolemic effect of soy, *Life Sci* **22**(11), 947-52 (1978)].

The efficacy of total substitution of animal proteins with a textured soybean protein in hypercholesterolemic individuals was assayed. It was inferred from the study that treatment with the soybean diet is an effective regimen for inducing a significant cholesterol reduction in type II patients refractory to standard low lipid regimens. [Sirtori CR, Gatti E, Mantero O, Conti F, Agradi E, Tremoli E, Sirtori M, Fraterrigo L, Tavazzi L, Kritchevsky D; Clinical experience with the soybean protein diet in the treatment of hypercholesterolemia, *Am J Clin Nutr* **32**(8), 1645-58 (1979)].

Substituting soya oil for lard considerably reduced hypercholesterolemia in the male rat with induced hypercholesterolemia due to a dietary overload of cholesterol and sodium deoxycholate. The decrement was more marked when a mixture of soya oil and sardine oil replaced the lard. [Durand G, Pascal G, Gounelle de Pontanel H; Treatment of hypercholesterolemia in the male rat by introduction of soya oil supplemented or not with sardine oil in the diet, *Ann Nutr Aliment* **33**(5), 687-706 (1979) [Article in French].

Soybean diet induced a significant decrease of plasma cholesterol levels from 314 ± 24 to 267 ± 30 mg/100 ml, when administered to patients with type II hyperlipoproteinemia. Triglycerides levels remained unchanged. LDL-cholesterol decreased significantly from 241 ± 26 to 194 ± 32 mg/100 ml, whereas HDL-cholesterol increased only slightly and not significantly from 38 ± 7 to 40 ± 8 mg/100 ml. [Noseda G, Fragiacomo C, Bosia C, Ramelli F, Sirtori CR; Treatment of hyperlipidemia type II with soybeans, *Schweiz Med Wochenschr* **109**(47), 1852-3 (1979) [Article in German].

Feeding of diet containing soya proteins to rats enhanced neutral sterol excretion without affecting cholesterolemia. Dietary fibres, phytosterols and phytic acid rather than soya saponins might be responsible for such an effect. Incorporation of saponins from *Saponaria officinalis* in diet lowered the aortic and hepatic cholesterol contents without influencing serum cholesterol levels. Such an effect could be attributed to increased excretion of neutral sterols and bile acids. [Sautier C, Doucot C, Flament C, Lemonnier D; Effect of soya protein and saponins on serum, tissue and faecal steroids in rats, *Atherosclerosis* **34**(3), 233-41 (1979)].

Rats fed 15% soybean protein with 1% cholesterol had fatty livers, which were prevented by 30 and 45% soybean protein. Again rats fed with 15%casein with 1%

cholesterol did not cause fatty livers but fatty livers developed with 30 or 45% casein. Rats fed with soybean protein had less serum cholesterol than casein-fed rats. The hypocholesterolemic action of soybean protein was comparable to that of replacing sucrose by dextrin. Raising the quantity of dietary casein with sucrose was more hypercholesterolemic than raising soybean protein with sucrose. Increasing the concentration of casein with dextrin did not change serum cholesterol but increasing the concentration of soybean protein with dextrin was slightly hypocholesterolemic. These changes in serum cholesterol were paralleled by serum phospholipids. Serum triglycerides were unchanged by the source of dietary protein but decreased if dietary sucrose was decreased. Casein and soybean protein apparently influenced liver and serum lipids differently and their effects were influenced by dietary carbohydrate. [Hevia P, Clary RA, Visek WJ; Serum and liver lipids in rats fed with casein or soybean protein with sucrose or dextrin or sucrose and cholesterol, *Nutr Reports International* **20**(4), 539-48 (1979)].

Feeding of reconstituted milk with soya bean oil or corn oil or vegetable shortening or tallow to different groups of two weeks old calves increased the plasma cholesterol levels in all groups. At the end of 15 weeks, the blood or hepatic cholesterol content were higher in soya bean and corn oil-fed animals compared to vegetable shortening or tallow fed calves. Low density lipoprotein was identified as the carrier of the increased amounts of cholesterol noted in the blood. [Richard MJ, Stewart JW, Heeg TR, Wiggers KD, Jacobson NL; Blood plasma lipoprotein and tissue cholesterol of calves fed soya bean oil, corn oil, vegetable shortening or tallow, *Atherosclerosis* **37**(4), 513-20 (1980)].

Adult male rats were maintained on one of two diets containing 0.5% cholesterol and soy flour high or low in endogenous saponins. In high and low saponin fed rats, plasma cholesterol was significantly lower than those fed chow and the hypercholesterolemia, normally observed with high cholesterol diets, was absent. In high saponin-fed rats, biliary bile acid secretion and faecal bile acid and neutral sterol excretion were raised relative to low saponin-fed animals. The proportion of primary acids excreted increased. The results confirmed the role of soy saponins in enhancing bile acid excretion. The role of other factors in the observed hypocholesterolemic effect, particularly the composition of plasma amino acids, has been discussed. [Topping DL, Trimble RP, Illman RJ, Potter JD, Oakenfull DG; Prevention of dietary hypercholesterolemia in the rat by soy flour, high and low in saponins, *Nutr Reports International* **22**(4), 513-20 (1980)].

An experiment was conducted to study whether the hypocholesterolemic action of soy products is due to the presence of saponins. Soy flour with or without endogenous saponins was added to the diet of normocholesterolemic, young adult males. Plasma cholesterol and lipoproteins remained unchanged in both groups, though the levels were above that on the usual diet. Faecal primary bile acid concentration was significantly increased during the first fortnight of the group receiving soy flour with endogenous saponins compared with the saponin deficient group. Saponins favourably altered bile acid excretion but failed to modify plasma cholesterol in this group of free-living subjects with no other dietary modification. The atherogenic potential of the diet was also discussed. [Potter JD, Illman RJ, Calvert GD, Oakenfull DG, Topping DL; Soy saponins, plasma lipids, lipoproteins and faecal bile acids: A double blind crossover study, *Nutr Reports International* **22**(4), 521-28 (1980).

The mechanism of hypocholesterolemic action of soy protein products (A having 62.2% protein and B having 92% protein) was studied in young male Yorkshire swine and compared with that of casein. Neither of the soy protein products, A or B, affected serum cholesterol levels when added to mash. No changes were noted when casein was added to mash. Total hepatic microsomal HMG-CoA reductase activities were not altered by the addition of either soy protein A or casein to mash. The activities of the enzyme were reduced by 70% in the group in which soy protein was used in a high cholesterol diet as compared to the activities of the enzyme with the groups fed mash alone or mash plus soy protein A. Soy protein products were hypocholesterolemic when added to high-cholesterol diet. The effect of soy protein on lowering serum cholesterol levels as compared with casein in swine fed high cholesterol diet may be due to the increases in faecal steroid excretions, not counter balanced by a concomitant increase in cholesterol synthesis. [Kim DN, Lee KT, Reiner JM, Thomas WA; Increased steroid excretion in swine fed high fat cholesterol diet with soy protein, *Exp Mol Pathol* **33**(1), 25-35 (1980)].

The effect of dietary soybean protein on plasma lipids in hyperlipoproteinemic individuals was compared with that of dietary meat. The mean total plasma cholesterol was reduced by 13% during the first 3 weeks of dietary sequence using a prudent low-fat, low cholesterol diet containing meat. Substituting soybean protein for the meat protein in the second dietary sequence had little additional effect. The major cholesterol changes occurred in the low density lipoprotein and very low density lipoprotein fractions. Complete replacement of all animal proteins with soybean protein without any appreciable changes in all other dietary components showed similar results. Soybean protein diet apparently has hypocholesterolemic activity and may be of benefit in the treatment of human atherosclerosis. [Holmes WL, Rubel GB, Hood SS; Comparison of the effect of dietary meat vs. soybean protein on plasma lipids of hypercholesterolemic individuals, *Atherosclerosis* **36**(3), 379-88 (1980)].

The hypolipidemic effect of soy and casein protein was determined in propylthiouracil induced hypothyroid chicks at the dietary protein level of 40 or 62%. Soy protein and casein at each level of administration had a significant hypocholesterolemic and hypotriglyceridemic effect. Soy may be a better protein supplement than casein for its hypolipidemic effect because it also decreases liver triglycerides. [Raheja KL, Linscheer WG; Hypolipidemic effect of casein vs. soy protein in the hyperlipidemic hypothyroid chick model, *Nutr Reports International* **21**(4), 497-504 (1980)].

Effects of low fat (1% corn oil) diets containing an isonitrogenous level (3.2%) of either casein, soybean protein isolate or three soybean globulin fractions (total, 11S and 7S globulins) on plasma and liver lipids and on the excretion of faecal neutral sterols were examined in rats. From the results of the investigation it was inferred that the antihypercholesterolemic effect of soybean protein was attributable to protein *per se*, and not to the carbohydrate components which were associated with the protein preparation. [Okita T, Sugano M; Effects of dietary soybean globulins on plasma and liver lipids and on faecal excretion of neutral sterols in rats, *J Nutr Sci Vitaminol* (Tokyo) **27**(4), 379-88 (1981)].

Rats, fed high cholesterol diets containing soy protein or the amino acid mixture simulating soy protein, produced lower levels of serum cholesterol throughout the experiments, as compared with those on the corresponding casein type diets. Feeding soy protein resulted in a significant decrease in serum apoA-I and apoB, but the relative concentration of high density lipoprotein-cholesterol was kept at the higher level. The concentration of liver cholesterol was also lower in rats fed the plant protein. Soy protein exhibited its hypocholesterolemic effect even when a diet rich in cholesterol was fed. The cholesterol-lowering effect of soy proteins appears to be a phenomenon common to rodents. [Nagata Y, Tanaka K, Sugano M; Serum and liver cholesterol levels of rats and mice fed soy-bean protein or casein, *J Nutr Sci Vitaminol* (Tokyo) **27**(6), 583-93 (1981)].

Feeding of soybean protein or its amino acid mixture to rats, showed decrease of high density lipoprotein, very low density lipoprotein as well as low-density-lipoprotein-cholesterol to a similar extent; the concentration of serum apolipoprotein A-I also decreased but that of apolipoprotein B increased. Although rats given soybean protein excreted more neutral and acidic steroids than casein fed animals, the difference disappeared when the amino acid mixture was fed, indicating that the hypocholesterolemic effect of the vegetable protein is not ascribed only to the increased elimination of steroids. The difference in the amino acid composition between animal and vegetable proteins probably is responsible for the different response of serum cholesterol. [Nagata Y, Tanaka K, Sugano M; Further studies on the hypocholesterolemic effect of soybean protein in rats, *Brit J Nutr* **45**(2), 233-42 (1981)].

The effect of substituting soy for animal protein in mixed diets was determined in young men with mildly elevated plasma cholesterol. The hypocholesterolemic effects were similar for both animal and soy protein diets. [Shorey RL, Bazan B, Lo GS, Steinke FH; Determinants of hypocholesterolemic response to soy and animal protein based diets, *Am J Clin Nutr* **34**(9), 1769-78 (1981)].

The hypothesis that soybean saponins, by binding bile salts in the gastrointestinal lumen, are responsible for some of the plasma cholesterol-lowering effect of soybean preparations was tested. Results of the investigation, however, indicate that soybean saponins are not responsible for the hypocholesterolemic effect of soybean products. [Calvert GD, Blight L, Illman RJ, Topping DL, Potter JD; A trial of the effects of soybean flour and soybean saponins on plasma lipids, faecal bile acids and neutral sterols in hypercholesterolemic men, *Brit J Nutr* **45**(2), 277- 82 (1981)].

The serum cholesterol-lowering effect of dietary soy protein was examined in hypercholesterolemic rats. The inclusion of soy protein in a diet containing cholesterol and casein brought about a reduction in the serum cholesterol levels. A further cholesterol-lowering effect was achieved by increasing the proportion of soy protein in the diet. The study clearly demonstrated the ability of dietary soy protein to reduce the levels of cholesterol in the serum and the liver. [Terpstra AH, van Tintelen G, West C E; The hypocholesterolemic effect of dietary soy protein in rats, *J Nutr* **112**(4), 810-17 (1982)].

Rats fed atherogenic diet and plant proteins (10% protein derived from soy bean, wheat gluten, or wheat gluten supplemented with lysine and threonine) were found to have lower serum cholesterol and triglyceride levels, no detectable amounts of low density lipoprotein, a smaller amount of very low density lipoprotein and a higher concentration of high density lipoprotein (HDL) as compared to the control animals, receiving 10% protein derived from casein. [Mokady S, Liener IE; Effect of plant proteins on cholesterol metabolism in growing rats fed atherogenic diets, *Ann Nutr Metab* **26**(2), 138-44 (1982)].

The decreased intestinal absorption of cholesterol and increased faecal steroid excretion were proved to be primarily responsible for the antihypercholesterolemic effect of soy protein compared with casein. The faecal loss of steroids far outweighs the activation of hepatic steroidogenesis. In the case of the soy protein-type amino acid mixture, the depression of hepatic cholesterol synthesis seems accountable for reducing serum cholesterol levels. [Nagata Y, Ishiwaki N, Sugano M; Studies on the mechanism of antihypercholesterolemic action of soy protein and soy protein-type amino acid mixtures in relation to the casein counterparts in rats, *J Nutr* **112**(8), 1614-25 (1982)].

The faecal steroid elimination profile was studied in 7 type II hyperlipoproteinemic patients given a low-lipid diet with textured soybean proteins, in order to define the mechanism of the hypocholesterolemic activity of this new dietary regimen. The reported results failed to provide a definitive contribution to the mode of action of the soybean protein diet. A redistribution of cholesterol from plasma to tissue pools was, however, considered to be a possibility. [Fumagalli R, Soleri L, Farina R, Musanti R, Mantero O, Noseda G, Gatti E, Sirtori CR; Faecal cholesterol excretion studies in type II hypercholesterolemic patients treated with the soybean protein diet, *Atherosclerosis* **43**(2-3), 341-54 (1982)].

The soy isoflavones (genistein, daidzein), their glucosides (genistin and daidzin) and coumestrol, were reported to contribute to the hypocholesterolemic response to soy-protein foods. Examination of several soy-based diets for laboratory animals showed the diets to have a highly variable content of isoflavones. [Murphy PA, Farmakalidis E, Johnson LD; Isoflavone content of soy-based laboratory animal diets, *Food Chem Toxicol* **20**(3), 315-18 (1982)].

The normal diet of six healthy volunteers was supplemented by 21 g of dietary fibre from two different soybean seed fibre preparations (a nonpurified and never-dried soya pulp A or a purified soya fibre B), for 3 weeks each. Mean daily faecal wet weight increased by 19 and 38% in the fibre periods A and B as compared to a two-week control period. Faecal fibre increased by 52% only during period B. Neither fibre changed serum triglycerides, but fibre B increased low density lipoprotein-cholesterol and low density lipoprotein-phospholipids. The ratio of high density to low density lipoprotein-cholesterol, however, did not change significantly. Thus, dietary fibres from soybean do not seem to contribute to the hypocholesterolemic effect of soya. The results of this study also demonstrate that two apparently similar dietary fibres, coming from a single source, can exert distinctly different metabolic effects. [Schweizer TF, Bekhechi AR, Koellreutter B, Reimann S, Pometta D, Bron BA; Metabolic effects of dietary fibre from dehulled soybeans in humans, *Am J Clin Nutr* **38**(1), 1-11 (1983)].

Administration of soya polysaccharide for 18 days to healthy human volunteers did not affect the serum lipid levels. However, faecal wet weight and faecal water contents were significantly increased without any change in total dry faecal weight, faecal neutral steroids, bile salts, protein and mineral contents following soya polysaccharide supplementation. [Tsai AC, Mott EL, Owen GM, Bennick MR, Lo GS, Steinke FH; Effect of soya polysaccharide on gastrointestinal function, nutrient balance, steroid excretion, glucose tolerance, serum lipids and other parameters in humans, *Am J Clin Nutr* **38**(4), 504-11 (1983)].

The effect of the purified unsaponifiable fraction of soybean, given in large dose over 24 weeks to 19 patients with primary types IIa and IIb hyperlipoproteinemia was studied. The reduction of plasma cholesterol in types IIa and IIb were 13.2% and 11.5%, respectively. The unsaponifiable fraction of soybean significantly reduced LDL cholesterol levels with little effect on VLDL or HDL-cholesterol. The triglyceride/cholesterol ratio in HDL-c fraction was also significantly reduced, suggesting its role in the catabolism of HDL-c. The hypocholesterolemic effect of the unsaponifiable fraction of soybean is considered to be a summation effect of plant sterols and tocopherols present in the fraction. [Nakashima Y, Nakamura T, Aramaki Y, Kuroiwa A Effect of the purified unsaponifiable fraction of soybean on primary type II hyperlipidemia, *Artery* **12**(3), 199-211 (1983)].

In hypercholesterolemic human volunteers, incorporation of soya bean protein in the diet significantly lowered the plasma cholesterol levels. [Beynan AC, West CE, Soyabean protein: A hypocholesterolemic drug, *Trends Pharmacol Sci* **4**(2), 61-62 (1983)].

The plasma cholesterol level of rats fed with the triterpene alcohol fraction, obtained by chromatographic resolution of the unsaponifiable matter of soybean oil, was significantly lower and the effect was synergistic with soysterol. Both cycloartenol and 24-methylenecycloartenol, the main constituents of triterpene alcohols in soybean oil unsaponifiable matter, in combination with soysterol greatly reduced the plasma cholesterol and enhanced cholesterol excretion. [Kiribuchi M, Miura K, Tokuda S, Kaneda T; Hypocholesterolemic effect of triterpene alcohols with soysterol on plasma cholesterol in rats, *J Nutr Sci Vitaminol* **29**(1), 35- 44 (1983)].

A study was undertaken to compare the effects of sodium phytate and dietary proteins of vegetable (*Glycine max* and *Helianthus annuus*) and animal (casein and whey) origin on the lipoprotein and cholesterol metabolism in albino rats. The results of this investigation indicated that the cholesterol and lipoprotein lowering effects of these proteins depended on the different amino acid proportions and not on the source of protein. The metabolism of sterols was not affected by sodium phytate. [Sautier C, Dieng K, Flament C, Doucet C, Lemonnier D; The influence of four dietary proteins and sodium phytate on the metabolism of cholesterol and the lipoproteins in rat, *Plant Food Human Nutr* **33**(2&3), 193–96 (1983)].

In albino rats, administration of soya saponins caused slight hyperlipemia and lowered the serum lipid levels. It also exhibited an increase of transaminases. [Ohminami H, Kimura Y, Okuda H, Arichi S, Yoshikawa M, Kitagawa I; Effect of soya saponins on liver injury induced by highly peroxidised fat in rats, *Planta Med* **50**(5), 440-41 (1984)].

The effect of substitution of animal protein with soybean protein and addition of soybean protein to low lipid diet on hypercholesterolemia was studied in 57 patients. Both types of diets reduced the serum cholesterol, triglyceride and LDL-cholesterol levels at the end of 16 weeks. These diets did not affect the HDL-cholesterol levels. However, the low lipid diet with soybean protein was relatively more effective in lowering lipids in hypercholesterolemic patients. [Verrillo A, de Teresa A, Giarruso PC, La Rocca S; Soya bean protein diets in the management of type II hyperlipoproteinemia, *Atherosclerosis* **54**(3), 321-31 (1985)].

Piglets aged 8 weeks and weighing 12-18 kg were fed semi-purified casein or soy protein diets, with or without cholesterol and soy hull fibre, for 2 months. Dietary soy fibre-fed simultaneously with cholesterol decreased the cholesterol-induced hypercholesterolemia, but the reduction was significantly greater with soy protein than with casein in the diet. Analyses of the lipoprotein cholesterol indicated that LDL-cholesterol was much more sensitive to the changes induced by feeding cholesterol and soy fibre than either HDL or VLDL-cholesterol. The findings suggested a beneficial role of dietary soy fibre in hypercholesterolemia. [Cho BH, Egwim PO, Fahey GC Jr; Plasma lipid and lipoprotein cholesterol levels in swine: Modification of protein-induced response by added cholesterol and soy fibre, *Atherosclerosis* **56**(1), 39-49 (1985)].

Analyses of gastrointestinal contents of rats, fed soybean protein isolate and casein, showed that soybean protein was readily digested in the stomach but migrated slowly to the small intestine. Fractionation of the stomach contents of rats fed soybean protein led to separation of large and low molecular weight fractions, the latter being absent in rats-fed casein. In rats the peptic digest of soybean protein was found to be as hypocholesterolemic as intact soybean protein. However, it was the large molecular fraction of the peptic digest that showed greater cholesterol lowering effect than that of the small molecular fraction in mice. Peptic digestion was thus proved to play a significant role in the cholesterol-lowering action of soybean protein. [Yashiro A, Oda S, Sugano M; Hypocholesterolemic effect of soybean protein in rats and mice after peptic digestion, *J Nutr* **115**(10), 1325-36 (1985)].

Soya bean protein and casein were treated with pepsin to develop a protein hydrolysate with molecular weights 200-1500 daltons and arginine / lysine ratio greater than 0.6. In this process, soya protein was dissolved in water, treated with pepsin at pH 1.6 for 24 hrs at 37^0C and then heated to inactivate enzyme and finally centrifuged. The supernatant was concentrated and freeze dried. This hydrolysate elicited potent anticholesterolemic activity. [Fugi oil company Ltd.; Anticholesterolemic protein hydrolysate, *Japan Kokai Tokkyo Koho JP* 60,11,425 (Cl. A 61K37/18) (1985)].

The effects of casein, soy protein and their combination with egg yolk or crystalline cholesterol on blood and liver lipids were studied in one-week-old broiler chickens. Serum cholesterol and phospholipids were the lowest in chicks, fed the diets of combined soyprotein with egg yolk. There were no significant differences in HDL-cholesterol between the casein and soyprotein groups, however, VLDL + LDL-cholesterol was lower in soyprotein groups than in casein groups. Feeding soyprotein and egg yolk resulted in a lower concentration of cholesterol in liver than feeding casein and crystalline cholesterol. No differences were found in triglycerides and phospholipids in liver among treatment groups. The results suggest that soyprotein acts strongly as a hypocholesterolemic factor in diets containing egg yolk. [Kim KN, Han IK; Effects of different dietary sources of cholesterol, protein and fibre on lipid metabolism in broiler chicks 2: Effects of casein, soy protein and their combination with egg yolk or crystalline cholesterol on blood and liver lipids in chicks, *Korean J Animal Sci* **27**(6), 367-73 (1985)].

The fish and soybean protein feedings significantly increased the faecal excretions of cholesterol and coprostanol, respectively, and lowered the plasma cholesterol level, as compared to casein feeding. In addition, both fish and soybean protein feedings increased the excretion of bile acids. The stimulation of cholesterol metabolism and the increased excretions of cholesterol and its metabolites by feeding fish or soybean protein appear to play important roles in their hypocholesterolemic effects. [Iritani N, Narita R, Fujita T, Tanaka T; Effects of dietary fish protein, soybean protein and casein on cholesterol turnover in rats, *J Nutr Sci Vitaminol* **31**(3), 385-92 (1985)].

Young Sprague-Dawley litters were fed with diets containing different percentage of soy protein, casein or a mixture of both from weaning to six weeks of age. The litters showed higher plasma cholesterol levels at the weaning than at six weeks. Increase in the cholesterol levels at weaning was ascribed to a rise of LDL-cholesterol accompanied by lowering of HDL-cholesterol. As such no hypocholesterolemic effect of soy protein or casein was observed at the weaning stage. However, at the end of six weeks, the plasma LDL-cholesterol levels were significantly decreased in these animals. [Egwim PO; Plasma and lipoprotein cholesterol in weanling and post-weaning rats fed casein and soy protein diets, *Nutr Res* **5**(11), 1237-46 (1985)].

The effect of substitution of a significant portion of meat proteins in diets by soybean proteins was studied in patients with hyperlipidemia, type IIa, and in experimental rats. Soybean proteins included into the diet were found to induce blood plasma amino acid imbalance, change in the excretion of some amino acids with urine, and significantly diminish the blood plasma cholesterol level. From the results of the investigation, it was inferred that the hypocholesterolemic effect of soybean proteins is caused by decreased apoprotein E synthesis and metabolism due to low levels of blood plasma lysine and arginine. [Lyapkov BG, Yatsyshina TA, Fedotova NYu, Kalamkarova OM; Clinical and experimental approaches to the study of hypocholesteremic effects of soybean proteins, *Vopr Pitan* (2), 39-43 (1986) [Article in Russian].

From the results of an investigation, it was suggested that supplementing the diet with soy fibre might be beneficial in dietary management of hyperlipidemia in patients with hypercholesterolemia and particularly in hyperlipidemic patients with hyperinsulinemia and impaired glucose tolerance. [Lo GS, Goldberg AP, Lim A, Grundhauser JJ, Anderson C, Schonfeld G; Soy fibre improves lipid and carbohydrate metabolism in primary hyperlipidemic subjects, *Atherosclerosis* **62**(3), 239-48 (1986)].

The effects of dietary animal protein (casein) or soy protein (soy isolate) on plasma lipids and hormones were investigated in gerbils. Plasma total cholesterol concentrations were lower in gerbils fed with the soy protein diet than in those fed the casein diet. Absolute HDL-cholesterol concentrations were unaffected by the protein source, but LDL-cholesterol concentrations were lower in the soy-fed gerbils. Thus, the ratio of LDL to HDL-cholesterol was lower in the soyfed gerbils (0.42) compared to the casein-fed gerbils (0.70). The changes in plasma thyroxine levels may, in part, account for the hypocholesterolemic effect of soy protein. [Forsythe WA III, Comparison of dietary casein or soy protein effects on plasma lipids and hormone concentrations in the gerbil (*Meriones unguiculatus*), *J Nutr* **116**(7), 1165-71 (1986)].

In twelve male vegetarians, the effect of consumption of isocaloric Tofu (a soy product) and cheese for three weeks on plasma lipids was studied. Total cholesterol and LDL-cholesterol levels were significantly decreased during Tofu intake. However, no changes in the plasma lipids were observed during cheese consumption. [Dunn C,

Liebman M, Plasma lipid alterations in vegetarian males resulting from the substitution of Tofu for cheese, *Nutr Res* **6**(12), 1343-52 (1986)].

See *Oenothera biennis* (Evening primrose): [Sugano *et al.*; *Agric Biol Chem* **50**(9), 2335-40 (1986)].

See Saponins and sapogenins in Appendix: [Sidhu & Oakenfull; *Brit J Nutr* **55**(3), 643-50 (1986)].

The contribution of enterohepatic circulation of cholesterol and bile acids in the hypocholesterolemic activity of soybean protein isolate was compared with the activity of casein on intact, sham-operated, jejunectomised or ileectomised adult rats. In intact rats the plasma cholesterol concentration was significantly higher when casein diet was fed than when soybean protein isolate diet was fed. The findings from detailed investigation indicated that the differential effects of dietary proteins on plasma cholesterol concentration is not primarily due to interruption of enterohepatic circulation of cholesterol and bile acids. [Saeki S, Nishikawa H, Kiriyama S; Effects of casein or soybean protein on plasma cholesterol level in jejunectomized or ileectomized rats, *J Nutr* **117**(9), 1527-31 (1987)].

The dynamics of blood lipid values, activity of the kinin-kallikrein system and immunologic responsiveness were studied in coronary patients (males aged 43-56 years) who had survived myocardial infarction, during dietotherapy with rations in which 2/3, 1/3 and 1/2 protein were sequentially substituted for soybean protein. The hypocholesterolemic action of soybean protein correlated with its content in the ration, the kallikrein and prekallikrein levels in the blood serum rose simultaneously with a tendency to decrease in the tryptic and to increase in the inhibitory activity of the blood, positive shifts in the cellular immunity were recorded in the patients followed up during dietotherapy. [Meshcheryakova VA, Yatsyshina TA, Plotnikova OA, Tsagikyan TA, Voitko NE, Kalamkarova OM; The role of soy protein in the diet therapy of patients with ischemic heart disease, *Vopr Pitan* (No.**4**), 16-21 (1987) [Article in Russian].

See *Cicer arietinum* (Bengal gram): [Sharma RD, *Nutr Res* **7**(4), 351-64 (1987)].

Rabbits consuming soy fibre and/or isolated soy protein diets had lower plasma cholesterol levels and lower incidence of atherosclerotic lesions relative to the rabbits fed casein-based cellulose diet. Rabbits fed with soy fibre and/or isolated soy protein diets also had a lower cholesterol content in their liver and heart. Rabbits fed with isolated soy protein -based diets had consistently increased faecal bile acid excretion, whereas rabbits fed diets containing soy fibre had increased faecal cholesterol concentration. These results suggest a complementary role for soy fibre and isolated soy protein in preventing atherosclerosis in rabbits. [Lo GS, Evans RH, Phillips KS, Dahlgren RR, Steinke FH; Effect of soy fibre and soy protein on cholesterol metabolism and atherosclerosis in rabbits, *Atherosclerosis* **64**(1), 47-54 (1987)].

In conscious restrained baboons, intraduodenal infusion of isocaloric diets containing 45% amino acids (Soy or casein type), 50% glucose and 5% corn oil for 5 days or rapid and constant intraduodenal infusion of daily diet did not affect the cholesterol levels. Although, during rapid feeding the cholesterol levels did not change but the rate of cholesterol oxidation to bile acids was significantly decreased. However, in fed state, slow isocaloric intraduodenal infusion of diets containing soy protein produced significantly greater lowering of plasma cholesterol and triglyceride levels than the casein diet. It was suggested that the nutritional status (fasting or fed) of the animals and the rate of feeding (rapidly or slowly) markedly influenced the cholesterol and triglyceride reducing effect of soy protein and casein. [Wolfe BM, Grace DM; Substitution of mixed amino acids resembling soy protein for mixed amino acids resembling casein in the diet reduces plasma cholesterol in slowly but not rapidly fed nor fasted baboons, *Metab Clin Exp* **36**(3), 223-29 (1987)].

Soybean protein was exhaustively digested with endo and exo-type microbial proteases and the effect of the digestible low molecular fraction and the undigested high molecular fraction on the serum cholesterol level was compared to that of the intact protein in rats given a cholesterol-enriched diet. The high molecular fraction peptides, relatively abundant in hydrophobic amino acids, were found to be substantially hypocholesterolemic when fed at the nitrogen level equivalent to that of the 20% soybean protein diet, and not only serum but also liver cholesterol levels were similar to those usually encountered in rats given diets free of cholesterol. [Sugano M, Yamada Y, Yoshida K, Hashimoto Y, Matsuo T, Kimoto M; The hypocholesterolemic action of the undigested fraction of soybean protein in rats, *Atherosclerosis* **72**(2-3), 115-22 (1988)].

The influence of levels of soy protein on cholesterol metabolism and the development of atherosclerosis in Japanese quail were studied. The results of the investigation demonstrated that in quail, the presence of higher dietary levels of soy protein not only exhibited hypocholesterolemic action but also a preventive effect on cholesterol-induced atherosclerosis. Increased excretion of cholesterol was considered to be the mechanism. [McClelland JW, Shih JC; Prevention of hypercholesterolemia and atherosclerosis in Japanese quail by high intake of soy protein, *Atherosclerosis* **74**(1-2), 127-38 (1988)].

The effects of long-term (41 weeks) feeding of soybean phospholipid on the level of serum cholesterol and immunological and physiological parameters were compared with those of soybean oil. Body weight gain was lower in soybean phospholipid group when compared to soybean oil group although food intake was similar between the groups. The concentration of serum cholesterol was significantly lower in phospholipid group. Supplementation of soybean phospholipid did not affect urinary proteins and pH, serum immunoglobulins (IgG and IgM) and cutaneous delayed hypersensitivity. It is concluded that hypocholesterolemic effect by soybean phospholipid can be maintained for longterm period without any adverse effects on physiological functions. [Murata M, Imaizumi K, Sugano M; Hypocholesterolemic action of soybean phospholipid and its long-term effects on growth immunological and physiological parameters, *Sci Bull Faculty of Agric Kyushu Univ* **42**(3-4), 187-90 (1988)].

The degree of the contribution of the enterohepatic circulation of bile acids in the hypocholesterolemic activity of soybean protein isolate in comparison with the activity of casein in adult male Sprague-Dawley rats was determined. Rats were fed a cholesterol-free semipurified diet containing either 20% casein or 20% soybean protein isolate for 12 days. Then each group was divided into 3 subgroups, and fed the respective diets supplemented with 0, 2, or 4% of cholestyramine for 8 additional days. During the experimental period, the plasma cholesterol levels were always significantly higher when the casein diet was fed than when the soybean protein isolate diet was fed. At the end of the experiment, the liver cholesterol levels were also significantly higher in casein-fed rats than in soybean protein-fed rats. The casein induced higher cholesterol levels in plasma and liver could not be diminished by the administration of cholestyramine. Data from this study and those from previous study indicate that the interruption of the enterohepatic circulation of bile acids does not play an important role in the hypocholesterolemic activity of soybean protein isolate. [Saeki S; Kiriyama S; Conservation of hyper- and hypo-cholesterolemic activities of dietary casein and soybean protein isolate after the administration of cholestyramine in the rat, *Nutr Reports International* **37**(3), 565-74 (1988)].

The effect of partial replacement of meat protein with three different soyabean-protein products on bile acid and cholesterol excretion was studied in seven ileostomy subjects. Incorporation of moderate amounts of soybean products (soybean flour, soybean concentrate or soybean isolate) in solid diets does not seem to affect short-term sterol balance in man. [Bosaeus I, Sandstrom B, Andersson H; Bile acid and cholesterol excretion in human beings given soybean-based and meat-protein based diets: A study in ileostomy subjects, *British J Nutr* **59**(2), 215-22 (1988)].

See *Zea mays* (Corn): [Green and Green; *Nutr Res* **8**(11), 1265-76 (1988)].

The effects of a soya-based liquid formula were compared with that of a milk-based liquid formula in a weight loss program on eleven obese volunteers. The results of the investigation indicated that whereas moderate weight loss induced by a vegetable protein supplement was associated with a reduction in blood lipids, such weight loss on a control low calorie diet or milk based formula was not associated with a reduction in blood lipids. [Jenkins DJ, Wolever TM, Spiller G, Buckley G, Lam Y, Jenkins AL, Josse RG; Hypocholesterolemic effect of vegetable protein in a hypocaloric diet, *Atherosclerosis* **78**(2-3), 99-108 (1989)].

Direct introduction of an aqueous alcohol extract of a protein isolate (soy 500 E) into a culture of atherosclerotic plaques of human aorta intima caused decrease of the cholesterol content in the cells and their proliferation. The protein isolate (soy 500 E) thus produces an antiatherogenic effect in a cell culture and exhibits antiatherosclerotic properties. [Tutel'ian VA, Vasil'ev AV, Ren LH; Antiatherogenic properties of the soy protein isolate 500 E, *Patol Fiziol Eksp Ter* (4), 62-65 (1989) [Article in Russian].

Platelet lysosomal proteinase and phospholipase activity, cholesterol content in the blood serum and circulating immune complexes, as well as blood serum atherogenic potential were studied using human aortic intima atherosclerotic cell culture from patients with postinfarction cardiosclerosis, 1-3 h before and 2-6 h after a single intake of one of the different foods. The data obtained indicated that the soybean protein isolate produces hypolipidemic, hypocholesterolemic and pronounced antiatherosclerotic effects. [Vasil'ev AV, Li Hva Ren, Pokrovskaya GR, Pogozheva AV, Shimanovskaya NP, Samsonov MA,Tutel'yan VA; Antiatherosclerotic properties of certain food components: A clinico-experimental investigation, *Vopr Pitan* (5), 33-36 (1989) Article in Russian].

Hypocholesterolemic effects of soy protein and soy fibre, the effects of soy products upon glucose tolerance and the bioavailability of zinc and iron from soy foods have been reviewed. [Erdman JW Jr, Fordyce EJ; Soy products and the human diet, *Am J Clin Nutr* **49**(5), 725-37 (1989)].

Treatment of casein with formaldehyde changes its tertiary structure and makes it hypocholesterolemic. Whether formaldehyde-treated casein exerts its hypocholesterolemic effect in the same manner as soybean protein or not was investigated on rabbits. It was observed that while formaldehyde-treated casein exhibited its hypocholesterolemic activity only when fed to rabbits having low cholesterol diet, the hypocholesterolemic effect of soybean protein was independent of the amount of cholesterol included in the diet. From the results of the detailed investigation, it was inferred that the hypocholesterolemic action of dietary formaldehyde-treated casein does not resemble that of soybean protein. [West CE, Spaau CJK, Clous WM, Twisk HP, Goertz MPH, Hubbard RW, Kuyvenhoven MW, Van der Meer R, Roszkowski WF *et al.*; Comparison of the hypocholesterolemic effects of dietary soybean protein and those of formaldehyde-treated casein in rabbits, *J Nutr* **119**(6), 843-56 (1989)].

The effects of the levels of dietary proteins (soybean protein or casein) on various lipid parameters were examined in rats. The plasma and liver cholesterol level tended to decrease with an increasing dietary protein level, in particular when diets contained cholesterol. The hypocholesterolemic effect of soybean protein was evident with cholesterol-enriched diets. The faecal excretion of acidic but not neutral steroids increased with an increasing protein level and it was higher in rats fed with soybeans protein than in those fed casein. The ratio of arachidonate to linoleate in plasma and liver phosphatidylcholine tended to elevate accompanying with an increasing dietary protein level, although it was considerably higher in casein than in soybean protein diets. The results indicated that the hypocholesterolemic effect of soybean protein is influenced not only by the level but also by the presence or absence of dietary cholesterol. [Okita T, Sugano M; Effects of the type and level of dietary proteins on plasma lipids, fatty acid profiles and faecal steroid excretion in rats, *Agric Biol Chem* **53**(3), 659-66 (1989)].

In alcohol-fed rats, the effect of interaction of dietary protein and fat on lipid parameters was studied. Alcohol reduced the hypocholesterolemic effect of soy protein and whey protein compared with casein. Safflower oil lowered the plasma and liver cholesterol levels compared to palm olein. Casein enhanced the desaturation of linoleic acid in the hepatic phoshatidyl choline compared to soy protein. The aortic prostacyclin (PGI-2) production was significantly higher in the casein-fed animals than soy protein group. These results suggested that even in alcohol-fed rats dietary proteins differently affected the lipid parameters. [Koba K, Sugano M; Protein fat interaction on the cholesterol levels and fatty acid desaturation in rats consuming alcohol, *Agric Biol Chem* **53**(10), 2769-76 (1989)].

A decrease in serum cholesterol and a small increase in HDL-cholesterol in healthy female subjects were observed after ingestion of an egg and 3 g of soya lecithin. However, the hypocholesterolaemic effect of soya lecithin is not clearly proven. [Aloia S, Carbini L, Peretti M; Effects of soy lecithin on the lipid pattern of subjects with dyslipidemia after ingestion of one egg, *Clinica Dietologica* **16**(6), 275-82 (1989) Article in Italian].

In 10 normolipidemic adult women, the effect of alternate 3 weeks feeding of diets containing Tofu (a soy product) or cheese on plasma lipids was studied. In Tofu-fed women, the plasma cholesterol and LDL levels were significantly lower than the subject who consumed cheese diet. However, no significant difference in total triglycerides, VLDL-cholesterol and HDL-cholesterol was noted between the two groups. The above mentioned diet schedule modified by equilibrating the amount and type of fat also showed similar response in terms of plasma lipids changes. These observations suggested that the hypocholesterolemic action of Tofu might be attributed to its P/S ratio. [Meredith L, Liebman M, Graves K; Alteration in plasma lipid levels resulting from Tofu and cheese consumption in adult women, *J Am Coll Nutr* **8**(6), 573-79 (1989)].

In 10 hypercholesterolemic coronary artery disease patients, the resistance to warfarin therapy occurring during soy protein cholesterol lowering diet was studied. After bypass surgery all patients were given different doses of warfarin. The patients on soy protein diet showed pronounced increase in the prothrombin time. These observations suggested that soy protein diet produced resistance to warfarin therapy. [Gaddi A, Sangiorgi Z, Ciarrocchi A, Braiato A, Descovich GC; Hypocholesterolemic soy protein diet and resistance to warfarin therapy, *Curr Ther Res* **45**(6), 1006-10 (1989)].

Soy cotyledon fibre supplementation significantly lowered plasma total cholesterol by 7.7% (from 240 to 222 mg/dl) and LDL-cholesterol by 7.4% (from 159 to 145 mg/dl). Plasma HDL cholesterol and total triglycerides were not significantly affected. [Lo GS, Cole TG; Soy cotyledon fibre products reduce plasma lipids, *Atherosclerosis* **82**(1-2), 59-67 (1990)].

Effect of dietary Miso (a soy food) on the cholesterol metabolism was examined in rats fed with the diet containing 0.5% cholesterol and 0.15% sodium cholate. The inclusion of 20% desalted Miso to the atherogenic diet significantly decreased the concentration of serum cholesterol throughout the 30 days experimental period. The ingestion of the Miso preparation doubled the faecal excretion of acidic steroids, while the increase of neutral steroids was nominal. The dietary Miso appeared to exert the potent hypocholesterolemic activity primarily through the enhancement of the catabolism of cholesterol to bile acids in rats fed an atherogenic diet. [Hori M; Ide T, Kawashima K, Yamamoto T; Hypocholesterolemic activity of desalted Miso in rats fed an atherogenic diet, *J Jpn Soc Food Sci Technol* **37**(2), 148-53 (1990)].

Both goldthioglucose-treated and the genetically obese (ob/ob) mice were fed semisynthetic diets containing either soy protein isolate or casein as a protein source, or laboratory chow. In goldthioglucose -induced obese mice, no difference was observed in the plasma cholesterol level between soy protein and casein groups regardless of the fat content of the diet. Thus, in the goldthioglucose -treated mice, soy protein did not have a hypocholesterolemic effect while dietary fat had a hypercholesterolemic effect. Both neutral and acidic steroid contents in faeces of the soy protein group were not different from those of the casein group, and both groups of mice excreted a smaller amount of steroids than mice fed laboratory chow. The results strengthened the inverse correlation between the amount of faecal steroids and the plasma cholesterol level upon feeding various proteins, indicating that the former is one of the important factors that determine the latter. The ob/ob mice showed a marked hypercholesterolemia irrespective of the kind of diet. The amount of faecal steroids was highest in the laboratory chow group and lowest in the casein group. This indicates that some factor(s) other than faecal steroid excretion is dominantly responsible for their hypercholesterolemia. [Yamashita J, Hayashi S; The effect of dietary protein source on plasma cholesterol level and faecal steroid excretion in obese mice, *J Nutr Sci Vitaminol* **36**(6), 545-58 (1990)].

Heating the raw meal or germinated soybean meal did not affect cholesterol levels, though it suppressed the hypotriglyceridemic effect. The triglyceride-lowering effect of soybean was probably caused by the presence of thermolabile substances. [Chandrasiri V, Bau HM, Villaume C, Giannangeli F, Mejean L; Effect of germinated and heated soybean meals on plasma cholesterol and triglycerides in rats, *Reprod Nutr Dev* **30**(5), 611-18 (1990)].

In human beings, substitution of soy protein for dietary animal protein or addition of soy protein to the diet lowers total and low density lipoprotein cholesterol levels in individuals with hypercholesterolemia. Reductions of 20% or more have been obtained with diets high in protein (about 20% of total energy) and relatively low in fat. Triglycerides are also decreased, particularly in subjects with hypertriglyceridemia, but soy-protein diets appear to have little effect on high density lipoprotein cholesterol levels. The hypocholesterolemic effect is mainly attributable to the protein itself rather than to nonprotein components of soy-protein preparations [Carroll KK; Review of clinical studies on cholesterol-lowering response to soy protein, *Am Diet Assoc* **91**(70), 820-27 (1991)].

Familial hypercholesterolemia, one form of type IIa hyperlipidemia, usually responds poorly to standard low-lipid diets. Substitution of animal protein from traditional hypocholesterolemic diet with texturized soy protein caused a marked decrease in total (-20.8%) and low densitylipoprotein (-25.8%) cholesterol and in apolipoprotein B (-14.1%). The plasma cholesterol reduction was higher in patients with apolipoprotein E3/E3 or E3/E4 vs an almost negligible effect on E3/E2. These results confirm that soy-protein diets can lower cholesterol in type IIa patients with familial disease. [Gaddi A, Ciarrocchi A, Matteucci A, Rimondi S, Ravaglia G, Descovich GC, Sirtori CR; Dietary treatment for familial hypercholesterolemia-differential effects of dietary soy protein according to the apolipoprotein E phenotypes, *Am J Clin Nutr* **53**(5), 1191-96 (1991).].

Golden Syrian hamsters fed a cholesterol-free diet containing 25% casein had higher plasma total triglyceride and cholesterol levels and VLDL + LDL-cholesterol levels than animals fed a 25% soybean protein diet. Addition of cholesterol to the diets caused even greater mean differences between the animals fed different types of protein, but the increased inter-animal variablity of response to the added cholesterol resulted in less statistically significant differences. Although less responsive than the nonhybrid Golden Syrian hamsters, hybrid F1B hamsters showed similar effects of dietary casein vs. soybean protein on plasma lipids. These results indicate that the hamster may be a useful model to examine the effect of different types of protein and the interaction with dietary cholesterol on various plasma lipids and lipoproteins. [Terpstra AHM, Holmes JC, Nicolosi RJ; The hypocholesterolemic effect of dietary soybean protein vs. casein in hamsters-fed cholesterol-free or cholesterol enriched semipurified diets, *J Nutr* **121**(7), 944-47 (1991)].

The effects of diets containing either cow's milk or soy protein beverage on plasma lipids and lipoproteins were studied in children with familial hypercholesterolemia. The soy protein beverage, compared to cow's milk, induced significant reductions in plasma triglycerides and very low density lipoprotein cholesterol, as well as a significant increase in high density lipoprotein cholesterol, indicating that consumption of soy protein beverage may be beneficial for the prevention of coronary heart disease in children with familial hypercholesterolemia. [Jacques H, Laurin D, Moorjani S, Steinke FH, Gagne C, Brun D, Lupien PJ; Influence of diets containing cow's milk or soy protein beverage on plasma lipids in children with familial hypercholesterolemia,

J Am Coll Nutr **11** Suppl: 69S-73S (1992)].

An experiment carried on male Wistar rats showed that a diet containing 22.5 or 23.5g soybean protein /100g of diet was hypocholesterolemic compared with a diet containing 20.0 g casein/100 g diet. A comparison of serum amino acids in soybean protein-fed vs. casein-fed rats showed that, whereas concentrations of many amino acids were lower in the soybean protein-fed rats compared with the casein-fed groups, glycine was the only amino acid having a higher concentration. Further, alanine was significantly lower in the soybean protein-fed rats compared with the casein-fed rats. [Horigome T, Cho YS, Dietary casein and soybean protein affect the concentrations of serum cholesterol, triglyceride and free amino acids in rats, *J Nutr* **122**(11), 2273-82 (1992)].

The liver microsomal diacylglycerol acyltransferase activity was decreased in rats, fed with diet containg 10% soybean oil, soybean phospholipid and egg yolk phospholipid. In comparison to soybean oil, the two phospholipids were more effective in decreasing the enzyme activity. Soybean phospholipid also significantly reduced the hepatic triglycerides content. [Ide T, Murata M, Moriuchi H; Microsomal triacyl glycerol synthesis and diacyl glycerol concentration in the liver of rats fed with Soyabean and egg yolk phospholipids, *Biosci Biotechnol Biochem* **56**(5), 732-35 (1992)].

The hypocholesterolemic activity of the undigested fraction (UDF) from soybean protein was significantly greater than that of the parent protein even when rats were fed no cholesterol. This fraction prevented the rise of serum cholesterol during a feeding period of 4 months. Compared with the results obtained with soybean protein, UDF increased faecal excretion of both neutral and acidic steroids and it seemed to interfere with the metabolism of linoleic acid to arachidonic acid more than soyben protein. The results showed that UDF was hypocholesterolemic when the diet was cholesterol-free, and that the effect on linoleic acid metabolism was specific. [Ogawa T, Gatchallan YM, Sugano M, Kimoto M, Matsuo T, Hashimoto Y; Hypocholesterolemic effect of undigested fraction of soybean protein in rats fed no cholesterol, *Biosci Biotechnol Biochem* **56**(11), 1845-48 (1992).

The value of serum cholesterol in rats fed with soy milk was significantly lower than that of rats fed milk. The nutritive value of soy milk protein was found to be lower than that of milk, but the hypocholesterolemic effect of soy milk was more than that of milk. [Ishii T, Yamaguchi M; Nutritive value of soy milk protein and hypocholesterolemic effect of soy milk in growing rats, *Japanese J Nutr* **50**(6), 347-53 (1992)].

Effects of protein source, protein content and soybean saponins in the diet on the plasma cholesterol concentration of chicks were investigated. Soybean protein isolate fortified with methionine or casein with arginine, methionine and glycine was used as protein source. Dietary protein source did not affect the plasma total cholesterol when chicks were fed with 18% protein diet without added cholesterol.

Supplementation of 1% cholesterol significantly elevated the plasma total cholestrol in chicks fed with the casein diet, but the replacement of casein with soybean protein suppressed that elevation. The plasma total and high density lipoprotein (HDL)-cholesterol remained unaffected on addition of soybean saponins (1%) to the casein diet containing 18% protein, irrespective of dietary cholesterol addition. The results of the detailed investigation indicate that the hypocholesterolemic effect of soybean protein cannot be attributed to saponins or non-protein portions. [Ueda H; Effects of dietary protein and soybean saponins on plasma cholesterol concentration in chicks, *Animal Sci Technol* **63**(8), 793-99 (1992)].

See *Medicago sativa* (Alfalfa): [Ueda & Ohshima; *Animal Sci Technol* **63**(10), 1032-37 (1992)].

Sitosterol isolted from *Glycine max* and saponins from *Dioscorea* species, *Trigonella foenum-graecum, Medicago sativa* and *Panax* species lowered cholesterol by competing with cholesterol at binding site or by interfering with hepatic cholesterol biosynthesis. Soluble fibres like gums, pectins and mucilage exert hypolipidemic effect by blocking intestinal cholesterol absorption, whereas *Curcuma longa* loweres cholesterol by stimulating bile flow. [Lanksy PS; Plants that lower cholesterol, *Acta Horticulturae* (332), 131-36 (1993)].

Experiments were designed and undertaken to investigate the hypocholesterolemic effect of prepared soy milk. From the results of the investigation, it was inferred that prepared soy milk is capable of alleviating exogenous hypercholesterolemia, but not of improving endogenous hypercholesterolemia. [Ishii T, Yamaguchi M; Effect of prepared soy milk on dietary or hypothyroid hypercholesterolemia in rats, *Japanese J Nutr* **51**(2), 73-79 (1993)].

The hypocholesterolemic effect of soy protein is mediated through thyroxine (T4). [Ham JO, Chapman KM, Essex Sorlie D, Bakhit RM, Prabhudesai M, Winter L, Erdman JW, Jr, Potter SM; Endocrinological response to soy protein and fibre in mildly hypercholesterolemic men, *Nutr Res* **13**(8), 873-84 (1993)].

The effects on growth rate, serum and liver lipids of peanut meal and soy protein, were compared to those of two animal proteins (casein and fish protein) in rabbits fed with purified diets for 30 days. Total serum, low density lipoprotein (LDL) and high density lipoprotein (HDL)-cholesterol levels were significantly lower in rabbits fed with vegetable protein diets than in those fed animal protein diets. However, peanut meal, which may induce serum cholesterol level as low as that obtained by soy protein, is unable to maintain low serum and hepatic triglyceride levels in the rabbit. [Jacques H, Chaumette P, Lavigne C; Further investigation on the hypocholesterolemic effect of vegetable proteins in the rabbit, *Nutr Res* **13**(8), 969-77 (1993)].

The interaction of dietary protein (casein or soybean protein), and fats (α-linolenic acid rich perilla oil or linoleic acid rich safflower oil) on various lipid parameters and plasma amino acids was studied in a rat model sensitive to dietary cholesterol. The hypolipidemic effect of soybean protein in comparison with that of casein was confirmed in this model irrespective of the fat source. Thus, the hypocholesterolemic effect of soybean protein appeared to be intrinsic. An analysis of plasma amino acids suggested a regulatory role of specific amino acid(s) in the hypocholesterolemic effect of soybean protein. [Ikeda A, Imaizumi K, Sugano M; Interaction of dietary protein and fat on plasma cholesterol and amino acid levels, fatty acid desaturation, and prostacyclin production in exogenous hypercholesterolemic rats, *Biosci Biotechnol Biochem* **57**(11), 1867-72 (1993)].

The effects of dietary soy protein isolate (SPI) and casein on plasma cholesterol level and faecal steroid excretion in rats, mice and hamsters were studied. In rats, SPI significantly stimulated, in comparison to casein, faecal steroid excretion in 9 out of 12 experiments with or without dietary cholesterol, whereas it suppressed plasma cholesterol level in 5 experiments and tended to suppress that, though not significantly, in 4 experiments. In mice, however, no significant difference was observed between the effects of casein and SPI on either the faecal steroid excretion or plasma cholesterol level in most of 12 experiments. The species-dependent difference indicated the existence of inverse correlation between faecal steroid excretion and plasma cholesterol level and supported the view that in species like rat and hamster, but not mice, SPI lowers plasma cholesterol level by stimulating faecal steroid excretion. [Hayashi S, Miyazaki Y, Yamashita J, Nakagawa M, Takizawa H; Soy protein has no hypocholesterolemic action in mice because it does not stimulate faecal steroid excretion in that species, *Cell Mol Biol* (Noisy-Le-grand) **40**(7), 1021-28 (1994)].

The undigested fraction of soybean protein exerts a markedly greater hypocholesterolemic effect than soybean protein itself in rats. The hypocholesterolemic effect of the undigested fraction of soybean protein was apparently reproduced even in hamsters, a more appropriate animal model for human cholesterol metabolism.. [Gatchalian Yee M, Imamura M, Nonaka M, Gu JY, Sugano M; Effect of dietary fats on cholesterol metabolism and eicosanoid production in hamsters fed with undigested fraction of Soybean protein, *J Nutr Sci Vitaminol* **40**(5), 499-504 (1994)].

Feeding the guinea pigs on soybeans significantly reduced the level of serum free, esterified and total cholesterol. [Bagalote SG, Okelo RO, Okelo O, Akhulia J, Jumbe J; Hypocholesterolaemic and hypolipaemic effects of soybeans (*Glycine max*) in guinea pigs, *Discovery and Innovation* **6**(4), 397-400 (1994)].

The metabolic changes that have been observed on soy protein feeding in a variety of animal models, include increased cholesterol synthesis, increased bile acid synthesis (or faecal bile acid excretion), increased apolipoprotein B or E receptor activity and decreased hepatic lipoprotein secretion and cholesterol content, which are associated with an increased clearance of cholesterol from the blood. Whether protein amino acids or non-protein compounds present in soy protein are responsible for this activity is not yet settled. [Potter SM; Overview of proposed mechanisms for the hypocholesterolemic effect of soy, *J Nutr* **125**(3 Suppl), 606S- 611S (1995)].

The per cent reduction in plasma cholesterol levels was found to be greater when the hypercholesterolemic men were placed on a soy protein diet than on an animal protein diet. [Wong WW, Hachey DL, Clarke LL, Zhang S; Cholesterol synthesis and absorption by $^{2}H_2O$ and ^{18}O-cholesterol and hypocholesterolemic effect of soy protein, *J Nutr* **125**(3 Suppl), 612S- 618S (1995)].

An experiment designed to study the effect of the undigested high molecular fraction (HMF) of soybean protein confirmed that HMF increases faecal steroid excretion and reduces serum cholesterol levels in humans. [Wang MF, Yamamoto S, Chung HM, Chung SY, Miyatani S, Mori M, Okita T, Sugano M; Antihypercholesterolemic effect of undigested fraction of soybean protein in young female volunteers, *J Nutr Sci Vitaminol* (Tokyo) **41**(2), 187-95 (1995)].

Effect of a low soy protein isolate (SPI) diet supplemented with methionine on hyperlipidemia, proteinuria, and hypoalbuminemia was studied in rats with nephrotoxic serum nephritis (NSN). Rats were fed experimental diets for 14 days after an injection of nephrotoxic serum. An 8.5%-SPI diet (8.5S), as compared to a basal 20% SPI diet (20S), improved the hyperlipidemia, proteinura, and hypoalbuminemia secondary to NSN but retarded the growth of rats. The addition of 0.3% methionine to 8.5S (8.5SM) alleviated the growth retardation without loss of the above mentioned beneficial effects. 8.5SM was found to suppress hepatic cholesterol synthesis compared with 20S. These results suggest that the methionine supplemented low-SPI diet has a beneficial effect on hyperlipidemia, proteinuria, and hypoalbuminemia without inducing either growth retardation or severe fatty liver in nephritis. The hypocholesterolemic effect of 8.5SM in nephritic rats may be partly attributable to reduced hepatic cholesterol synthesis. [Fujisawa K, Yagasaki K, Funabiki R; Reduction of hyperlipidemia and proteinuria without growth retardation in nephritic rats by a methionine supplemented, low soy protein diet. *Am J Clin Nutr* **61**(3), 603-06 (1995)].

The effects of freeze-dried soybean milk (20%), 20% equivalents of soybean milk lipid extract and defatted soybean milk on serum and hepatic lipids were investigated in rats. The cholesterol-induced increase of liver weight was inhibited only by soybean milk. All the three soybean milk preparations prevented the serum total cholesterol levels; the effect being most pronounced in the group of rats receiving the soybean milk. The serum triglyceride levels were also decreased in soybean milk fed animals. An increase in the faecal neutral steroid excretion was also observed in all the three groups of animals. [Tuzuki K, Iino H, Asao H, Honda Y, Fukuba H; Effects of Soybean milk intake on serum and liver cholesterols of rats, *Japanese J Nutr* **53**(2), 127-34 (1995) [Article in Japanese].

Soybean protein in comparison to casein has selective effects on various parameters of lipid metabolism when added in cholesterol-enriched diets. [Gatchalian Yee M, Imamura M, Nonaka M, Gu JY, Sugano M; Effects of different fats and proteins on cholesterol metabolism and eicosanoid production in hamsters, *Nutr Res* **15**(8), 1149-58 (1995)].

The effects of soy fibres on blood lipid concentration, platelet aggregation and clotting time were studied in Sprague-Dawley rats. Results of investigation showed that soy fibres not only significantly lowered serum total cholesterol (TC), LDL-cholesterol, atherosclerotic index, but also increased the ratio of HDL-c/TC. Soy fibre also significantly lowered serum fibrinogen and platelet aggregation and prolonged clotting time. [Wang C, Zhao L, Chen Y; Hypolipidemic action of soy fibre and its effects on platelet aggregation and coagulation time in rats, *Zhonghua Yufang Yixue Zazhi* **30**(4), 205-08 (1996) [Article in Chinese].

Both isolated soy protein (ISP) and soy protein concentrate were found effective in lowering blood cholesterol concentrations, whereas only ISP increased thyroxine concentrations. Therefore, the concept that modulation of thyroid hormone status is responsible for the cholesterol-lowering effect of soy protein appears to have no basis. [Potter SM, Pertile J, Berber-Jimenez MD; Soy protein concentrate and isolated soy protein similarly lower blood serum cholesterol but differently affect thyroid hormones in hamsters, *J Nutr* **126** (8), 2007-11 (1996)].

The role of soybean saponin in the hypocholesterolemic effect of soybean protein was studied in chicks, fed with diets containing 1% cholesterol. Seven-day-old White Leghorn male chicks were fed diets with different composition for 10 days. Addition of 12% beef tallow to the basal diet containing casein increased cholesterol and triglyceride concentrations of the serum and liver. Supplementation of 1.5% soybean saponin was effective in lowering cholesterol and triglyceride concentrations of the serum and liver in chicks given the beef tallow diet, whereas it did not show significant effects in chicks fed with beef tallow-free diet. When soybean protein isolate was used to substitute casein in the diet, the hypocholesterolemic effect of soybean protein isolate was more manifested in chicks fed with beef tallow-free diet than those fed with beef tallow diet. These results indicated that the hypocholesterolemic effects of soybean saponin and soybean protein isolate were differently affected by the diet composition. Results of this work show that high levels of soybean saponin potentially have the hypocholesterolemic effect. However, it seems unlikely that saponin in the diet containing soybean protein isolate is a primary determinant factor in the cholesterol-lowering effect of soybean protein. [Ueda H, Matsumoto A, Goutani S; Effects of soybean saponin and soybean protein on serum cholesterol concentration in cholesterol-fed chicks, *Animal Sci Technol* **67**(5), 415-22 (1996)].

Effects of dietary protein on oxidised cholesterol-induced alterations in linoleic acid and cholesterol metabolism were studied in 4-weeks-old male Sprague-Dawley rats.

Soybean protein significantly increased the faecal excretion of neutral and acidic steroids and tended to reduce the accumulation of oxidised cholesterols in the liver. Thus, soybean protein partly modified some of the undesirable effects of oxidised cholesterol through its hypocholesterolemic effect and possibly through the modulation of hepatic Δ^6 desaturase (the rate-limiting enzyme in the metabolism of linoleic acid to arachidonic acid) activity. [Osada K, Kodama T, Minehira K, Yamada K, Sugano M; Dietary protein modifies oxidized cholesterol-induced alterations of linoleic acid and cholesterol metabolism in rats, *J Nutr* **126**(6), 1635-43 (1996)].

The serum cholesterol level in rats was significantly decreased in a group fed on a soyprotein peptic hydrolyzate (SPH) when compared with a group fed on a casein tryptic hydrolyzate (CTH). The faecal excretion of total steroids was significantly greater with rats fed on the SPH diet when compared with the CTH diet. The suppression of cholesterol absorption in the intestinal epithelia was considered to be part of the mechanism for the hypocholesterolemic action induced by SPH. [Nagaoka S, Awano T, Nagata N, Masaoka M, Hori G, Hashimoto K; Serum cholesterol reduction and cholesterol absorption inhibition in CaCo-2 cells by a soyprotein peptic hydrolyzate, *Biosci Biotechnol Biochem* **61**(2), 354-56 (1997)].

Antiatherosclerotic effect of soy protein and casein was studied in hypervitamin D2 and hypercholesterolemic diet-induced aortic atherosclerosis. Soy protein was found to be comparatively more effective in reducing the degree of severity of atherosclerotic lesions than casein. In casein treated rats, the serum cholesterol particularly triacyl glycerol- rich lipoprotein remained elevated. It was suggested that soy protein produced less atherosclerotic lipoprotein by partitioning cholesterol into triacyl glycerol poor lipoprotein. [Sakano M, Fukuyama T, Ni WH, Nagao K, Ju HR, Sato M, Saketa N, Iwamoto H, Imaizumi K; Comparison between dietary soy bean protein and casein of the inhibitory effect on atherogenesis in the thoracic aorta of hypercholesterolemic (Ex Hc) rats treated with hypervitamin D2, *Biosci Biotechnol Biochem* **61**(3), 514-19 (1997)].

Rats were fed cholesterol-free purified diets containing casein, rice, potato or soybean proteins having different amounts of methionine (25.9, 21.3, 16.2 and 10.9 g methionine/kg, respectively). Each protein was fed with 250g/kg diet for 14 days. Growth rates of rats were the same in all groups. Serum total cholesterol concentrations were lower in rats fed with soybean, potato and rice proteins than in those fed casein. Faecal bile acid plus neutral steroid excretion was significantly higher in rats fed with the above protein diets compared to those fed casein. These results of the investigation supported the view that soybean, potato and rice proteins lower serum cholesterol concentration in a similar manner. [Morita T, Oh-hashi A, Takei K, Ikai M, Kasaoka S, Kiriyama S; Cholesterol-lowering effects of soybean, potato and rice proteins depend on their low methionine contents in rats fed with a cholesterol-free purified diet, *J Nutr* **127**(3), 470-77 (1997)].

The effects of dietary protein types and methionine supplementation on phospholipid metabolism were investigated to clarify the mechanism of the hypocholesterolemic action of soybean protein in rats fed with a cholesterol-free diet. Feeding of soybean protein diet led to significantly higher proportions of linoleic acid and linoleic acid containing molecular species in plasma and liver microsomal phosphatidylcholine in comparison to casein diet. In addition, significantly lower plasma cholesterol levels, hepatic S-adenosylmethionine concentration and liver microsomal phosphatidylcholine-phosphatidylethanolamine ratio resulted. These alterations were significantly suppressed by supplementing methionine in the diet. These results indicated that about 40% of the hypocholesterolemic action of soybean protein was due to its low methionine content. [Sugiyama K, Yamakawa A, Kumazawa A, Saeki S; Methionine content of dietary proteins affects the molecular species composition of plasma phosphatidylcholine in rats fed a cholesterol-free diet, *J Nutr* **127**(4), 600-7 (1997)].

The undigested fraction (UDF) of soybean protein exerts a marked hypocholesterolemic effect in relation to soybean protein (SOY) in rats. The present study was conducted to confirm whether UDF was effective in hamsters as in rats in combination with different fat sources. Because the hamster, unlike the rat, disliked the bitter taste of UDF, the effect of debittering UDF also was studied. Debittered UDF, similar to UDF, exerted a distinct influence on the various parameters of lipid metabolism in relation to SOY. [Gatchalian Yee M, Arimura Y, Ochiai E, Yamada K, Sugano M; Soybean protein lowers serum cholesterol levels in hamsters: Effect of debittered undigested fraction, *Nutrition* **13**(7-8), 633-39 (1997)].

In order to specify the amino acids responsible for the hyper and hypocholesterolemic effects, respectively of casein and soybean protein isolate (SPI), an experiment was conducted on chicks. In the preliminary trials, 18 amino acids were individually supplemented to the cholesterol-free SPI diet, and the relative toxicity was compared on the equimolar basis. Among the toxic amino acids, lysine and cystine affected the serum cholesterol concentrations; lysine was hypercholesterolemic in SPI-fed chicks, whereas cystine was hypocholesterolemic in casein-fed chicks. The addition of arginine, glycine, aspartic acid, tyrosine and valine to the casein diet also lowered the serum cholesterol concentrations. However, casein itself contains less arginine, glycine, aspartic acid and cystine, but more tyrosine and valine than SPI does. These results indicated that the hyper and hypocholesterolemic effects of certain amino acids were not related to their toxicity, indispensability for the growth, and difference in the amino acid composition between the two proteins. In conclusion, the different effects of casein and SPI on the serum cholesterol concentrations were not accounted for by the method used in the present experiment. [Ueda H; Effects of 18 amino acids individually added to the diet containing casein or soybean protein isolate on the serum cholesterol concentrations in chicks, *Animal Sci Technol* **68**(10), 926-33 (1997)].

The effects of partial substitution of amino acid mixture for dietary proteins on the serum and liver cholesterol concentrations were investigated in chicks. Chicks given soybean protein isolate (SPI) diets had lower serum and liver cholesterol concentrations as compared with those given casein diets, regardless of the dietary protein content. However, the hypocholesterolemic effect of SPI was partly lost when half of SPI in the diet was replaced with the amino acid mixture equivalent to SPI. Partial substitution of the casein-type amino acid mixture for the casein diet had little effect on the serum and liver cholesterol concentrations. The results of the investigation indicated that the differential effects of soybean protein isolate and casein on the serum and liver cholesterol concentrations were not only due to the different amino acid composition in the two proteins. [Ueda H, Fujisawa Y; Partial substitution of amino acid mixture for soybean protein isolate or casein modifies the effects on serum and liver cholesterol concentrations in chicks, *Animal Sci Technol* **68**(11), 1032-38 (1997)].

Two groups of Golden Syrian hamsters were fed cholesterol-enriched semipurified diets containing either 40% casein or soybean protein concentrate for a period of 8 weeks. Compared to casein-containing diet, animals fed with soybean protein concentrate had significant reductions in plasma total cholesterol (TC) and very low density and low density lipoprotein cholesterols (VLDL-c + LDL-c) with no significant effects on high density lipoprotein cholesterol. Plasma triglycerides were also significantly reduced in the soybean protein concentrate-fed with hamsters compared to the casein-fed animals. The degree of aortic fatty streak involvement was reduced by 76% in the soybean protein concentrate-fed hamsters compared to the casein-fed hamsters. There was a significant correlation between TC and aortic fatty streak area as well as between VLDL-c + LDL-c and aortic fatty streak area. The hypocholesterolemic properties of soybean protein concentrate were thus found to be associated with a striking reduction in aortic fatty streak formation. [Nicolosi RJ, Wilson TA; The anti-atherogenic effect of dietary soybean protein concentrate in hamsters, *Nutr Res* **17**(9), 1457-67 (1997)].

See *Cocos nucifera* (Cocoanut): [Nicolosi *et al.*; *Med Sci Sports Exerc* **29**(11), 1422-28 (1997)].

The ability of alcohol extract of isolated soy protein to contribute to the hypochoesterolemic effect mediated by the intake of soy protein was tested in gerbils. The results suggest that in gerbils, consumption of an isoflavone-containing extract does not contribute to the hypocholesterolemic effect of alcohol-extracted soy, but may influence lipid metabolism by altering gene expression for lipid-related genes. [Tovar Palacio C, Potter SM, Hafermann JC, Shay NF; Intake of soy protein and soy protein extracts influences lipid metabolism and hepatic gene expression in gerbils, *J Nutr* **128**(5), 839-42 (1998)].

The specific effects of soybean protein on lipid metabolism were determined with highly purified soybean protein. Growing rats were fed with diets containing 20%

highly purified soybean protein or casein supplemented or not with 0.1% cholesterol for 2 months. Plasma and liver lipid composition, faecal steroid excretion and several hepatic enzyme activities were measured. There were no significant dietary protein-related differences in plasma and liver cholesterol concentrations. When diets were cholesterol-free, highly purified soybean protein stimulated faecal neutral and acidic steroid excretion associated with concomitantly higher HMG-CoA reductase but lower cholesterol 7α-hydroxylase activities. Soybean protein lowered the linoleate desaturation index in liver microsomal lipids and phospholipids. Cholesterol supplementation (0.1%) did not affect plasma cholesterol but increased liver cholesterol and triacylglycerol concentrations and reduced HMG-CoA reductase activity; this latter effect was greatest in rats fed with soybean protein. Desaturase activities were lowered by cholesterol supplementation in rats fed with both protein diets. Thus although dietary proteins have no effect on serum cholesterol in rats, they affect enzyme activities involved in cholesterol metabolism and fatty acid desaturation. [Madani S, Lopez S, Blond JP, Prost J, Belleville J; Highly purified soybean protein is not hypocholesterolemic in rats but stimulates cholesterol synthesis and excretion and reduces polyunsaturated fatty acid biosynthesis, *J Nutr* **128**(7), 1084-91 (1998)].

Soy protein is known to lower blood cholesterol concentrations in animals but its effect in humans has yielded less consistent results. The presence or absence of the soybean isoflavone fraction is an important factor. This fraction, consisting primarily of genistein, daidzein and glycetein, has been shown to have a hypocholesterolemic effect in animals and humans. Potential mechanisms by which soy protein and/or isoflavones induce lowering of blood cholesterol concentrations include thyroid status, bile acid balance and the estrogenic effects of genistein and daidzein. Some studies have suggested that isoflavones exhibit antioxidant properties and have favourable effects on arterial compliance. Further, the increased consumption of products containing soy protein may displace foods relatively high in saturated fat and cholesterol from the diet and hence have an indirect blood cholesterol-lowering effect. [Lichtenstein AH; Soy protein, isoflavones and cardiovascular disease risk, *J Nutr* **128**(10), 1589-92 (1998)].

The effect of soy protein and casein on the levels of plasma glucose and lipids in hamsters with streptozotocin-induced diabetes was investigated. Streptozotocin-induced diabetic hamsters were divided into two groups; one group was fed with casein and the other with soy protein isolate. After 4 weeks, plasma levels of glucose, triglycerides and total cholesterol were significantly lower in the diabetic soy protein group than in the diabetic casein group. Soy protein was thus found to exert hypocholesterolemic effects in this diabetic model system, and had favorable effects on lowering plasma glucose and triglycerides. The soy protein diet, however, did not affect lipid peroxide production or the erythrocyte antioxidant enzyme activities. [Yeh SL, Hsu CY, Shieh MJ; Effect of dietary casein and soy protein on plasma lipids in streptozotocin-induced diabetes model in hamsters, *Nutr Res* **18**(10), 1757-68 (1998)].

The hypocholesterolemic and anti-atherogenic properties of soy lecithin were investigated on cynomolgus monkeys. It was concluded from the investigation that the cholesterol-lowering efficacy of Step I diet recommended by the American Heart Association can be enhanced with the addition of soy lecithin without reducing plasma HDL-c levels. Further, the hypocholesterolemic, and in particular, the anti-atherogenic properties of soy lecithin cannot be attributed solely to its linoleate content. [Wilson TA; Meservey CM; Nicolosi RJ; Soy lecithin reduces plasma lipoprotein cholesterol and early atherogenesis in hypercholesterolemic monkeys and hamsters: Beyond linoleate, *Atherosclerosis* **140**(1), 147-53 (1998)].

Activation of low density lipoprotein receptors has been described in a human hepatoma cell line exposed to the 7S globulin from soy. In order to ascertain whether α or α′ subunits from 7S globulin, or both, are responsible for this biochemical effect, a mutant soy cultivar, devoid of the α′ subunit (Keburi), as well as a commercial isoflavone-poor, heat-hydrolyzed soy preparation (Croksoy) were evaluated in the *in vitro* human liver cell model. While Croksoy proved to have a similar activity as the whole 7S globulin, the α′-free Keburi variant showed no effect on LDL receptor activation. The findings support the reliability of the human liver cell model in predicting a human hypocholesterolemic activity and suggest that specific peptide(s) may be responsible for the activity. [Manzoni C, Lovati MR, Gianazza E, Morita Y, Sirtori CR; Soybean protein products as regulators of liver low density lipoprotein receptors: II. α- α′ rich commercial soy concentrate and α′ deficient mutant differently affects low density lipoprotein receptor activation, *J Agric Food Chem* **46**(7), 2481-84 (1998)].

In 13-*cis*-retinoic acid-induced hypertriglyceridemic rats, partial replacement of casein with soy protein isolate, resulted in lowering of serum cholesterol levels. The observation indicated that isonitrogenous replacement of casein with soy protein improved retinoid-induced hypertriglyceridemia and decreased the serum cholesterol levels. [Radcliffe JD, Czaika Narins DM; Partial replacement of dietary casein with soy protein isolate can reduce the severity of retinoid induced hypertriglyceridemia, *Plant Foods Human Nutr* **52**(2), 97-108 (1998)].

Dietary soybean protein alleviated the deleterious actions of exogenous oxidized cholesterol on hepatic cholesterol and linoleic acid metabolism, although these efficacies were not necessarily significant. A great part of these moderations may be exerted by the specific hypocholesterolemic function of soybean protein, such as the stimulation of faecal oxidized cholesterol excretion, the change of hormonal release and modulation of lipoprotein catabolism. [Osada K, Inoue T, Nakamura S, Sugano M; Dietary soybean protein moderates the deleterious disturbance of lipid metabolism caused by exogenous oxidized cholesterol in rats, *Biochim Biophys Acta* **1427**(3), 337-50 (1999)].

The effects of casein, soy protein, soy protein with bound phospholipids (SP), soy protein peptic hydrolysate (SPH) or soy protein peptic hydrolysate with bound phospholipids (SPHP) on the micellar solubility of cholesterol and the taurocholate binding capacity were studied *in vitro*. The effects of various proteins on cholesterol metabolism in rats and Caco-2 cells were also evaluated. SPHP had a significantly greater bile acid-binding capacity than that of SPH *in vitro*. Micellar cholesterol solubility *in vitro* was significantly lower in the presence of SPHP compared to casein tryptic hydrolysate. The cholesterol micelles containing SPHP and SPH significantly suppressed cholesterol uptake by Caco-2 cells compared to the cholesterol micelles containing casein tryptic hydrolysate. These findings were consistent with results obtained by *in vivo* studies. Faecal excretion of total steroids was significantly greater in rats fed with the SPHP diet compared to those fed with the casein, soy protein, SP and SPH diets. Serum total cholesterol was significantly lower in rats fed SPHP than in those fed casein. The concentrations of total lipids and cholesterol in liver were significantly lower in the SPHP-fed group compared to all other groups. These results suggest that the suppression of cholesterol absorption by direct interaction between cholesterol-mixed micelles and SPHP in the jejunal epithelia is part of the mechanism underlying the hypocholesterolemic action of SPHP. [Nagaoka S, Miwa K, Eto M, Kuzuya Y, Hori G, Yamamoto K; Soy protein peptic hydrolysate with bound phospholipids decreases micellar solubility and cholesterol absorption in rats and Caco-2 cells, *J Nutr* **129**(9), 1725-30 (1999)].

In weanling albino rats, soy milk decreased serum total cholesterol, triacyl glycerol and phosphoplipid levels alongwith enhancement of HDL-cholesterol levels. [Njoku OU, Nagandu FT, Alumunah EO; Effect of soybean milk on rat serum lipid levels, *J Food Sci Technol* **36**(1), 53-57 (1999)].

The effects of soymilk and fermented soymilk on lipid metabolism were studied in ovariectomized Syrian hamsters. The results of the investigation demonstrated that bifidobacterium-fermented soymilk had a hypolipidemic effect in ovariectomized hamsters. [Kikuchi Hayakawa H, Onodera Masuoka N, Kano M, Matsubara S, Yasuda E, Ishikawa F; Effect of soymilk and bifidobacterium-fermented soy milk on plasma and liver lipids in ovariectomized Syrian hamsters, *J Nutr Sci Vitaminol* (Tokyo) **46**(2), 105-08 (2000)].

The effect of soymilk supplementation, a whole soy product, with usual diet on serum lipids was assessed in normolipidemic subjects. A randomised controlled trial was conducted on 60 premenopausal normolipidemic Japanese women. After the trial, a significant decrease in serum concentration of total cholesterol in the soy milk-supplemented group was observed. The results suggest the hypocholesterolemic effect of soymilk, a traditional whole soy product, in normolipidemic subjects. [Takatsuka N, Nagata C, Kurisu Y, Inaba S, Kawakami N, Shimizu H; Hypocholesterolemic effect of soymilk supplementation with usual diet in premenopausal normolipidemic Japanese women, *Preventive Med* **31**(4), 308-14 (2000)].

Dietary intake of soy protein is associated with reductions in plasma cholesterol. Isoflavones are thought to be active components of soy and responsible for the beneficial effects because of their structural similarities to estrogen. The investigation undertaken to settle this point, however, leads to the conclusion that the hypocholesterolemic effect of soy protein is mediated, in part, by decreased cholesterol absorption. The semipurified soy extract, rich in isoflavones, added to casein protein did not have lipid-lowering effects. Other components of soy such as saponins, phytic acid or the amino acid composition may be involved in the hypocholesterolemic effects seen in the study. [Greaves KA, Wilson MD, Rudel LL, Williams JK, Wagner JD; Consumption of soy protein reduces cholesterol absorption compared to casein protein alone or supplemented with an isoflavone extract or conjugated equine estrogen in ovariectomized cynomolgus monkeys, *J Nutr* **130**(4), 820-26 (2000)].

The antiatherogenic effect of soy protein with intact isoflavones is well established, but the effects of isoflavones without soy protein have not been determined. The antiatherogenic effect of an isoflavone aglycone-rich extract without soy protein was studied in cholesterol-fed rabbits. Immunohistochemical analysis revealed fewer oxidized LDL-positive macrophage derived foam cells in atherosclerotic lesions in the aortic arch of isoflavone groups compared with that of the cholesterol group. From the results of the investigation, it was suggested that antioxidative action of isoflavones and their antioxidative metabolites inhibited the oxidation of LDL, and thereby exerted an antiatherosclerotic effect. [Yamakoshi J, Piskula MK, Izumi T, Tobe K, Saito M, Kataoka S, Obata A, Kikuchi M; Isoflavone aglycone-rich extract without soy protein attenuates atherosclerosis development in cholesterol-fed rabbits, *J Nutr* **130**(8), 1887-93 (2000)].

Soy protein diets lower plasma cholesterol in hyperlipoproteinemic human subjects, as well as in animal models. Addition of the isoflavones extract to the atherogenic diet lowered the liver triglyceride concentration by 33% relative to the atherogenic diet without isoflavones. The study suggests that the hypocholesterolemic mechanism of dietary soy protein involves a cooperative interaction between the protein and isoflavone-enriched fraction that lowers hepatic lipid concentrations. [Peluso MR; Winters TA, Shanahan MF, Banz WJ; A cooperative interaction between soy protein and its isoflavone-enriched fraction lowers hepatic lipids in male obese Zucker rats and reduces blood platelet sensitivity in male Sprague-Dawley rats, *J Nutr* **130**(9), 2333-42 (2000)].

The investigation points out the importance of experimental conditions such as nutritional status of animals when blood samples are taken in studies of the hypocholesterolemic effect of soy protein compared to casein. [Guermani Nicolle L, Villaume C, Bau HM, Schwertz A, Nicolas JP, Mejean L; The cholesterol-lowering property of soybeans fed to rats is related to the fasting duration, *Plant Foods Hum*

Nutr **56**(3), 239-49 (2001)].

Isoflavones or other nonprotein components of soybean, perhaps in combination with soy protein, play an important role in exerting hypocholesterolemic effect in ovariectomized hamsters, taken as a model of postmenopausal hypercholesterolemia. [Lucas EA, Khalil DA, Daggy BP, Arjmandi BH; Ethanol-extracted soy protein isolate does not modulate serum cholesterol in golden Syrian hamsters: A model of postmenopausal hypercholesterolemia, *J Nutr* **131**(2), 211-14 (2001)].

The effects of vitamin C and soybean oil on vitamin C concentration, total cholesterol, trigliycerides, low density lipoprotein cholesterol (LDL-c), high density lipoprotein cholesterol (HDL-c) and total lipids were examined in chickens. The results of the investigation confirm the hypochlesterolemic effect of soybean oil and vitamin C on chickens. Because soybean oil decreased the level of vitamin C when applied per os, it would be advisable to increase doses of vitamin C as a preventive, when the former is being administered. [Badzian B, Nagorna Stasiak-B, Kowalczyk M; The effect of soybean oil and vitamin C on lipid levels in the blood serum of chickens, *Medycyna Weterynaryjna* **57**(12), 921-23 (2001) Article in Polish].

The effects of three different proteins (whey protein concentrate, soy protein isolate and casein) on the growth and lipid concentration on rat liver and blood serum were compared in a 45 days feeding experiment. Blood serum and liver cholesterol was significantly higher for rats on the casein diet than for the rats on whey protein and soy protein diets. Soy protein isolate diet was relatively more hypocholesterolemic than whey protein diet. None of the dietary proteins was able to maintain blood serum triacylglycerols at or near reference levels. [Jacobucci HB, Sgarbieri VC, Dias Nadia FGP, Borges P, Tanikawa C; Impact of different dietary protein on rat growth, blood serum lipids and protein and liver cholesterol, *Nutr Res* **21**(6), 905-15 (2001)].

The effects of soy isoflavone supplementation on plasma lipids, erythrocyte antioxidant enzyme activities and bone mineral density were investigated in postmenopausal women. The results of the investigation indicate the antioxidant effect of isoflavones in normal postmenopausal women is not obvious and supplementation with isoflavone alone may not have a hypocholesterolemic effect. [Hsu CS, Shen WW, Hsueh YM, Yeh SL; Soy isoflavone supplementation in postmenopausal women: Effects on plasma lipids, antioxidant enzyme activities and bone density, *J Reproductive Med* **46**(3), 221-26 (2001)].

Clinical trial data suggest a hypocholesterolemic effect of soy protein. The effect may be attributable, at least partly, to the isoflavones present in soy. Separate effects of soy protein and isoflavones are also on record. With an objective to study the effect of soy protein and isoflavones on plasma lipid concentrations in postmenopausal, moderately hypercholesterolemic women, a randomized, double blind, placebo-controlled clinical trial was made with 3 treatment groups (milk group, soy protein group, soy protein +isoflavone group). LDL-cholesterol concentrations were found to decrease more in the soy protein +isoflavone group than in the soy-protein group.

This difference in total and LDL-cholesterol lowering between the two soy-protein supplements suggests an effect attributable to the isoflavone containing fraction. [Gardner CD, Newell KA, Cherin R, Haskell W; The effect of soy protein with or without isoflavones relative to milk protein on plasma lipids in hypercholesterolemic postmenopausal women, *Am J Clin Nutr* **73**(4), 728-35 (2001)].

Effects of genistein and its glycoside genistin, isolated from soybean, were studied in nephritic rats with endogenous hyperlipidemia. These isoflavones suppressed nephritis-induced severe hypercholesterolemia and hypertriglyceridemia; and their hypolipidemic action was almost identical. From the results of investigation it was suggested that genistin is hydrolyzed to genistein in the system and that the suppression of hepatic lipid synthesis may be one mechanism of the hypolipidemic action of genistein. [Kojima T, Uesugi T, Toda T, Miura Y, Yagasaki K; Hypolipidemic action of the soybean isoflavones genistein and genistin in glomerulonephritic rats, *Lipids* **37**(3), 261-65 (2002)].

Postmenopausal women are at an increased risk of developing coronary artery disease (CAD). This increase is considered primarily due to elevated cholesterol concentrations accompanying the loss of endogenous estrogen secretion. The consumption of soy foods is claimed to reduce serum cholesterol concentrations and this is supposed to be due to phytoestrogens, present in soy foods. However, phytoestrogens supplementation with 150 mg/d over a 6-month period did not significantly alter serum lipoproteins in postmenopausal women and, therefore, might not effectively reduce the risk of CAD in this population. [Dewell A, Hollenbeck CB, Bruce B; The effects of soy-derived phytoestrogens on serum lipids and lipoproteins in moderately hypercholesterolemic postmenopausal women, *J Clin Endocrinol Metab* **87**(1), 118-21 (2002)].

The claimed hypocholesterolemic effects of soy can be attributed solely to the isoflavones. Several studies found no changes in serum LDL-cholesterol concentrations after consumption of isolated soy isoflavones without soy protein, indicating that a combination of soy protein and isoflavones may be needed for eliciting a cholesterol-lowering effect of soy. The exact combination of active ingredients in soy products requires identification. [Kerckhoffs DA, Brouns F, Hornstra G, Mensink RP; Effects on the human serum lipoprotein profile of β- glucan, soy protein and isoflavones, plant sterols and stanols, garlic and tocotrienols, *J Nutr* **132**(9), 2494-505 (2002)].

The effect of isoflavone-free soy protein on plasma cholesterol was studied in cholesterol-fed Sprague Dawley albino rats. The rats were given diets containing either 20 % casein or 20% soy protein isolate or 20 % flavone-free soy protein isolate. Rats fed with soy protein isolate or isoflavones-free soy protein isolate exhibited comparable plasma cholesterol level but the levels were significantly lower than casein-fed rats. The plasma cholesterol levels remained unaffected following addition of isoflavones- concentrate to isoflavone-free soy protein isolate or casein diet. Soy protein isolate also enhanced faecal steroid excretion, as compared to casein. The cholesterol lowering activity of soy protein isolate was suggested to be due to its protein contents though isoflavones and other constituents might have some contributing roles. [Fukui K, Tachivana N, Wanezaki S, Tsuzaki S, Takamatsu K, Yamamoto T, Hashimoto Y, Shimoda T; Isoflavone free soy protein prepared by column chromatography reduces cholesterol in rats, *J Agric Food Chem* **50**(20), 5717-21 (2002)].

The effect of diets with different protein sources (soy protein isolate, casein and casein added with soy isoflavones) on plasma triglyceride levels and post heparin plasma lipoprotein lipase activity was investigated in rats. The animals fed with soy protein and casein plus isoflavones (1.82mg/g) exhibited a reduction in plasma triglyceride levels. However, these diets did not affect liver triglyceride concentration, hepatic triglyceride secretion rate and the post heparin plasma lipoprotein lipase activity. Hypotriglyceridemic effect of soy protein isolates was more marked and it was attributed partly to its isoflavones contents. [Demonty I, Lamarche B, Deshaies Y, Jacques H; Role of soy isoflavones in the hypotriglyceridemic effect of soy protein in the rat, *J Nutr Biochem* **13**(11), 671-77 (2002)].

The mechanisms by which dietary soy favourably influences lipoprotein metabolism and inhibits atherosclerosis are uncertain. Studies of blood mononuclear cells and cultured hepatocytes have indicated that certain soy peptides (i.e., 7S globulins) stimulate expression of LDL receptors. This pathway represents a hypothetical mechanism by which soy's hypocholesterolemic and antiatherosclerotic effects may be mediated. However, direct evidence supporting this hypothesis is lacking. To address this, the effects of dietary soy protein isolate in two genetically engineered mouse models of atherosclerosis were compared, atherosclerosis being assessed by quantifying the aortic content of esterified cholesterol. The results of the investigation provide direct evidence for the existence of LDL receptor and plasma lipoprotein-independent pathways by which dietary soy protein inhibits atherosclerosis. [Adams MR, Golden DL, Anthony MS, Register TC, Williams JK; The inhibitory effect of soy protein isolate on atherosclerosis in mice does not require the presence of LDL receptors or alteration of plasma lipoproteins, *J Nutr* **132**(1), 43-49 (2002)].

The beneficial effects of soy protein on lipid metabolism are modulated, in part, by hepatic sterol regulatory element binding protein-1. However, in rats with nephrotic syndrome, the benefit may be through a direct effect of this protein on kidney rather than mediated by changes in expression of hepatic lipid metabolism genes. [Tovar AR, Murguia F, Cruz C, Hernandez P, Rogelio AS, Carlos A, Pedraza Chaverri J, Correa RR, Torres N; A soy protein diet alters hepatic lipid metabolism gene expression and reduces serum lipids and renal fibrogenic cytokines in rats with chronic nephrotic syndrome, *J Nutr* **132**(9), 2562-69 (2002)].

Soy isoflavones have been shown to improve lipid metabolism, produce antidiabetic effect, and activate PPAR (Peroxisome-proliferator activated receptors). [Mezei O, Banz WJ, Steger RW, Peluso MR, Winters TA, Shay N; Soy isoflavones exert antidiabetic and hypolipidemic effects through the PPAR pathways in obese Zucker rats and murine RAW 264.7 cells, *J Nutr* **133**(5), 1238-43 (2003)].

Epidemiologic data suggest an inverse relationship between the consumption of soy isoflavones and cardiovascular disease risk. However, in most studies, beneficial effects could not be attributed with certainty to soy isoflavones. There are currently not enough data to recommend the consumption of isoflavone supplements to lower plasma cholesterol levels. [Demonty I, Lamarche B, Jones PJ; Role of isoflavones in the hypocholesterolemic effect of soy, *Nutr Rev* **61**(6 Pt 1), 189-203 (2003)].

The beneficial effects of soy protein and flaxseed meal on hypertriglyceridemia and liver steatosis associated with obesity and diabetes were evaluated. Both soy protein and flaxseed meal significantly decreased plasma total cholesterol, compared to casein in lean rats. In obese rats flaxseed meal had significant cholesterol-lowering effect compared to control rats. While soy protein significantly lowered both plasma LDL-cholesterol and HDL-cholesterol in lean phenotypes, flaxseed meal showed the same effects even in obese phenotypes compared to casein-fed rats. Flaxseed meal also significantly lowered plasma triglyceride in both lean and obese rats compared to casein-fed rats. There was significantly greater fat accumulation in livers of obese rats than lean rats regardless of dietary protein type. Flaxseed meal significantly lowered fat deposition in livers of both lean and obese rats compared to rats fed with casein or soy protein. Dietary component(s) present in flaxseed meal or soy protein responsible for hypolipidemic effects is not clear. The marked hypotriglyceridemic and hypocholesterolemic effects of flaxseed meal may have important therapeutic implications in patients with hypertriglyceridemia and hypercholesterolemia and deserve further study in humans with these disorders. Flaxseed meal supplementation may provide a new therapeutic strategy to reduce hypertriglyceridemia and fatty liver. [Bhathena SJ, Ali AA, Haudenschild C, Latham P, Ranich T, Mohamed AI, Hansen CT, Velasquez MT; Dietary flaxseed meal is more protective than soy protein concentrate against hypertriglyceridemia and steatosis of the liver in an animal model of obesity, *J Am Coll Nutr* **22**(2), 157-64 (2003)].

Semen Sojae Preparatum (fermented soybean) lowered serum oxidised-low density lipoprotein cholesterol, triglyceride and malondialdehyde, and enhanced serum high density lipoprotein cholesterol, a polipoprotein A I and superoxide dismutase activity. The preparation had effects on regulating lipid and antioxidation and therefore, it was expected to inhibit atherosclerosis in ovariectomized rats. [Wang X, Ge X, Bai X, Song C, Niu L, Xu H; Effects of Semen Sojae Preparatum on lipid metabolism in ovariectomized rat, *Zhong Yao Cai* **26**(9), 652- 54 (2003) [Article in Chinese].

The antioxidant and atherogenic effects of soya isoflavones and of the synthetic organic compounds of selenium on the primary cell culture of human aortic subendothelial intima and on macrophage cell culture were investigated. Soya isoflavones were found to exhibit mainly antiatherogenic effect while organic compounds of selenium exhibited mainly antioxidant effect. [Khachaturova VR, Suprun IV, Vasiljev AV;

Comparative evaluation of antioxidant and antiatherogenic effects of naturally occuring compounds and synthetic organic compounds of selenium, *Biomeditsinskaya Khimiya* **49**(2), 201-07 (2003) [Article in Russian].

Having estrogen and antioxidant activities, soybean isoflavones are usable in prevention and treatment of common diseases such as atherosclerosis, cancer, osteoporosis and others. Biological activity of isoflavones and prospects of their therapeutical use have been discussed in the review. [Kaprelynts LV, Kisilev SV, Iorgachova EG; Soybean isoflavones and prospects of their therapeutic application, *Vopr Pitan* **72**(4), 36-41 (2003) [Article in Russian].

The effects of isoflavones on blood LDL-cholesterol concentration independently of soy protein level were studied by meta analysis of 8 randomized controlled trials. It was observed that intake of soy protein with high isoflavone content led to significantly greater decreases in serum LDL-cholesterol than that having low isoflavone content, demonstrating that isoflavones have LDL-cholesterol-lowering effects independent of soy protein. [Zhuo XG, Melby MK, Watanabe S; Soy isoflavone intake lowers serum LDL cholesterol: A meta-analysis of 8 randomized controlled trials in humans, *J Nutr* **134**(9), 2395-400 (2004)].

In order to elucidate antioxidative action and regulation of lipid metabolism by soy isoflavones, male Sprague Dawley rats, 4 weeks of age, were fed with purified diets either with or without 0.2% soy isoflavone-rich powder for 5 weeks. Dietary soy isoflavones decreased serum lipid peroxide level in rats. Levels of liver and serum α-tocopherol were higher in the rats fed isoflavone than in those fed isoflavone-free diet. Thus, dietary soy isoflavones exhibited mild antioxidative function in this animal experiment. Dietary soy isoflavones lowered hepatic 3-hydroxy-3-methylglutaryl CoA reductase activity although liver cholesterol level was not modulated. However, the levels of serum cholesterol and triglyceride decreased by consumption of soy isoflavones exhibiting hypocholesterolemic and hypolipidemic functions. Based on this study soy isoflavones are expected to reduce the risk of some cardiovasucular diseases through their radical scavenging function and hypocholesterolemic action. [Kawakami Y, Tsurugasaki W, Yoshida Y, Igarashi Y, Nakamura S, Osada K; Regulative actions of dietary soy isoflavone on biological antioxidative system and lipid metabolism in rats, *J Agric Food Chem* **52**(6), 1764-68 (2004)].

The effect of soy protein isolate (SPI) and isoflavones on hepatic thyroid hormone receptors (TRs) was studied in rats. The study demonstrated for the first time that SPI upregulates hepatic TR β1 expression, and that isoflavones reduce the hepatic TR α1 level in young male rats. The SPI-induced TR β1 may play a role in mediating the hypocholesterolemic and lipid-lowering actions of soy protein. [Xiao CW, L'Abbe MR, Gilani GS, Cooke GM, Curran IH, Papademetriou SA; Dietary soy protein isolate and isoflavones modulate hepatic thyroid hormone receptors in rats, *J Nutr* **134**(4), 743-49 (2004)].

The effects of soybean isoflavones with or without probiotics on tissue fat deposition, plasma cholesterol, and steroid and thyroid hormones were studied in SHR/N-cp rats, an animal model of obesity and were compared to lean phenotype. In both phenotypes, isoflavones lowered fat deposition in several fat depots. Isoflavones lowered total, LDL,-and HDL-cholesterol in lean rats, but in obese rats isoflavones lowered only total and LDL-cholesterol. Isoflavones also lowered many of the steroid hormones involved in lipid metabolism but had no significant effect on thyroid hormones. Probiotics had no significant effect on cholesterol or hormones. Soy isoflavones were proved to lower plasma cholesterol and that this hypocholesterolemic effect appeared to be due, in part, to the modulation of steroid hormones. Probiotics do not seem to enhance the effect of isoflavones. [Ali AA, Velasquez MT, Hansen CT, Mohamed AI, Bhathena SJ; Effects of soybean isoflavones, probiotics, and their interactions on lipid metabolism and endocrine system in an animal model of obesity and diabetes, *J Nutr Biochem* **15**(10), 583-90 (2004)].

Epidemiologic studies have shown that women with a higher dietary intake of plant-derived compounds with estrogen-like properties have a lower incidence of cardiovascular disease than women with a lower dietary intake of these substances. The most studied category of phytoestrogens is the isoflavones found in soybeans, chickpeas and other legumes. Genistein and daidzein are the two major isoflavonoides that have demonstrated lipid-lowering properties, especially in hypercholesterolemic subjects. The mechanism for the hypocholesterolemic effects is considered to involve altered hepatic metabolism, antioxidant properties, tyrosine kinase inhibition, and improved vascular reactivity. Other phytoestrogens like coumestans and lignans have shown unfavourable results with regard to their role in the prevention of coronary artery disease. It would be sensible not to recommend phytoestrogens as cardioprotective substances until adequate safety and efficacy studies are completed. [Park D, Huang T, Frishman WH; Phytoestrogens as cardioprotective agents, *Cardiol Rev* **13**(1), 13-17 (2005)].

Glycine tomentella: Administration of aqueous extract of *G. tomentella* root to hyperlipidemic hamsters leads to a decrease of high serum cholesterol and triglyceride levels induced by high fat diet. The extract also increased serum high density lipoprotein (HDL)-cholesterol and decreased serum low density lipoprotein (LDL)-cholesterol. The reduction of serum triglyceride levels was accompanied by a significant decrease in the hepatic triglyceride content, while the cholesterol content was not changed. [Ko YJ, Wu YW, Lin WC; Hypolipidemic effect of *Glycine tomentella* root extract in hamsters, *Am J Chin Med* **32**(1), 57- 63 (2004)].

Glycyrrhiza glabra (Licorice, H. Mulhatti, S. Yashti-madhu)**:** The licorice root extract manifested a hypolipidemic effect on various models of atherosclerosis. The effect is considered to be due to the presence of triterpene glycyrrhizinic acid, which can bind cholesterol into an insoluble complex and retard its absorption as well as inhibit the cholesterol biosynthesis. [Mezenova TD; Hypolipidemic effect of the licorice root extract, *Khim Farma Zh* **17**(4), 432-35 (1983)].

The hypolipidemic activity of fine licorice root powder, licorice extract, glycyram (3β-Hydroxy-11-oxo-olean-12-en-30-oic acid), glycyrenate and liquiriton (a preparation containing the sum of flavanoids of *G. glabra* and *G. uralensis*) was studied and compared with that of miscleron. While the preparations were administered with food in case of rabbits, these were given by ip injections in case of rats. All the preparations showed pronounced hypolipidemic activity. The hypolipidemic effect of these compounds exceeded that of miscleron. Licorice extract possessed the highest hypocholesterolemic activity combined with antiatherogenic properties. [Vasilenko Yu K, Mezenova TD, Skulte IV, Kozharskii VV; Comparative evaluation of the hypolipidemic effect of some licorice preparations, *Izvestiya Severo Kavkazskogo Nauchnogo Tsentra Vysshei Shkoly Estestvennye Nauki* (4), 83-87 (1984) [Article in Russian].

Drugs obtained from the overground part and roots of *Glycyrrhiza* were found to possess hypolipidemic activity despite a variation in their triterpene constituents. The biogenesis of triterpenes occurs mainly in its overground part. A relationship between the drugs' biological activity and biosynthesis of triterpenes has been drawn. [Vasilenko YK, Stepanova EF, Skul'te IV, Mezenova TD; Hypolipidemic activity of *Glycyrrhiza* preparations in relation to the biogenesis of its triterpene compounds, *Farmatsiya* (Moscow) **37**(6), 9-13 (1988)].

See Flavonoids in Appendix: [Khushbaktova *et al.*; *Khim Farma Zh* **25**(4), 53-57 (1991)].

Ammonium salts of glycyrretic acid and 18-dehydroglycyrretic acid effectively reduced the concentration of total cholesterol, triglycerides, and atherogenic lipoproteins in blood serum of rabbits with modeled cholesterol atherosclerosis. The compounds reduced significantly the content of malonic dialdehyde and raised the activity of superoxide dismutase in the animals' organs. The compounds also significantly reduced atherosclerotic changes in the aorta of the animals. [Zakirov UB, Abdullaev AK; The hypolipidemic and antiatherosclerotic properties of the ammonium salt of glycyrrhetic acid and of 18-dehydroglycyrrhetic acid, *Eksp Klin Farmakol* **59**(5), 53-55 (1996) [Article in Russian].

The beneficial effects of dietary flavonoids, derived from the ethanolic extract of licorice root, against atherosclerotic lesion development in association with inhibition of low density lipoprotein (LDL) oxidation in atherosclerotic mice were demonstrated. Administration of licorice extract to normolipidemic subjects also inhibited LDL oxidation. Dietary consumption of licorice-root extract by hypercholesterolemic patients may act as a moderate hypocholesterolemic nutrient and a potent antioxidant agent and, hence against cardiovascular disease. [Fuhrman B, Volkova N, Kaplan M, Presser D, Attias J, Hayek T, Aviram M; Antiatherosclerotic effects of licorice extract supplementation on hypercholesterolemic patients: Increased resistance of LDL to atherogenic modifications, reduced plasma lipid levels and decreased systolic blood pressure, *Nutrition* **18**(3), 268-73 (2002)].

***Glycyrrhiza uralensis*:** Hypolipidemic, antiulcer effect, glucocorticoid like activity, hepatic activity and antitussive effect of *Glycyrrhiza uralensis*, a traditional Chinese medicine, have been summarised. [Zia Guoyuan, Yao Yajuan; The action mechanism of *Glycyrrhiza uralensis*, *Chinese J Hospital Pharm* **12**(9), 423-24 (1992)].

***Gossypium hirsutum*:** See Polysaccharides in Appendix: [Khushbaktova et *al.*; *Khim Farm Zh* **21**(11), 1348-52 (1987)].

***Guatteria gaumeri*:** The effect of α-asarone, the known hypolipidemic principle of *G. gaumeri*, was studied on hepatic lipid metabolism using adult rat hepatocytes cultured on a feeder layer of 3T3 cells. These cultures synthesise and secrete for at least two weeks various lipids from 14C-acetic and 14C-oleic acid. Exposure for one or two weeks to 10 μg/ml of α- asarone decreased the secretion of various lipids to the culture medium; triacylglycerol secretion was inhibited by 80-97%, phospholipid secretion by 70-87%, cholesterol by 64-70%, and cholesterol esters by 50-92%. The results suggest that the hypolipidemic effect of α- asarone could be due to a decrease in the secretion of lipids (i.e., lipoproteins) by the hepatocytes. [Hernandez A, Lopez ML, Chamorro G, Mendoza-Figueroa T; Inhibition of lipid synthesis and secretion in long-term cultures of adult rat hepatocytes by α-asarone, *Planta Med* **59**(2), 121-24 (1993)].

Bark infusion of the plant is used in the traditional Mexican medicine for the treatment of hypercholesterolemia and cholelithiasis. α-Asarone, the main component of the extract, did not produce any toxic effect after oral administration to rats at a dose of 10 or 50 mg/kg for 28 days, or genotoxicity by the dominant lethal test. However, long-term exposure of cultivated hepatocytes to micromolar concentrations produced morphological and ultrastructural alterations. The toxic effects of α-asarone in animals suggest caution in the use of this plant. [Chamorro G, Salazar M, Salazar S, Mendoza T, Pharmacology and toxicology of *Guatteria gaumeri* and α-asarone, *Rev Invest Clin* **45**(6), 597-604 (1993) [Article in Spanish].

Long-term exposure to micromolar concentrations of α-asarone produces morphologic and ultrastructural alterations, triacylglycerol accumulation (fatty liver), and inhibition of protein synthesis and secretion. [Lopez ML, Hernandez A, Chamorro G, Mendoza-Figueroa T; α- Asarone toxicity in long-term cultures of adult rat hepatocytes, *Planta Med* **59**(2), 115-20 (1993)].

The hypolipidemic activity of α-asarone (2,4,5-trimethoxy propenyl benzene), isolated from *G. gaumeri* was investigated in mice. α-Asarone caused significant lowering of lipoprotein and other lipid parameters. [Garduno L, Salazar M, Salazar S, Morelos ME, Labarrias F, Tamariz J, Chamorro GA, Hypolipidemic effect of α asarone in mice, *J Ethnopharmacol* **55**(2), 161-63 (1997)].

The mutagenicity of α-asarone, a hypolipidemic drug obtained from *Guatteria gaumeri*, was investigated in rats. The dominant lethal assay, a test, which detects agents producing chromosomal aberration in sperm and thereby affecting the viability of progeny, was used. Sexually mature male or female Wistar rats received 0, 5, 10 or 20 mg/kg of α-asarone orally for 5 days. In a male dominant lethal phase, each treated male was allowed to mate with two untreated virgin females each week for eight consecutive weeks; and in a female dominant lethal phase untreated males were allowed to mate with treated females. In both cases their foetuses were evaluated 14 days after the mid-point of the week of cohabitation. Examination of uteri and ovaries of pregnant females showed pre-and post-implantation losses, indicating genotoxic activity. Use of extracts and products from *Guatteria gaumeri* is, therefore, not considered safe for humans. [Chamorro G, Madrigal E, Ruiz LE, Salazar M; Dominant lethal study of α-asarone in male and female rats after short-term treatment, *Medical Sci Res* **27**(5), 337-39 (1999)].

***Gymnema montanum*:** Ethanolic extract of *G. montanum* leaves at doses of 50, 100 and 200 mg/kg body weight for 3 weeks suppressed the elevated blood glucose and lipid levels in diabetic rats. At a dose of 200mg/kg body weight, it was found to be comparable to glibenclamide, a reference drug. [Ananthan R, Latha M, Ramkumar KM, Pari L, Baskar C, Narmatha Bai V; Effect of *Gymnema montanum* leaves on serum and tissue lipids in alloxan diabetic rats, *Exp Diabesity Res* **4**(3), 183-89 (2003)].

Gymnema sylvestre (H. Gurmar, S. Meshashringi)**:** Oral administration of of *G. sylvestre* leaf extract for two weeks inhibited high fat diet-induced increase of serum triglycerides, total cholesterol, LDL and VLDL-cholesterol. HDL-cholesterol level was increased alongwith an improvement in the antiatherogenic index in these animals. It was suggested that this drug might be useful in cases of coronary heart disease, in which hyperlipidemia is considered as one of the causative factors. [Bishayee A, Chatterjee M; Hypolipidemic and antiatherosclerotic effect of *Gymnema sylvestre* leaf extract in rats fed on a high fat diet, *International Seminar onTraditional Medicine*, Calcutta, p. 157 Nov 7- 9, (1992)].

Leaf extract of *Gymnema sylvestre* (25-100 mg/kg) reduced the elevated serum triglycerides, total cholesterol, LDL–c and VLDL-c levels in hyperlipidemic rats at the end of two weeks. Hyperlipidemia-induced lowering of HDL-c levels and antiatherogenic index were also reversed back to normalcy after treatment with this drug. The hypolipidemic activity of *G. sylvestre* leaf extract was found to be comparable to that of clofibrate. [Bishayee A, Chatterjee M; Hypolipidemic and antiatherosclerotic effect of *Gymnema sylvestre* R.Br.leaf extract in albino rats fed on a high fat diet, *Phytother Res* **8**(2), 118-20 (1994)].

See *Cyamopsis tetragonoloba* (Cluster bean, Guar): [Bharadwaj *et al.*; *J Indian Med Assoc* **92**(3), 80-81 (1994)].

See *Coccinia indica:* [Annapurna *et al.*; *Indian J Exp Biol* **39**(5), 500-02 (2001)].

See *Allium sativum* (Garlic): [Chander *et al.*; *Ethnobotany* **14**(1-2), 123-28 (2001)].

The antidiabetic and hypolipidemic potential of dried powdered leaves of *Gymnema sylvestre* was investigated. From the results of the investigation, it was not possible to recommend the dried powdered leaves of the plant for treatment of diabetes and hyperlipidemia without further experimental and clinical trials. [Galletto R, Siqueira VLD, Ferreira EB, Oliveira AJB, Bazotte RB; Absence of antidiabetic and hypolipidemic effect of *Gymnema sylvestre* in non-diabetic and alloxan-diabetic rats, *Braz Arch Biol Techn* **47**(4), 545-51 (2004)].

***Gypsophylla* species:** The interaction between bile salts and saponins from *Gypsophylla* was investigated *in vitro*. The results suggest that despite the protective effect of bile salts, *Gypsophylla* saponins interact with the mucosa of the proximal small intestine *in vivo*, but at the dietary level used in this study the mucosa was protected by an enhanced rate of cell replacement. The loss of cholesterol *via* exfoliated mucosal cells may contribute to the hypocholesterolemic effect of saponins in rats. [Gee JM, Johnson IT; Interactions between hemolytic saponins, bile salts and small intestinal mucosa in the rat, *J Nutr* **118**(11), 1391-97 (1988)].

Saponins from *Gypsophylla* species elicited hypocholesterolemic activity. A method for the assay of saponins from *Gypsophylla* species has been described. [Henry M, Panthe Dayde D, Rochd M; Extraction and high performance liquid chromatographic determination of gypsogenin 3-O-glucuronide, *J Chromatogr* **477**(2), 413-19 (1989)].

H

Haplophyllum perforatum: See Flavonoids in Appendix: [Khushbaktova *et al.*; *Khim Farma Zh* **25**(4), 53-57 (1991)].

Helenium amarum: See *Balduina angustifolia*: [Hall *et al.*; *J Pharm Sci* **69**(6), 694-97 (1980)].

Helianthus annuus (Sunflower, H. Surajamukkhi, S. Suryamukhi): In tests conducted on rats kept for 60 days on a complete standard ration that included one of the several fat varieties (sunflower, cotton oils, butter, mutton fat, margarine), a hypocholesterolemic effect of the diet with sunflower oil was recorded, which was attended by an increased excretion of bile acids and cholesterol in the bile. With the rats fed on a low protein or fat-rich diet that included sunflower oil (30 and 60%, respectively) a marked change in the ratio between the bile acids and cholesterol, in favour of cholesterol, was noted. [Nesterin MF, Markova MN, Narodetskaya RV; Effect of different fat products on bile composition and blood cholesterol level, *Vopr Pitan* (4), 9-13 (1976)].

See *Olea europea* (Olive): [Siddique *et al.*; *Planta Med* **1**, 46-49 (1986)].

Patients with ischemic heart disease with type II hyperlipidemia received diets containing sunflower oil (group I) or margarine "Zdorovie" (group II) as a source of polyunsaturated fatty acids. Pronounced reduction of the blood cholesterol level was recorded in both groups of patients studied. [Meshcheriakova VA, Samsonov MA, Levachev MM, Iazeva LI, Stetsenko AV; Comparative evaluation of the hypolipidemic action of sunflower oil and "Zdorovie" margarine incorporated into the anti-atherosclerotic diet of ischemic heart disease patients, *Vopr Pitan* (1), 10-13 (1987) [Article in Russian].

See *Zea mays* (Corn): [Green and Green; *Nutr Res* **8**(11), 1265-76 (1988)].

See *Brassica napus:* [McDonald *et al.*; *Am J Clin Nutr* **50**(6), 1382-8 (1989)].

Addition of 45 g sunflower oil daily to the diet of moderate hypertensive patients for 8 weeks reduced blood lipids, mainly cholesterol, in 9 out of 19 patients. A decrease in the body mass index was also noted in sunflower oil-fed hypertensive subjects. This study showed a remarkable decrease in systolic and diastolic blood pressure in these treated hypertensive patients. [Hidalgo XP, Caballero MDP, Batard GA, Viera IR, Hernandez AC, Castellanos NM; Treatment of arterial hypertension with vegetable oil, *Rev Cubana Med* **28** (6), 622-31 (1989)].

The hypocholesterolemic effect of sunflower oil-fried sardines in cholesterol-enriched diet-fed Wistar rats was investigated. Feeding of sardines fried in sunflower oil reduced the cholesterol contents of lower density lipoproteins (LDL + VLDL) in hypercholesterolemic animals. [Sanchez Muniz, Fransicisco J, Higon Enrique, Cava Fernando, Viejo Jesus M; Prevention of dietary hypercholesterolemia in rats using sunflower oil-fried sardines; Effects on cholesterol and serum enzymes, *J Agric Food Chem* **40**(11), 2226-31 (1992)].

See *Rosa canina* [Gonzalez *et al.*; *Rev Esp Fisiol* **53**(2), 199-204 (1997)].

In different groups of hyperlipidemic subjects, substitution of normally consumed oil by sunflower oil (*H. annuus*), gingelly oil (*Sesamum indica*) and groundnut oil (*Arachis hupogaea*) showed that groundnut oil (rich in monounsaturated fatty acids) significantly reduced all lipid fractions unlike sunflower and gingelly oil (both rich in polyunsaturated fatty acids), which only decreased cholesterol levels. Maximum reduction of cholesterol levels was noted in the subjects who consumed sunflower oil followed by groundnut and gingelly oils. [Krishnakumar C, Vasanthamani G; Impact of oil-rich in mono and poly unsaturated fatty acids on hyperlipidemia *Indian J Nutr Diet* **35**(11), 287-293 (1998)].

See *Brassica campestris:* [Trautwein *et al.*; *Ann Nutr Metab* **43**(3), 159-72 (1999)].

Feeding of sunflower seed protein fraction to rats led to significant lowering of plasma cholesterol and triglyceride levels. The treated animals also showed significant change in the erythrocyte membrane phospholipids and phosphatidylcholin / phosphatidyl ethanolamine ratio. However, the protein fraction did not affect liver and brain lipids, organ weights and plasma protein contents. [Sen M, Bhattacharya DK; Hypolipidemic effect of enzymatically extracted sunflower seed protein fraction, *J Sci Food Agric* **81,** 347-52 (2000)].

See *Brassica campestris* (Rapeseed): [Gorinstein *et al.*; *Nutr Res* **23**(3), 317-30 (2003)].

Helicteres isora (H. Marorphali, S. Mrigashinga): Ethanolic extract of *H. isora* root caused significant reduction in plasma glucose and triglyceride levels at 300mg/kg dose after 9 days of administration to insulin resistant diabetic C57BL/KsJdb/db mice. In normoglycemic and mildly hypertriglyceridemic Swiss albino mice, the extract also showed significant reduction in plasma triglyceride. In high fat-fed hamster model, the extract showed significant reduction in plasma lipid levels. [Chakrabarti R, Vikramadithyan RK, Mullangi R, Sharma VM, Jagadheshan H, Rao YN, Sairam P, Rajagopalan R; Antidiabetic and hypolipidemic activity of *Helicteres isora* in animal models, *J Ethnopharmacol*, **81**(3), 343-49 (2002)].

Hemidesmus indicus (H. Magrabu, S. Ananta): See *Commiphora mukul:* [Mary et al., *Phytomedicine* **10** (6-7), 474-82 (2003)].

Hibiscus rosa-sinensis (H. Gurhal, S. Japakusum): Administration of a polyherbomineral formulation, "Anna Pavala Sindhooram" (containing *Hibiscus rosa-sinensis, Corallium rubrum, Lawsonia alba* leaves, *Cyanodon dactylon* whole plant and ferrous sulphate) to 30 patients of Ischemic heart disease significantly reduced plasma cholesterol, LDL and VLDL- cholesterol, triglycerides, phospholipids and free fatty acids levels. The levels of HDL2 and HDL–cholesterol increased in these patients following treatment. A slow increase in the lipid levels was noted after withdrawl of this drug. No adverse or side effect was observed. [Shanmugasundaram ERS, Sundaram P, Srinivas K, Shanmugasundaram KR, Shankaran JR; Double blind crossover study of modified "Anna Pavala Sindhooram" in patients with hyperlipidemia and Ischemic heart disease, *J Ethnopharmacol* **31**, 85-89 (1991)].

Hibiscus sabdariffa (Karkade, H. Lalambera): Administration of the plant drug at 5 and 10% for 9 weeks to hypercholesterolemic albino rats, fed on a mixture of cholesterol and cholic acid for 12 weeks, showed remarkable progress (lowering effect) in the level of different lipid fractions inspite of the continued cholesterol and cholic acid loading during the treatment. Although the administration of the plant drug at 5 and 10%, induced a significant decrease in the activity of serum GOT and serum GPT, alkaline and acid phosphatase as well as total serum protein, the values nearly returned to the initial levels after 9 weeks of drug administration. [el- Saadany SS, Sitohy MZ, Labib SM, el-Massry RA; Biochemical dynamics and hypocholesterolemic action of *Hibiscus sabdariffa* (Karkade), *Nahrung* **35**(6), 567-76 (1991)].

White rabbits were fed with a high cholesterol diet (normal diet + 1.3% cholesterol + 3% lard) with or without 0.5 or 1% *H. sabdariffa* extract for 10 weeks. The levels of triglyceride, cholesterol, and low density lipoprotein cholesterol (LDL-c) were lower in the serum of rabbits fed with high cholesterol diet plus *H. sabdariffa* extract than in the serum of rabbits fed only high cholesterol diet. Feeding *H. sabdariffa* extract (0.5 and 1% in the diet) to rabbits significantly reduced severe atherosclerosis in the aorta. Histopathological examination showed that the extract reduced foam cell formation and inhibited smooth muscle cell migration and calcification in the blood vessel of rabbits. An antiatherosclerotic activity of the plant extract was thus verified. [Chen CC, Hsu JD, Wang SF, Chiang HC, Yang MY, Kao ES, Ho YC, Wang

CJ, *Hibiscus sabdariffa* extract inhibits the development of atherosclerosis in cholesterol-fed rabbits, *J Agric Food Chem* **51**(18), 5472-77 (2003)].

Hordeum vulgare (Barley, H. Jau, S. Divya): Hypocholesterolemic effects of green juice from young barley leaves were investigated on high cholesterol diet-induced hypercholesterolemic rats. The n-hexane extract from a water insoluble fraction of green juice, which showed hypocholesterolemic activity yielded, on chromatography, β-sitosterol and n-hexacosyl alcohol. Addition of n-hexacosyl alcohol in high cholesterol diet at a concentration of 1%, lowered the plasma cholesterol level of rats hardly on day 3 but markedly on day 9. In a similar experiment, β-sitosterol markedly lowered the plasma cholesterol level of rats both on day 3 and day 9. The compounds, β-sitosterol and n-hexacosyl alcohol, present in barley leaves, are responsible for the hypocholesterolemic activity. [Ohtake H, Nonaka S, Sawada Y, Hagiwara Y, Hagiwara H, Kubota K; Studies on the constituents of green juice from young barley leaves: Effect on dietarily induced hypercholesterolemia in rats, *Yakugaku Zasshi* **105**(11), 1052-57 (1985)].

The cholesterol lowering activity of *Hordeum vulgare* in birds, animals and humans was reviewed. Possible mechanism of action with regard to hypocholesterolemic activity of *H. vulgare* has been discussed. [Mc Intosh GH, Oakenfulle D; Possible health benefits from barley grain, *Chemistry in Australia* **57**(9), 294-96 (1990)].

The structure of mixed-linked β-glucans was studied in three hull-less barley cultivars (Arizona, Washonupana and Franubet). Arizona, a waxy-starch genotype with a higher content of mixed-linked β-glucan exhibited hypocholesterolemic responses in chickens. Washonupana, also a waxy-starch type, with normal mixed-linked β-glucan contents was found to reduce blood cholesterol whereas the other, Franubet, showed no effect. When a ground sample was suspended in water, Arizona and Washonupana gave highly viscous slurries whereas Franubet gave low viscosity. This viscosity was greatly reduced by addition of endo- β-glucanase. Gel filtration established that the water-soluble mixed-linked β-glucans in Washonupana had the highest average molecular weight and Franubet the lowest. The hypocholesterolaemic responses observed in chickens were attributed to viscous conditions within the gastrointestinal tract, and this was a function of the content and molecular weight of the mixed-linked β- glucans and of endogenous β-glucanase activity in the barleys. [Bengtsson S, Aman P, Graham H, Newman CW, Newman RK; Chemical studies on mixed-linked β-glucans in hullless barley cultivars giving different hypocholesterolemic responses in chickens, *J Sci Food Agric* **52**(4), 435-46 (1990)].

Three hull-less barleys (Washonupana, Waxbar and Bangsa) were fed to broiler chicks in 21% protein diets containing 0.5% cholesterol in replicate trials. A corn-based diet, with added cholesterol, served as a control. Alternative diets were supplemented with β-glucanase and soluble dietary fibre. Chicks fed with barley diets had lower total serum cholesterol and LDL-cholesterol than those fed corn diets, regardless of β-glucanase supplementation. The Bangsa variety of hull-less barley + β-glucanase lowered total serum cholesterol by 30% from the corn control compared to 10.7% and 18% for the other two varieties suggesting the presence of additional hypocholesterolemic factors, possibly tocotrienol and soluble dietary fibre other than β-glucans in this variety. [Newman RK, Newman CW, Hofer PJ, Barnes AE; Growth and lipid metabolism as affected by feeding of hull-less barleys with and without supplemental β- glucanase, *Plant Foods Hum Nutr* **41**(4), 371-80 (1991)].

A crossover design studying lipid and apoprotein levels in serum and excretion of sterols, nitrogen and fat in ileostomy effluent was performed in 10 subjects, fed diets with or without supplementation with brewer's spent grain, which is the residue of barley after the brewing of beer. More cholesterol, nitrogen, fat and energy were excreted in the ileostomy effluents when the subjects consumed a brewer's spent grain supplemented, high fibre diet than when they consumed a low fibre diet. No significant change was found in the daily net sterol excretion. The six subjects with low daily excretion of bile acids had increased cholesterol and decreased bile acid excretion per day, and lowered serum LDL-cholesterol and apoprotein B levels after supplementation with brewer's spent grain. Increased faecal cholesterol excretion is suggested to be the primary mechanism for the serum LDL-cholesterol lowering effect of brewer's spent grain. [Zhang JX, Lundin E, Andersson H, Bosaeus I, Dahlgren S, Hallmans G, Stenling R, Aman P; Brewer's spent grain, serum lipids and faecal sterol excretion in human subjects with ileostomies, *J Nutr* **121**(6), 778-84 (1991)].

The effects of barley and wheat diets supplemented with five fat sources (palm oil, dehydrated egg yolk, butter, tallow or corn oil) on lipid metabolism were studied in chicks. All chicks, fed with red spring wheat, grew faster and had greater food efficiency than those fed hull-less barley. All barley-fed chicks had lower total plasma cholesterol concentration (3.1 to 4.0 mmol/L) than those fed wheat (6.0 to 11.3 mmol/L). Liver cholesterol concentration was higher for all wheat-fed chicks (22.8-86.4 mmol/g) compared with those fed barley (6.7 to 12.2 mmol/g). Faecal crude fat was higher for chicks fed barley, and excreta dry matter was lower for barley-fed chicks. Results indicate that the high soluble fibre content of this barley exerts a hypocholesterolemic effect in chicks regardless of dietary fat source, possibly mediated through lowered fat absorption. [Martinez VM, Newman RK, Newman CW; Barley diets with different fat sources have hypocholesterolemic effects in chicks, *J Nutr* **122**(5), 1070-76 (1992)].

Ground meal of two barley cultivars (Waxbar and Prowashonupana) was compared with oat bran and wheat red dog for their cholesterol-lowering effects in chicks and rats. In both chicks and rats, oat bran and Waxbar barley demonstrated a significant lowering effect on total and low density lipoprotein (LDL)-cholesterol levels, but high density lipoprotien cholesterol was not decreased. Soluble β-glucan appeared to be the strongest predictor of the serum cholesterol response in both species. Barley grain can offer a high-fibre, cholesterol-lowering alternative to oat bran. [Newman RK, Klopfenstein CF, Newman CW, Guritno N, Hofer PJ; Comparison of the cholesterol lowering properties of whole barley, oat bran and wheat red dog in chicks and rats, *Cereal Chem* **69**(3), 240-44 (1992)].

See Tocotrienols in Appendix: [Pearce *et al.*; *J Med Chem* **35**(2), 3595-606 (1992)].

Barley oil (10% in diet) decreased total plasma cholesterol and plasma low density lipoprotein cholesterol (LDL-c) in chicks compared to margarine. The oil also reduced plasma LDL-c without affecting plasma high density lipoprotein cholesterol (HDL-c) in chicks compared to corn oil. α-Tocotrienol and γ-tocotrienol contents of barley oil were 24 and 17 times more than those of corn oil. Similarly polyunsaturated fatty acids contents of barley oil were also three times higher than that of margarine. These observations suggested that higher content of α-tocotrienol and polyunsaturated fatty acid of barley oil are responsible for its hypocholesterolemic activity. [Wang L, Newman RK, Newman CW, Jackson LL, Hofer PJ; Tocotrienol and fatty acid composition of barley oil and their effect on lipid metabolism, *Plant Food Hum Nutr* **43**(1), 9-17 (1993)].

Of the raw grain (barley, oat and wheat) diets, only the barley diet had a hypocholesterolemic effect when compared to the casein-based control diet. Rats fed with extruded barley (with husks) had lower serum and liver cholesterol than any other grain-fed group. Factors contributing to the greater hypocholesterolemic effects of barley diets could be the higher total and soluble β-glucan contents and higher viscosities of the barley diets *versus* the oat, wheat, and control diets. [Wang WM; Klopfenstein CF; Effect of twin-screw extrusion on the nutritional quality of wheat, barley, and oats, *Cereal Chem* **70**(6), 712-15 (1993)].

Barley (*H. vulgare*) elicited hypocholesterolemic and hypoglycemic activity. History, chemistry, pharmacology and toxicology of barley have also been described. [Olin BR, Dombek C, Rubber D, Liberty L; Barley- a monograph, *Lawrence Review of Natural Products* p.1-2 (1994)].

An aggravated dose of food fibres from barley has been shown to reduce deviations from the reference level brought about by administration of exogenous cholesterol. [Yatskovskaya-NY, Solov'eva VF, Solomko GI, Pliss MB, Veprinskaya NI, Dem'yanchuk TM, Gulich MP; Study of a possible hypolipidemic effect of food fibre from barley, *Likars'ka Sprava* Nos. (9-12), 106- 09 (1995) Article in Ukrainian].

Dietary β-D-glucan is associated with low blood cholesterol levels. Increased excretion of bile acids is considered to be the reason for blood cholesterol lowering effect but there is little evidence for the mechanism involved in enhanced bile acid clearance. To investigate the possibility of specific binding between a representative bile acid salt, glycocholic acid, and barley β-glucan, solid-state ^{13}C NMR spectroscopy was used but the observation failed to suggest that the hypocholesterolemic property of β-D-glucan involves a simple binding of bile acid salt molecules to specific sites on the β-D-glucan polymer. [Bowles RK, Morgan KR, Furneaux RH, Coles GD; ^{13}C CP/MAS NMR study of the interaction of bile acids with barley β-D-glucan, *Carbohydrate Polymers* **29**(1), 7-10 (1996)].

In normolipidemic subjects, feeding of boiled barley-rice (50/50w/w) for 2-4 weeks did not affect the serum lipids. However, the hypercholesterolemic men and women showed a fall in the serum total cholesterol, LDL-cholesterol, phospholipid and LDL and VLDL following ingestion of barley-rice. The results suggested that barley–rice could be safely used to lower the lipids in hypercholesterolemic individuals. [Ikegami S, Tomita M, Honda S, Yamaguchi M, Mizukawa R, Suzuki Y, Ishi K, Ohsawa S, Kiyooka N, Higuchi M, Kobayashi S; Effect of boiled barley–rice feeding in hypercholesterolemic and normolipidemic subjects, *Plant Foods Human Nutr* **49**(4), 317-28 (1996)].

See Plant fibres in Appendix: [Ismail *et al.*; *Biochem Arch* **13**(3), 161-70 (1997)].

Feeding of diet containing different percentage (0, 25, 50 and75 %) of barley powder (rich in soluble fibre and β-glycan) to hamsters showed that the hypocholesterolemic effect of barley was not dose-dependant. However, serum triglyceride lowering effect of barley exhibited a dose dependant pattern. The ratios of serum total cholesterol to high density lipoprotein cholesterol (HDL-c) and low density lipoprotein cholesterol to HDL-c were not affected by barley content of diets. [Ranhotra GS, Gelroth JA, Leinen SD, Bhatty RS; Dose response to soluble fibre in barley in lowering blood lipids in hamsters, *Plant Foods Hum Nutr* **52** (40), 329-36 (1998)].

Feeding of flour tortillas (containing extract of β-glycan from barley-56% fibres) to rats decreased the plasma low density lipoprotein cholesterol compared to cellulose fed animals, although total cholesterol and triglyceride levels did not differ much between these two groups of rats. However, β-glycan-fed rats exhibited comparatively higher faecal fat excretion. The hepatic total lipids and cholesterol levels were also decreased in β.glycan-treated rats. [Hacker KD, Meier ML, Newman RK, Newman CW; Barley β.glycan is effective as a hypocholesterolemic ingredient in foods, *J Sci Food Agric* **77**(2), 179-83 (1998)].

The glucose and lipid responses of three barley cultivars (Glacier, covered high-amylose Glacier and hull-less high-amylose Glacier) were investigated with chicks. All the cultivars, particularly, high amylose varieties showed lower total and LDL plasma cholesterol, higher HDL-cholesterol values and lower LDL/HDL-cholesterol ratios than controls. The results suggest that the soluble fibre, mainly β-glucan and starch structures, in barley may be responsible for the hypocholesterolaemic effect. [Sundberg B, Xue Qi, Newman RK, Newman CW; Glycaemic responses and hypocholesterolaemic effects of high-amylose barley diets on broiler chicks, *J Sci Food Agric* **76**(3), 457-63 (1998)].

The antioxidative and hypolipidemic effects of barley leaf essence, investigated in a rabbit model of atherosclerosis, revealed its ability to lower the plasma levels of total cholesterol, triacylglycerol, lucigenin-chemiluminescence and luminol-chemiluminescence. The value of T50 of red blood cell hemolysis and the lag phase of low density lipoprotein oxidation increased in the barley leaf group compared to the control animals, fed on chow containing 0.5% cholesterol and 10% corn oil.

Ninety per cent of the intimal surface of the thoracic aorta was covered with atherosclerotic lesions in the control group, but only 60% of the surface was covered in the barley leaf group. This 30% inhibition of hyperlipidemic atherosclerosis by barley leaf was associated with a decrease in plasma lipids and an increase in antioxidative abilities (as measured by T50, lag phase and chemiluminescence). [Yu YM, Wu CH, Tseng YH, Tsai CE, Chang WC; Antioxidative and hypolipidemic effects of barley leaf essence in a rabbit model of atherosclerosis, *Jpn J Pharmacol.* **89**(2), 142-48 (2002)].

The hypocholesterolemic effect of barley is thought to be due to the presence of soluble dietary fibres, particularly β-glucan. The hypocholesterolemic effects.of waxy barley and the extent of its dependence on β-glucan were evaluated using male Sprague-Dawley rats, which were fed control (fibre-free) diets, diets with the addition of 2.5% refined β-glucan or 30% waxy barley (equivalent to 2.5% β-glucan) for 2 weeks. β-Glucan and waxy barley decreased serum levels of total cholesterol by 13.5% and 18.9%, and also decreased LDL-cholesterol by 19.4% and 24.3%, respectively. Addition of refined β-glucan or waxy barley to the diet resulted in greater bile acid excretions compared to the control group. The waxy barley diet upregulated the activity of cholesterol 7α-hydroxylase by 2.3 times, while β-glucan up-regulated cholesterol 7α-hydroxylase only by 1.5 times. Hepatic cholesterol 7α-hydroxylase mRNA level paralleled the increases in enzyme activity. The hypocholesterolemic effects of both β-glucan and a waxy barley diet were considered to be due to the enhancement of cholesterol 7α- hydroxylase expression resulting from increased faecal excretion of bile acids. [Yang JL, Kim YH, Lee HS, Lee MS, Moon YK; Barley β-glucan lowers serum cholesterol based on the upregulation of cholesterol 7 α-hydroxylase activity and mRNA abundance in cholesterol-fed rats, *J Nutr Sci Vitaminol* (Tokyo) **49**(6), 381-87 (2003)].

An indigenously developed and sequentially fermented (*Saccharomyces boulardii* + *Lactobacillus casei*) cereal-pulse food mixture, containing barley flour, sprouted green gram paste, milk co-precipitate and tomato pulp (in the ratio 2:1:1:1 w/w) was fed to mice for 42 days. The fermented food mixture significantly decreased the mean values for serum cholesterol and LDL-cholesterol concentrations in mice. HDL cholesterol and triglycerides were less affected. The food was wholesome, nutritious with therapeutic applications. [Sindhu SC, Khetarpaul N; Effect of feeding probiotic fermented indigenous food mixture on serum cholesterol levels in mice, *Nutr Res* **23**(8), 1071-80 (2003)].

The hypolipidemic effect of barley leaf extract was evaluated in 40 smoker and non-smoker hyperlipidemic patients. The patients were administered 15g young barley leaf extract or 60 g adlay (*Coix lachryma jobi*) once daily for 4 weeks. The plasma cholesterol and LDL-cholesterol levels were significantly lowered following treatment with both barley leaf extract and adlay. Further, these drugs also enhanced the lag phase of LDL oxidation. However, barley leaf extract exhibited comparatively better antioxidative effect on the prevention of LDL oxidation than adlay. Such an antioxidative effect of barley leaf extract was more pronounced in non-smokers compared to smokers. [Yu YM, Chang WC, Liu C, Tsai CM, Effect of young barley leaf extract and adlay on plasma lipids and LDL oxidation in hyperlipidemic smokers, *Biol Pharm Bull* **27**(6), 802-05 (2004)].

Humulus lupulus (Hop): The peroxisome proliferator-activated receptors (PPARs) are dietary lipid sensors that regulate fatty acid and carbohydrate metabolism. The hypolipidemic effects of fibrate drugs are due to their activation of PPAR-α. Isohumulones, the bitter compounds derived from hops that are present in beer, were found to activate PPAR- α and - γ in transient co-transfection studies. Among the three major isohumulone homologs, isohumulone and isocohumulone were found to activate PPAR-α and γ. Diabetic KK-Ay mice that were treated with isohumulones (isohumulone and isocohumulone) showed reduced plasma glucose, triglyceride, and free fatty acid levels. C57BL/6N mice fed with a high fat diet that were treated with isohumulones showed increased liver fatty acid oxidation and a decrease in size and an increase in apoptosis of their hypertrophic adipocytes. [Yajima H, Ikeshima E, Shiraki M, Kanaya T, Fujiwara D, Odai H, Tsuboyama-Kasaoka N, Ezaki O, Oikawa S, Kondo K; Isohumulones, bitter acids derived from hops, activate both peroxisome proliferatoractivated receptor α and γ and reduce insulin resistance, *J Biol Chem* **279**(32), 33456-62 (2004)].

Hydnocarpus wightiana: Hydnowightin, hydnocarpin, and neohydnocarpin, the flavonolignans from *H. wightiana* seeds, demonstrated potent hypolipidemic activity in mice, when administered 8mg/kg/day ip. Hydnowightin was most active of the three compounds. [Sharma DK, Hall IH; Hypolipidemic, anti-inflammatory and antineoplastic activity and cytotoxicity of flavonolignans isolated from *Hydnocarpus wightiana* seeds, *J Nat Prod* **54**(5), 1298-302 (1991)].

Hypericum perforatum (H. Bassant): See Proanthocyanidin polymer in Appendix: [Khushbaktova *et al.*; *Khim Farma Zh* **23**(9), 1111-15 (1989)].

The hypocholesterolemic effects of a flavonoid-rich extract of *H. perforatum* were tested in rats fed a cholesterol-rich diet. Administration of this flavonoid-rich extract at a moderate dose (75 mg/kg bw/d) and a high dose (150 mg/kg bw/d) significantly lowered the serum levels of total cholesterol, total triglycerides, and LDL- cholesterol, while increasing the serum level of high density lipoprotein cholesterol. Also, the content of malondialdehyde in serum and liver decreased significantly after oral administration of this extract compared with those fed a cholesterol-rich diet. The flavonoid-rich extract of *H. perforatum* also increased the activity of superoxide dismutase in serum and liver, but the activity of catalase was significantly elevated only in liver. [Zou Y, Lu Y, Wei D; Hypocholesterolemic effects of a flavonoid-rich extract of *Hypericum perforatum* L. in rats fed a cholesterol-rich diet, *J Agric Food Chem* **53**(7), 2462-66 (2005)].

I

Ilex cornuta**:** The glycoside 3- β-O-[β-D-glucopyranosyl- (1→2)- α -L-arabinopyranosyl pomolic acid and its analogues, isolated from dried leaves of *Ilex cornuta,* showed antithrombotic and anticholesterolemic activities. The process of isolation and purification of above compounds was described and patented. [Otsuka Pharmaceutical Company Ltd. Pomolic acid derivatives from *Ilex cornuta*, *Japan kokai Tokkyo Koho JP* 58,146,600(Cl Co_7 J 63/00) 8pp (1983)].

Ilex doniana**:** Dietary administration of pedunculoside, an ester glycoside of 3β, 19α, 23– trihydroxy- urs-12-en-28-oic acid, isolated from *Ilex doniana,* to hyperlipidemic albino rats showed significant hypocholesterolemic activity. [Jahromi MAF, Gupta M, Manickam M, Ray AB, Chansouria JPN; Hypolipidemic activity of Pedunculoside, a constituents of *Ilex doniana, Pharm Biol* **37**(1), 37-41(1999)].

Ilex paraguariensis**:** The passive diffusion of cholic acid through dialysis membranes was significantly inhibited by saponins isolated from *Ilex paraguariensis*. Such an activity of this plant was attributed to the formation of large macromolecular mixed miscelles between cholic acid and the saponins. These saponins also elicited antihypercholesterolemic activity *in vivo* possibily by increasing sterol excretion. [Ferreira F, Vazquez A, Gurtner C, Moyna P; Inhibition of the passive diffusion of cholic acid by *Ilex paraguariensis* St. Hil. Saponins, *Phytother Res* **11**(1), 79-81 (1997)].

Inula racemosa (S. Pushkarmul)**:** See *Commiphora mukul:* [Tripathi *et al.*; *Ancient Sci Life* **4**(1), 9-19 (1984)].

Administration of Pushkar guggulu- *Inula racemosa* powder (6-8g/d) for 6 months to 150 patients of coronary heart disease effectively lowered the blood lipid contents. [Singh R, Singh RP, Batliwala PG, Upadhya BN, Tripathi SN; Puskar guggulu an antianginal and hypolipidemic agent in coronary heart disease (CHD), *J Res Ayur and Siddah* **12**(1-2), 1-18 (1991)].

The effect of a combination of *I. racemosa* and *Commiphora mukul* (Pushkar guggulu) was studied in two hundred cases of Ischemic heart disease. Following treatment, an improvement in the precardial pain and dyspnea and restoration of normal ECG pattern was observed. Serum cholesterol, triglycerides and total lipids levels were also significantly decreased after treatment with this combined drug. [Singh RP, Singh R, Ram P, Batliwala PG; Use of Pushkar guggulu, an indigenous anti-ischemic combination in the management of ischemic heart disease, *Int J Pharmacogn* **31**(2), 147-60 (1993)].

See *Allium sativum* (Garlic): [Dwivedi S; *Ann Natl Acad Med Scs* (India) 32(3&4), 159- 175(1996)].

See *Allium sativum* [Sharma & Dwivedi; *Indian Drugs* **34**(5), 242-51 (1997)].

Irvingia gabonensis (Dikanut): The effects of Dikanut (*Irvingia gabonensis*), an African viscous preparation, as supplement (4g/d) in the diet of eleven Type II diabetics were studied. Levels of plasma lipids and glucose were monitored for one month. The dikanut supplement elicited hypolipidemic activity. The reduction in plasma lipids was primarily due to a decrease in LDL + VLDL-cholesterol and triglycerides levels. HDL-cholesterol was increased. [Adamson I, Okafor C, Abu-Bakare A; A supplement of Dikanut (*Irvingia gabonensis*) improves treatment of type II diabetics, *West Afr J Med* **9**(2), 108-15 (1990)].

Ixeris dentata: In streptozotocin-induced diabetic rats, intraperitoneal administration of methanolic extract of *I. dentata* whole plant caused a significant reduction of total blood lipids alongwith lowering of blood sugar levels. However, cynaroside, the main component of of the plant, exhibited significant lipid lowering activity without hypoglycemic action in diabetic rats. [Choi JS, Young HS, Kim BW; Hypoglycemic and hypolipidemic effects of *Ixeris dentata* in diabetic rats, *Arch Pharmacol Res* **13**(3), 269-73 (1990)].

Juglans regia (Walnut, H. Akhrot, S. Akschota): Walnut kernel and its oil were found to reduce serum cholesterol, triglycerides, phospholipids and total lipids in cholesterol-induced hypercholesterolaemic rats. Both refined and unrefined oils, having different contents of unsaponifiable matter and sterols, behaved in a similar way indicating that unsaponifiable matter and sterol contents of oil were not responsible for their efficacy. [George G, Bhar KK, Murti IAS, Sen DP; Hypolipidemic effect of walnut (*Juglans* regia) kernel and its oil in rats, *Fette Seifen Anstrichmittel* **88**(6), 238-43 (1986)].

J

Kalopanax pictus: Kalopanax saponin A and hedearagenin, isolated from the plant, showed significant hypocholesterolemic and hypolipidemic activities in addition to potent anti-diabetic activity. [Park HJ, Kim DH, Choi JW, Park JH, Han YN; A potent anti-diabetic agent from *Kalopanax pictus*, *Arch Pharm Res*, **21**(1), 24-9 (1998)].

K

L

***Lactuca indica*:** Methanolic extract of *L. indica* lowered the serum total cholesterol and LDL-cholesterol levels significantly. A chloroform soluble fraction of this extract also elicited similar activity. Chromatographic separation showed that it contained a mixture of triterpene alcohols and their acyl derivatives. [Park HJ, Lee MS, Choi Y, Cha BC, Junj WT, Young HS; Serum cholesterol lowering effect and triterpenoids of the herbs of *Lactuca indica, Korean J Pharmacogn* **26**(1), 40-46 (1995)].

Incorporation of triterpenoids isolated from *L. indica* in diet, fed to cholesterol-induced hyperlipidemic rats, significantly altered the metabolism of lipoprotein cholesterol alongwith lowering of atherogenic index. Considerable hypocholesterolemic activity was observed following administration of acetates of β-amyrin, α-amyrin, pseudotaraxasterol, lupeol, taraxasterol and germanicol. [Kim MJ, Lee E, Cha BC, Hoi MY, Rhim TJ, Park HJ; Serum cholesterol lowering effect of triterpene acetate obtained from *Lactuca indica, Korean J Pharmacogn* 28(1), 21-25 (1997)].

Ladyginia buchrica: A saponin, isolated from the ethanolic extract of the plant, exhibited potent hypolipidemic activity. [Ismailov II, Mamadov YM, Azizova SS, Khodzhear KN, Mamatkhanov AU, Shamstudinov MI, Saponins with hypolipidemic activity, USSR SU 1,130,348 (Cl. A61K35/78) (1984)].

***Lagonychium faretum*:** See Flavonoids in Appendix: [Khushbaktova *et al.*; *Khim Farma Zh* **25**(4), 53-57 (1991)].

***Laminaria digitata*:** Administration of *L. digitata* powder (1g/d) for 14 days to experimentally induced hyperlipoproteinemic rabbits caused a significant lowering of total cholesterol-lipoproteins and triglycerides. This drug also enhanced the levels of HDL-cholesterol and HDL2–cholesterol. Relative blood and plasma viscosity, reduction viscosity and fibrinogen were significantly decreased following *L digitata* treatment. [Zhaoh T, Shitang S; A study of *Laminaria digitata* powder on experimental hyperlipoproteinemia and its hemorrheology, *Chin J Integ Trad West Med* **9**(4), 223-25 (1989)].

Larix gmelinii: Dihydroquercetin, isolated from *L. gmelinii,* exhibited antioxidant and hypolipidemic activity. Dihydroquercetin decreased the lipid peroxidation in rat liver in a dose dependant manner. The hypolipidemic action of this compound (200mg/kg) was comparable to polysaponins [Kolhir VK, Bykov VA, Baginskaja AI, Sokolov SY, Glazova NG, Leskova TE, Sakovich GS, Tjukavkina NA, Kolesnik YA, Rulenko IA; Antioxidant activity of dihydroquercetin isolated from *Larix gmelinii* (Rupr.), *Phytother Res* **10**(6), 478-82 (1996)].

Lathyrus sativus (H. Khesari dhal, S. Sándika): See *Cicer arietinum* (Bengal gram): [Sharma RD; *Nutr Res* **7**(4), 351-64 (1987)].

Lawsonia alba (H. Mehandi, S. Mendika): See *Hibiscus rosasinensis* [Shanmugasundaram *et al.*; *J Ethnopharmacol* **31**, 85-89 (1991)].

Lens culinaris (Lentils, H & S. Masur): See *Vigna subterranea* (Bambara groundnuts): [Dabai *et al., British J Nutr* **75**(4), 557-71 (1996)].

Lens esculenta: See *Cicer arietinum:* [Soni *et al.*; *Indian J Nutr Dietet* **19**(6), 184-90 (1982)].

Leucaena leucocephala: Effect of *L. leucocephala* seeds on serum cholesterol and blood sugar level was studied in rats. This investigation revealed that *L. leucocephala* possesses significant hypocholesterolemic and hypoglycemic activity. [Singhal PC, Gupta RK, Singh JB, Joshi LD; Preliminary studies on hypoglycemic and hypocholesterolemic activities of *Leucaena leucocephala, Indian J Med Res* **76**(Dec. suppl.), 119-23 (1982)].

Licium europium: Administration of chloroform extract of aerial parts of *L. europium* to rabbits elicited significant hypolipidemic activity. Petroleum ether, alcoholic and aqueous extracts of this plant also exhibited considerable antihyperlipidemic effect. {Kalhoro MA, Kapadia Z, Bader Y, Hasnain SN; Comparative study of various parameters for hypolipidemic activity of *Licium europium, Hamdard Medicus* **39**(4), 16-24 (1996)].

Linum usitatissimum (Flaxseed, H. Alsi, S. Atasi): Rats were fed with diets containing varying levels of flaxseed (10%, 15%, and 20% flaxseed oil), 0.5% cholesterol and 0.2% cholic acid. Serum cholesterol levels rose with increasing levels of fat, but HDL-cholesterol and triglycerides were unaffected. Considering the presence of both cholesterol and cholic acid in the diet, the elevations of serum cholesterol were modest, which may reflect a potent hypocholesterolemic effect of linolenic acid. Liver total cholesterol levels fell with increasing levels of dietary flaxseed. Since high levels of flaxseed reduced cholesterol deposition in liver, it might be useful to test in experimental atherosclerosis. [Kritchevsky D, Tepper SA, Klurfeld DM; Influence of flaxseed on serum and liver lipids in rats, *J Nutr Biochem* **2**(3), 133-34 (1991)].

Growing pigs receiving 8% supplement of flaxseeds in their fodder were found to have a significantly lower level of total cholesterol and its LDL fraction in blood serum at slaughter. Blood serum of these animals contained lower, but a statistically insignificant level of triglycerides and total fat content. It is supposed that the hypocholesterolemic effect observed in the blood serum of growing pigs results from the increased content of unsaturated fatty acids - mainly linolenic acid - in the feed. [Barowicz T, Brzoska F, Pietras M, Gasior R; Hypocholesterolemic effect of full-fat flax seeds in the diets of growing pigs, *Medycyna Weterynaryjna* **53**(3), 164-67 (1997) Article in Polish].

In view of the beneficial effects of whole flaxseed in the treatment of experimental renal disease, the effects of dietary low-lignan flax oil, a rich source of α-linolenic acid, were studied in experimental polycystic kidney disease. In addition to moderation of renal injury and reduction of oxidised LDL content, a small hypocholesterolemic effect was noted in all animals fed with dietary low-lignan flax oil. [Ogborn MR, Nitschmann E, Bankovic-Calic N, Weiler HA, Aukema H; Dietary flax oil reduces renal injury, oxidized LDL content, and tissue n-6/n-3 FA ratio in experimental polycystic kidney disease, *Lipids* 37(11), 1059-65 (2002)].

See *Glycine max* (Soya bean, soybean): [Bhathena *et al.*; *J Am Coll Nutr* **22**(2), 157-64 (2003)].

Flaxseed oil is the most abundant plant source of omega-3 fatty acid, α-linolenic acid, which is not equivalent in its biological effects to the long-chain omega-3 fatty acids found in marine fish oils. However, α-linolenic acid is metabolised to eicosapentaenoic acid, which may replace arachidonic acid in membrane phospholipides. Ingestion of flaxseed oil may alter the generation of eicosanoids, procoagulant activity and other membrane-dependent responses and exert antiallergic, antiatherosclerotic, antiarrhythmic effects. Beneficial effects of flaxseed oil have been shown in prevention and management of cardiovascular disease. [Ipatova OM, Prozorovskaia NN, Baranova VS, Guseva DA; Biological activity of linseed oil as the source of omega-3 α-linolenic acid, *Biomed Khim* **50**(1), 25-43. (2004) [Article in Russian].

Lignan complex isolated from flaxseed contains secoisolariciresinol diglucoside, 3-hydroxy- 3-methylglutaric acid and cinnamic acids. The lignan complex isolated from flaxseed reduced the extent of hypercholesterolemic atherosclerosis and this effect was associated with marked decreases in oxidative stress, serum total cholesterol, LDL-c and risk ratio, and elevation of serum HDL-c. Lignan complex may, therefore, be beneficial in preventing atherosclerosis and reducing risk factors for coronary artery disease and stroke. [Prasad K; Hypocholesterolemic and antiatherosclerotic effect of flax lignan complex isolated from flaxseed, *Atherosclerosis* **179**(2), 269-75 (2005)].

***Liriope platyphylla*:** In cholesterol-fed rats, the effect of aqueous and methanolic extracts of tubers of *L. platyphlla* on lipid metabolism was investigated. Administration of aqueous or methanolic extract of this drug to hyperlipidemic rats produced lowering of lipid contents of blood, liver and faeces, as compared to controlled groups. Aqueous extract was more effective than methanolic extract. [Rhee IJ, Kim EJ, Jeong SW, Yang JH, Lee IS; Effect of *Liriope* tuber extract on lipid metabolism in rats fed with high cholesterol diet, *Korean J Pharmacogn* **34**(1), 65- 69 (2003)].

***Litsea cubeba*:** The effect of oil of *L. cubeba* on lipid profile and isoprenaline induced myocardial infarction was evaluated in rabbits. The serum free fatty acid levels were decreased in treated animals alongwith an improvement in the ST segment of ECG and reduction of cardiac infarct size. [Chen X, Hu ZW, Tang XL, Shen N; Effects of essential oil of *Litsea cubeba* (Lour) on experimental myocardial infarction in rabbits and myocardial necrosis induced by isoprenaline in rats, *Acta Pharma Sin* **18**(5), 388-91 (1983)].

Lolium multiflorum (Italian ryegrass): The hypocholesterolemic activities of various leaf proteins, prepared from Italian ryegrass (*L. multiflorum* Lam.), were investigated by feeding low-fat, cholesterol-free diets containing 20% protein to rats. Whole leaf protein was obtained on a pilot scale and dried by spray drying. Green leaf protein was separated from the white leaf protein fraction by centrifugation. Whole and green leaf proteins were inferior to white leaf protein in nutritional value and in cholesterolemia level. The nutritional value and hypocholesterolemic activity of the white leaf protein were comparable to those of soy protein. Among the protein concentrates examined, the white leaf protein is the best protein source with the strongest hypocholesterolemic effect. [Hormone T, Cho YS, Ohshima M; A study on the hypocholesterolemic activity of various leaf proteins of Italian ryegrass (*Lolium multiflorum* Lam.) in the rat, *Italian J Food Sci* **2**(4), 227-34 (1990)].

See *Coix lachrymajobi* (Adlay): [Hwang et *al*.; *J Japanese Soc Grassland Sci* **39**(1), 7-15 (1993)].

Lonicera japonica (Nindo): See *Nelumbo nucifera* (Kayo): [Onishi et *al*.; *Chem Pharm Bull* (Tokyo) **32**(2), 646-50 (1984)].

Lupinus albus (H. Turmos): Feeding of diet containing sweet white lupin (SWL) to rats significantly decreased plasma triglycerides, LDL–triglyceride, unesterified cholesterol and insulin/glucagon ratio as compared to sweet yellow lupin (SYL) and casein diet-fed rats. On the contrary, diet supplemented with sweet yellow lupin (SYL) significantly increased plasma glucose, insulin and hepatic total cholesterol levels compared to casein and sweet white lupin. [Chango A, Villaume C, Bau HM, Schwertz A, Nicolas JP, Mejean L; Effect of casein, sweet white lupin and sweet yellow lupin diet on cholesterol metabolism in rats, *J Sci Food Agric* **76**(2), 303-308(1998)].

Lupin seeds have a very low content of isoflavones, and lupin protein isolates are essentially isoflavone-free. In rats fed with a casein-based cholesterol + cholic acid diet, a relatively low daily intake (50 mg/d by gavage for 2 weeks) of total lupin protein extract reduced plasma total and VLDL + LDL-cholesterol concentrations by 21 and 30%, respectively. This initial study indicated that lupin, although isoflavone-free, exhibited hypocholesterolemic activity similar to that of other leguminous proteins in an established animal model. [Sirtori CR, Lovati MR, Manzoni C, Castiglioni S, Duranti M, Magni C, Morandi S, D'Agostina A, Arnoldi A; Proteins of white lupin seed, a naturally isoflavone-poor legume, reduce cholesterolemia in rats and increase LDL receptor activity in HepG2 cells, *J Nutr* **134**(1), 18-23 (2004)].

In experimentally-induced hyperlipidemic rodents moderate intake of lupin protein isolate, caused reduction of total and low density lipoprotein cholesterol. The protein isolate was subjected to detailed two-dimensional electrophoresis and mass spectrometry to identify the exact hypocholesterolemic component. The lupin protein isolate contained fragments of β- conglutin, the 7S-globulin, comparable to 7S-globulin of Soya protein, which is known to be the most active hypocholesterolemic component. The study showed that at least 18 peptides derived from β-conglutin of lupin are the likely biologically active components. [Wait R, Ginazza E, Bramnilla D, Eberini I, Morandi S, Arnoldi A, Sirtori CR; Analysis of *Lupinus albus* storage proteins by two-dimensional electrophoresis and mass spectrometry, *J Agric Food Chem* **53**(11), 4599-606 (2005)].

Lupinus angustifolius (Sweet lupin): Feeding of *L. angustifolius* seed meal (full supplemented with amino acids and minerals) and its five fractions for 10 days to different groups of growing rats significantly reduced the total plasma cholesterol and liver lipids and cholesterol, compared to lactalbumin fed rats. The buffer-dialysed insoluble fraction of sweet lupin seed meal lowered plasma cholesterol by 34% in comparison to lactalbumin-fed animals. The hypocholesterolemic activity of *L. angustifolius* seed meal was attributed to the disproportionate value for arginine:lysine and/or cystine:methionine ratio in the protein. [Rahman MH, Hossain A, Siddiqua A, Hossain I; Hemato-biochemical parameters in rats fed *Lupinus angustifolius* L. (sweet lupin) seed protein and fibre fractions, *J Clin Biochem Nutr* **20**(2), 99-111 (1996)].

Lupinus termis (Termis): See *Aloe vera:* [Nada *et al.*; *Fitoterapia* **68**(3), 240-44 (1997)]. See *Zygophyllum coccineum:* [Newairy *et al.*; *J Environ Sci Health* **B. 37**(5), 475-84 (2002)].

Lycium barbarum (H. Chirchitta): Treatment of rabbits with aqueous decoction of *L. barbarum* fruits and its polysaccharide fractions for 10 days significantly reduced blood glucose levels and serum total cholesterol and triglyceride concentrations with concomitant increase in high density lipoprotein cholesterol (HDL-c) levels indicating substantial hypoglycemic and hypolipidemic effects of the plant extract and its polysaccharide fractions. *L. barbarum* fruit extracts and its polysaccharide fractions also possessed antioxidant activity. However, water and methanolic fruit extracts and crude polysaccharide extracts exhibited stronger antioxidant activity than purified polysaccharide fractions because crude extracts were identified to be rich in antioxidants (e.g., carotenoids, riboflavin, ascorbic acid, thiamine, nicotinic acid). Both polysaccharides and vitamin antioxidants from *L. barbarum* fruits were possible hypolipidemic principles. [Luo Q, Cai Y, Yan J, Sun M, Corke H; Hypoglycemic and hypolipidemic effects and antioxidant activity of fruit extracts from *Lycium barbarum*, *Life Sci* **76**(2), 137-49 (2004)].

Lycium chinensis: Oral administration of aqueous extracts of fruits, leaves and cortex of *L. chinensis* to cholesterol (1%) and fructose (75%)-fed hyperlipidemic rats, significantly decreased serum lipid levels. These extracts also elicited hypoglycemic effect in streptozotocin diabetic mice. [Kim NJ, Youn WG, Hong ND; Pharmacological effect of *Lycium chinensis, Korean J Pharmacogn* **25**(3), 264-71 (1994)].

Lycopersicon esculentum (Tomato, H. Tamatar)**:** Dietary supplementation of tomato's lycopene (60 mg/d) to 6 males for a period of 3 months resulted in a significant reduction in their plasma LDL-cholesterol concentrations. *In vitro* studies showed that the effect of lycopene and β-carotene is related to suppression of cholesterol synthesis and augmentation of LDL receptor activity. Dietary supplementation of carotenoids may thus act as moderate hypocholesterolemic agents. [Fuhrman B, Elis A, Aviram M; Hypocholesterolemic effect of lycopene and β-carotene is related to suppression of cholesterol synthesis and augmentation of LDL receptor activity in macrophages, *Biochem Biophys Res Commun* **233**(3), 658-62 (1997)].

See Pectin in Appendix: [Prasanna Kumar et *al.*; *J Food Sci Technol* **34**(2), 103-07 (1997)].

The relationship between serum cholesterol levels and the risk of coronary heart disease (CHD) is well known. More recently, oxidative stress induced by reactive oxygen species (ROS) is also considered to play an important part in the etiology of this disease. Oxidation of the circulating low density lipoprotein (ox-LDL) is thought to play a key role in the pathogenesis of atherosclerosis and CHD. According to this hypothesis, macrophages inside the arterial wall take up the ox-LDL and initiate the process of plaque formation. *In vitro* studies have shown that dietary antioxidants such as vitamin E and β-carotene prevent the formation of ox-LDL and their uptake by macrophages. Ingestion of lycopene, a carotenoid antioxidant, in the form of tomato juice, tomato sauce, and oleoresin soft gel capsules to healthy human subjects for 1 week significantly lowered the levels of ox-LDL compared with controls. Recent epidemiological studies have also shown an inverse relationship between tissue and serum levels of lycopene and mortality from CHD, cerebrovascular disease and myocardial infarction. [Rao AV, Lycopene, tomatoes, and the prevention of coronary heart disease, *Exp Biol Med* (Maywood). **227**(10), 908-13 (2002)].

M

Malus domestica (Apple, Syn. *Malus sylvestris*, *Pyrus malus*, H. Seb, S. Seba): In hypercholesterolemic hamsters, apples, in addition to their choleretic effect, increased the bile acids secretion by 100%. The amounts of all bile acids were augmented. The relative proportion of taurine and glycine conjugated acids and that of di- and tri-hydroxy acids were not significantly altered. A 100% decrease of the lithogenic index was noticed. The hypocholesterolemic effect of apples could be related to an enhanced degradation of cholesterol in liver. [Berry Lortsch E, Sable Amplis R; Qualitative and quantitative changes in biliary secretion induced by apple consumption in hamsters, *Nutr Reports International* **23**(3), 505-16 (1981)].

The potential of apple pomace as a hypocholesterolemic agent was evaluated in postadolescent baboons, placed on high fat diet. Apple pomace (20% of diet) elicited and sustained a reduction of about 11% in total cholesterol levels; some of this reduction being in the high density lipoprotein fraction. Serum triglycerides were not affected. Halving the amounts of dietary apple pomace did not diminish the hypocholesterolemic response. [Sly MR, Robbins DJ, Van-der Walt WH, Du Bruyn DB; Evaluation of apple pomace as a hypocholesterolemic agent in baboons given a high fat diet, *Nutr Reports International* **40**(3), 465-76 (1989)].

The hypocholesterolemic effects of dietary apple pomace powder and the blended powder of apple pomace and refined corn bran (1:1) were examined in rats fed with hypercholesterolemic diets containing 1% cholesterol and 0.25% sodium cholate. The blended powder at 5% as dietary fibre level in a diet exhibited the strengthened hypocholesterolemic activity compared to apple pomace powder and refined corn bran, each used alone at the same dietary level. This result indicates that dietary fibre prepared by blending apple pomace powder with refined corn bran is useful to regulate the development of hypercholesterolemia. [Ayano Y, Ohta F, Endoh N, Kokubu T; Effect of dietary apple pomace on the cholesterol metabolism in rats, *Technical Bulletin of Faculty of Horticulture Chiba University* (42), 123-28 (1989) Article in Japanese].

Water soluble and water insoluble dietary fibres were isolated from apple pomace. Water insoluble fibre or its mixture with refined corn bran in the experimental diet did not effectively prevent elevation of serum or liver cholesterol content in rats. However, water soluble fibre from apple pomace, refined corn bran and the mixture of the two all showed significant effects for preventing elevation of the serum cholesterol level on day 9; the mixture showing a tendency to exhibit a stronger hypocholesterolemic activity than when used alone. The mixture in the diet decreased liver cholesterol accumulation and dietary cholesterol absorption significantly. The results indicated that the hypocholesterolemic effect was probably due to prevention of dietary cholesterol absorption from the small intestine. [Egashira Y, Sanada H; Effect of dietary fibres derived from apple pomace and refined corn bran on cholesterol metabolism in rats, *Japanese J Nutr* **51**(4), 207-14 (1993)].

See *Diospyros virginiana:* [Gorinstein et *al.*; *J Agric Food Chem* **49**(2), 952-7 (2001)].

Mangifera indica (Mango, H. Am, S. Amra): The effect of mangiferin with exercise on blood lipids was studied in KK-Ay mice, an animal model of type 2 diabetes. Mangiferin (30 mg/kg) reduced the blood cholesterol and triglyceride level of KK-Ay mice with exercise 2 weeks after oral administration when compared with the control group. Mangiferin exhibits beneficial effects on hyperlipidemia in type II diabetes. [Miura T, Iwamoto N, Kato M, Ichiki H, Kubo M, Komatsu Y, Ishida T, Okada M, Tanigawa K; The suppressive effect of mangiferin with exercise on blood lipids in type 2 diabetes, *Biol Pharm Bull* **24**(9), 1091-92 (2001)].

See *Emblica officinalis:* [Anila & Vijayalakshmi; *J Ethnopharmacol* **79**(1), 81-87 (2002)].

Manihot utilisima (Syn, *M. esculenta*, H. Sakarkanda): See *Eleucine coracana:* [Kurup and Krishnamurthy, *Ind J Exp Biol* **31**(3), 291-93 (1993)].

Marsilea minuta (Chaupatia, S. Chatuspatri): Feeding fraction I of *M. minuta* leaf extract to atherogenic diet-fed gerbils reduced serum cholesterol and triglycerides by 31 and 63%, respectively. The fraction also lowered liver cholesterol and triglycerides by 71 and 27% respectively, in comparison to atherogenic diet-fed controls. Treatment with this fraction of plant extract also prevented accumulation of cholesterol and triglycerides in liver and aorta and was able to dissolve atheromatous plaques of thoracic and abdominal aorta. Faecal excretions of cholesterol and triglycerides were significantly increased in treated gerbils. [Gupta RS, Kumar P, Sharma A, Bharadwaj TN, Dixit VP; Hypocholesterolemic activity of *Marsilea minuta* in gerbils, *Fitoterapia* **71**(2), 113-17 (2000)].

Medicago sativa (Alfalfa): In semipurified high butter cholesterol diet-induced hyperlipidemic monkeys, alfalfa root saponins prevented the increase in cholesterol levels. In rats, alfalfa root saponins were shown to decrease intestinal cholesterol absorption. [Malinow MR, McLaughlin P, Kohler GO, Livingstone AL; Prevention of elevated cholesterolemia in monkeys, *Steroids* **29**(1), 105-10 (1977)].

The radioactive cholesterol absorption was decreased by 47% in alfalfa fed rats as compared to controls. Saponin-free *M. sativa* did not elicit cholesterol lowering effect and it was restored by adding 0.25% alfalfa saponins. These observations suggested that alfalfa saponins and not its fibres are responsible for hypocholesterolemic activity of *M. sativa*. [Malinow MR, McLaughlin P, Stafford C, Livingstone AL, Kohler GO, Cheeke PR; Comparative effects of alfalfa saponins and alfalfa fibres on cholesterol absorption in rats, *Am J Clin Nutr* **32**(9), 1810- 812 (1979)].

In rats the levels of plasma cholesterol were decreased alongwith a reduction in the intestinal absorption of exogenous and endogenous cholesterol and enhancement of faecal biliary excretion following ingestion of alfalfa seeds. Consumption of diet containing alfalfa seeds for three weeks by 3 human volunteers also lowered serum cholesterol levels without any toxicity. [Malinow MR, McLaughlin P, Stafford C, Alfalfa seeds; Effects on cholesterol metabolism, *Experientia* **36**(5), 562-64 (1980)].

Feeding of alfalfa seeds and its saponins to rabbits for 4 months decreased hypercholesterolemia, aortic sudanophilia and serum cholesterol levels. [Malinow MR, Mc Laughlin P, Stafford C, Livingstone AL, Kohle VO, Alfalfa saponin and alfalfa seeds: dietary effects in cholesterol-fed rabbits, *Atherosclerosis* **37**(3), 433-38 (1980)].

Cholesterol-saponin interactions have been suggested as mechanisms for the observed hypocholesterolemic effects of alfalfa as well as the changes in intestinal morphology. Alfalfa plant saponins bound significant quantities of cholesterol both from ethanol solution and from micellar suspension. Alfalfa sprout saponins interacted with cholesterol to a lesser but significant extent. Sprout saponins also inhibited growth of *Trichoderma viride* significantly, another measure of saponin-cholesterol interaction. Saponin-cholesterol interaction is an important part of the hypocholesterolemic action of alfalfa but interaction of bile acids with other components of alfalfa may be of equal importance. [Story JA, LePage SL, Petro MS, West LG, Cassidy MM, Lightfoot FG, Vahouny GV; Interactions of alfalfa plant and sprout saponins with cholesterol *in vitro* and in cholesterol-fed rats, *Am J Clin Nutr* 39(6), 917-29 (1984)].

Feeding alfalfa seed extract to chicks resulted in significant reduction of total cholesterol, phospholipid, triglyceride, LDL-cholesterol and VLDL-cholesterol. The increase in the ratio of HDL-cholesterol/total cholesterol and reduction in total cholesterol and phospholipid contents of liver and (ventricular) muscle of the heart were observed by feeding alfalfa seed extract. [Dixit VP, Joshi SC; Antiatherosclerotic effects of alfalfa meal ingestion in chicks: a biochemical evaluation, *Indian J Physiol Pharmacol* **29**(1), 47-50 (1985)].

Nutritive value and hypocholesterolemic effect of alfalfa leaf protein concentrate, prepared from two different varieties (Dupuits and Natsuwakaba), were determined in chicks. The two varieties were similar in their overall chemical composition, available energy content and digestibilities of dry matter but the content of medicagenic acid, the toxic alfalfa saponin, was much higher in the leaf protein concentrate of Dupuits than in that of the other variety. When one-third of crude protein in the casein-amino acid basal diet was replaced by either of the leaf protein concentrates, no adverse effect was observed if an adequate amount of methionine was added. When both the leaf protein concentrates were used as the sole protein source, plasma HDL- and LDL-cholesterols were reduced, regardless of the cholesterol addition, which were not related to the medicagenic acid content of the leaf protein concentrates. [Ueda H, Ohshim M, Akitomo; Nutritive value and hypocholesterolemic effect of alfalfa leaf protein concentrates prepared from two different varieties in chickens, *Japanese J Zootech Sci* **58**(4), 347-55 (1987)].

Adminstration of alcoholic extract of *M. sativa* seeds to hyperlipidemic rabbits reduced serum cholesterol (38-41%) and LDL-cholesterol (48-53%). Maximum reduction in the LDL-cholesterol (64%) was noted in animals fed with alfalfa meals without cholesterol. Increase in the HDL-c / total cholesterol ratio following alfalfa treatment may help in reducing the incidence of atherosclerosis. [Dixit VP, Jain P; Hypolipidemic effects of *Medicago sativa* seed extract (50% EtOH) in rabbits under experimental condition, *Ancient Sci Life* **10**(1), 52-55 (1990)].

Alfalfa seed extract markedly reduced the levels of triglycerides, phospolipids, LDL and VLDL-cholesterol levels and enhanced HDL-cholesterol / total cholesterol ratio in Triton– induced hyperlipidemic Rhesus monkeys. [Dixit VP, Jain P; Effects of *Medicago sativa* (50% EtOH) on the serum lipid in Triton-induced hyperlipidemic Rhesus monkeys (*Macaca mulata*), *Adv Biosci* **9**(2), 1-6 (1991)].

Hypocholesterolemic effect of alfalfa leaf protein concentrate and soybean protein isolate were evaluated in chicks and compared with that of casein. Without dietary cholesterol, plasma cholesterol level was always lower in chicks fed with the alfalfa leaf protein concentrate diet than those fed the soybean protein isolate diet. Alfalfa leaf protein with high saponin content significantly decreased both body weight gain and plasma cholesterol level as compared to that with low saponin content. Plasma cholesterol levels in chicks fed with the alfalfa leaf protein diet were also increased slightly by added cholesterol but the levels were comparable to those fed soy protein diet. Substitution of casein with soybean protein isolate or alfalfa leaf protein concentrate at the level of 25% and 50% on the crude protein basis suppressed the hypercholesterolemia induced by 1% cholesterol addition, but there was no difference in hypocholesterolemic effect between both plant proteins. [Ueda H, Ohshima M; Hypocholesterolemic effect of alfalfa leaf protein concentrate and soybean protein isolate in chicks, *Animal Sci Technol* **63**(10), 1032-37 (1992)].

See *Glycine max* (Soya bean, soybean): [Lanksy PS; *Acta Horticulturae* (332), 131-36

(1993)].

See *Coix lachryma jobi* (Adlay): [Hwang *et al.*; *J Jpn Soc Grassland Sci* **39**(1), 7-15 (1993)].

Alfalfa extract containing less than or equal to 1 ppm canavanine and less than or equal to 9 ppm coumesterol exhibited anticholesterolemic and hypocholesterolemic activities. A method of the preparation of this drug from leaf extract of alfalfa has been described. [Mate H; Alfaalfa extract as hypolipidemic drug *Gen. Offen* DF 4,242, 149, (cl. 07G3/00) 1993, 3pp.].

Growing chickens (7 day-old male birds) were fed a casein-based diet (control group) in which 50% casein protein was substituted by protein originated from a commercially manufactured Pigmented Leaf Extract (PLEX) from alfalfa. A significant reduction in total and high density lipoprotein-cholesterol in blood plasma was recorded after 14 days feeding the chickens with the PLEX-supplemented diet as compared to the control diet. The results of the detailed investigation indicated that by including pure leaf extract into formulations for growing chickens and laying hens, not only are the nutritional properties of the eggs improved with desired pigmentation of the egg yolks but there was a substantial reduction in the total cholesterol in egg yolks as well as lower cholesterol in chicken meat obtained from use of PLEX as a dietary supplement. [Ostrowski Meissner H, Ohshima M, Yokota HO; Hypocholesterolemic activity of a commercial high protein leaf extract used as a natural source of pigments for laying hens and growing chickens, *Jpn Poultry Sci* **32**(3), 184-93 (1995)].

Purified alfalfa saponin supplemented diet lowered total plasma cholesterol, the effect being prominent, when cholesterol was absent in the diet. The saponin appeared to be a potent antiatherogenic agent when supplemented with cholesterol-free and cholesterol containing Bengal gram diets. However, saponin supplementation did not exert any significant effect on total liver lipids. The hypocholesterolemic and antiatherogenic effect of saponin could be directly correlated with their ability to decrease intestinal cholesterol absorption and to increase the faecal excretion of bile acids. [Venugopalan C, Srivastava KN; Hypocholesterolemic activity of saponin on cholesterol-added Bengal gram (*Cicer arietinum*) diet in rats, *J Food Sci Technol* **33**(5), 389-92 (1996)].

See *Trifolium alexandrinum* (Egyptian clover): [Geetanjali and Kapoor; *J Food Sci Technol* **36**(2), 106-08 (1999)].

Melia toosendam: Administration of *M. toosendam* seed oil to hyperlipidemic rats significantly lowered the serum and hepatic lipids. The oil, was found to be nontoxic to liver. It is also known to be used as an hepatoprotective drug in oriental medicine. [Ryu MY, Kim BS, Choi JW, Lee CK; Effects of *Melia toosendam* fructus on liver function (II) – effects of seed oil on lipid metabolism in rats, *Korean J Pharmacogn* **25**(3), 272-77 (1994)].

Momordica charantia (Bitter gourd, Bitter melon, H. Karela, S. Sushavi): The effect of aqueous and ether extract of bitter gourd on serum cholesterol and blood glucose levels was investigated in albino rats. These extracts exhibited significant hypocholesterolemic activity at the end of 21 days. The cholesterol lowering effect was relatively more marked in case of aqueous extract. A reduction in the weight of treated rats was also noted. Hypoglycemic effect of these extracts became evident from second week onwards, maximum being at the end of 21 days. [Upadhayaya GL, Pant MC; Effect of water and ether extracts of bitter gourd on blood sugar and serum cholesterol levels in albino rats, *J Diabetic Assoc India* **26**(1), 17-19 (1986)].

Feeding of freeze-dried powder of *M. charantia* for 14 days at 0.5,1.0 and 3% dietary levels with diet containing cholesterol and diet without cholesterol led to an increase of HDL-cholesterol level. However, it had little or no effect on other serum lipid parameters. Blood sugar levels were consistently decreased by *M. charantia* in rats fed with cholesterol free diet. Besides this, treated rats exhibited marked reduction of hepatic total cholesterol and triglyceride levels both in the presence or absence of cholesterol in diet. [Jayasooriya AP, Sakono M, Yukizaki C, Kawano M, Yamamoto K, Fukuda N; Effects of *Momordica charantia* powder on serum glucose levels and various lipid parameters in rats fed with cholesterol-free and cholesterol-enriched diet, *J Ethnopharmacol* **72**(1-2), 331-36 (2000)].

See *Emblica officinalis:* [Anila & Vijayalakshmi; *Phytother Res* **14**(8), 592-95 (2000)].

The effects of long-term feeding (10 weeks) of *M. charantia* fruit extract on blood plasma and tissue lipid profiles in normal and streptozotocin (STZ)-induced Type 1 diabetic rats were studied. An increase in plasma cholesterol, triglycerides and phospholipids, accompanied by a decrease in high density lipoprotein cholesterol was observed in STZ-induced diabetic rats. A moderate increase in plasma lipid peroxidation product (LPO), malondialdehyde, and about two-fold increase in kidney LPO was also observed in STZ-induced diabetic rats. The treatment of diabetic rats with *M. charantia* fruit extract over a 10-week period returned these levels close to normal. [Ahmed I, Lakhani MS, Gillett M, John A, Raza H; Hypotriglyceridemic and hypocholesterolemic effects of anti-diabetic *Momordica charantia* (karela) fruit extract in streptozotocin-induced diabetic rats, *Diabetes Res Clin Pract* **51**(3), 155-61 (2001)].

See *Coccinia indica:* [Annapurna *et al.*; *Indian J Exp Biol* **39**(5), 500-02 (2001)].

See *Commiphora mukul:* [Raut *et al.*; *J Mahatma Gandhi Inst Med Sci* **7**(2), 10-16 (2002)].

Peroxisome proliferator-activated receptor *alpha* (PPAR-α) is a ligand-dependent transcription factor that regulates the expression of genes involved in lipid metabolism and transport. The ethyl acetate extract of *M. charantia* activated PPAR-α to an extent that was equivalent to or even higher than 10 μM Wy-14643, a known ligand of PPAR α. The ethyl acetate extract prepared from the whole fruit showed significantly higher activity than that from seeds or flesh alone. PPAR-associated health benefits of bitter gourd warrant further investigation. [Chao CY, Huang Ching-jang; Bitter gourd (*Momordica charantia*) extract activates peroxisome proliferator-activated receptors and upregulates the expression of the acyl CoA oxidase gene in H4IIEC3 hepatoma cells, *J Biomed Sci* **10**(6 Part 2), 782-91 (2003)].

The hypolipidemic effect of methanol-extracted fraction of bitter melon (Koimidori variety), at the levels of 0.5% and 1.0%, was examined in male golden Syrian hamsters fed diets supplemented with and without cholesterol. The effect of dietary bitter melon extract on serum triglyceride was not seen in hamsters fed diets free of cholesterol, while hypertriglyceridemia induced by dietary cholesterol was significantly lowered in a dose-dependent manner. Serum total cholesterol concentration also tended to decrease in a dose-dependent manner following feeding of increasing amounts of bitter melon extract in the presence or absence of cholesterol in the diet. The effects of dietary bitter melon extract on liver triglyceride and total cholesterol levels were marginal, although dietary cholesterol caused a marked accumulation of these lipid molecules in the liver. These results suggest that bitter melon extract contains some components that could ameliorate lipid disorders such as hyperlipidemia. [Senanayake GVK, Maruyama M, Sakono M, Fukuda N, Morishita T, Yukizaki C, Kawano M, Ohta H; The effects of bitter melon (*Momordica charantia*) extracts on serum and liver lipid parameters in hamsters-fed cholesterol-free and cholesterol-enriched diets, *J Nutr Sci Vitaminol* **50**(4), 253-57 (2004)].

The effects of treatment of *Momordica* fruit extract and sodium orthovanadate, separately and in combination, were studied on serum and tissue lipid profile and on the activities of lipogenic enzymes in alloxan-induced diabetic rats. The results suggest that *Momordica* fruit extract and sodium orthovanadate exhibit hypolipidemic as well as hypoglycemic effect in diabetic rats and their effect is pronounced when administered in combination. [Yadav UC, Moorthy K, Baquer NZ; Combined treatment of sodium orthovanadate and *Momordica charantia* fruit extract prevents alterations in lipid profile and lipogenic enzymes in alloxan diabetic rats, *Mol Cell Biochem* **268**(1-2), 111-20 (2005)].

Momordica cymbalaria: The effect of *M. cymbalaria* fruit powder on blood glucose and other biochemical parameters was studied using alloxan-induced diabetic rats. The fruit powder was shown to possess antidiabetic and hypolipidemic effects in alloxan-induced diabetic rats. [Rao BK, Kesavulu MM, Giri R, Appa Rao C; Antidiabetic and hypolipidemic effects of *Momordica cymbalaria* Hook. fruit powder in alloxan-diabetic rats, *J Ethnopharmacol.* **67**(1), 103-09 (1999)].

Oral administration of an aqueous extract of *M. cymbalaria* fruit (0.5 g/kg) for 6 weeks showed significant antihyperglycemic as well as antihyperlipidemic effects in alloxan-induced diabetic rats. [Kameswararao B, Kesavulu MM, Apparao C; Evaluation of antidiabetic effect of *Momordica cymbalaria* fruit in alloxan-diabetic rats, *Fitoterapia* **74**(1-2), 7-13 (2003)].

Moringa oleifera (H. Sahjan, S. Shobhanjana)**:** Administration of the crude leaf extract of *M. oleifera* alongwith high fat diet decreased the high fat diet-induced increases in serum, liver, and kidney cholesterol levels by 14.35%, 6.40% and 11.09%, respectively. The effect on the serum cholesterol was statistically significant. [Ghasi S, Nwobodo E, Ofili JO; Hypocholesterolemic effects of crude extract of leaf of *Moringa oleifera* Lam in high fat diet-fed Wistar rats, *J Ethnopharmacol* **69**(1), 21-25 (2000)].

Morus indica (Mulberry, S. Shalmali): Mulberry is known to possess hypoglycemic, hypotensive, and diuretic properties. Analysis of serum and erythrocyte membrane lipid profiles of the patients before and after the treatments with mulberry therapy revealed a significant decrease in the concentration of serum total cholesterol (12%), triglycerides (16%), plasma free fatty acids (12%), LDL-cholesterol (23%), VLDL-cholesterol (17%), plasma peroxides (25%), urinary peroxides (55%) and an increase in HDL-cholesterol (18%). The results of investigation clearly indicated potential hypoglycemic and hypolipidemic effects of Mulberry therapy in diabetic patients. [Andallu B, Suryakantham V, Lakshmi Srikanthi B, Reddy GK; Effect of mulberry (*Morus indica* L.) therapy on plasma and erythrocyte membrane lipids in patients with type 2 diabetes, *Clin Chim Acta* **314**(1-2), 47-53 (2001)].

Mucuna pruriens (H. Kawanch, S. Atmagupta): In diet and triton-induced hyperlipidemic rats, administration of a decoction of *M. pruriens* (dose equivalent to 0.5 g dry drug per day) significantly lowered plasma cholesterol and total lipid levels. [Iauk L, Galati EM, Foresteri AM, Kirjavainen S, Trovato A; *Mucuna pruriens* decoction loweres cholesterol and total lipids plasma levels in rats, *Phytother Res* **3**(6), 263-64 (1987)].

Murraya koenigii (H. Meethi Neem, S. Surabhinimba): Male albino rats were fed diet +20% cocoanut oil without any supplement or with addition of 10% *M. koenigii* leaves or 10% mustard seeds (*Brassica juncea*) for 90 days. Both *M. koenigii* leaves and *B. juncea* seeds lowered the serum cholesterol, LDL and VLDL-cholesterol along with enhancement of HDL-cholesterol levels. These spices also decreased the release of lipoprotein in the circulation and enhanced the Lecithin cholesterol acyltransferase (LCAT) activity. [Khan BA, Abraham A, Leelamma S; Biochemical response in rats to addition of curry leaf (*Murraya koenigii*) and mustard seeds (*Brassica juncea*) to the diet, *Plant Foods Hum Nutr* 49(4), 295-99 (1996)].

Leaves of *M. koenigii* and seeds of *Brassica juncea* at 10% levels were incorporated into a high fat cholesterol diet and fed to rats for 3 months. The results showed pronounced hypolipidemic effect. These spices reduced remarkably the levels of plasma cholesterol, triglycerides, phospholipids, low density lipoproteins and very low density lipoprotein fractions. [Khan BA, Abraham A, Leelamma S; Influence of spices: *Murraya koenigii* and *Brassica juncea* on rats fed with atherogenic diet, *J Food Sci Technol* **35**(1), 66-68 (1998)].

Musa sapientum (Plantain, H. Kela, S. Kadali): Administration of pectin, isolated from inflorescence stalk juice of of plantain (containing hexose 32.4% and uronic acid 52.5%), to rats maintained on cholesterol and cholesterol-free diets, significantly reduced the cholesterol and triglycerides. Hepatic bile acids and lipoprotein lipase activity was also significantly enhanced in these animals. [Gomathy R, Vijayalakshmi NR, Kurup PA; Hypoliopidemic principle of the inflorescence stalk of plantain (*Musa sapientum*), *J Biosci* **14**(3), 301-09 (1989)].

Musa sapientum var. ***cavendishii*** (Banana)**:** Freeze-dried banana pulp showed a marked cholesterol-lowering effect when incorporated into a diet at the level of 300 or 500 g/kg, while the banana pulp dried in a hot-air current (65°C) did not. Both soluble and insoluble fibres, with the exception of cellulose, fractionated from banana pulp showed a cholesterol-lowering effect. It was concluded that soluble and insoluble components of dietary fibre participate in the hypocholesterolaemic effect of banana pulp. [Horigome T, Sakaguchi E, Kishimoto C; Hypocholesterolemic effect of banana (*Musa sapientum* var. *Cavendishii*) pulp in the rat fed on a cholesterol-containing diet, *Brit J Nutr* **68**(1),: 231-44 (1992)].

Myristica fragrans (H. Jaiphal, S. Jatiphala): Administration of seed extract of *M. fragrans* to hypercholesterolemic rabbits significantly reduced serum cholesterol, LDL-cholesterol and cholesterol: phospholipids ratio alongwith a significant elevation of HDL-cholesterol levels. This drug also prevented deposition of cholesterol, phospholipids and triglycerides in liver, heart and aorta. This extract reduced aortic atheromatous plaques by 76% and enhanced the faecal excretion of cholesterol and phospholipids in hypercholesterolemic animals. [Sharma A, Mathur R, Dixit VP; Prevention of hypercholesterolemia and atherosclerosis in rabbits after supplementation of *Myristica fragrans* seed extract, *Indian J Physiol Pharmacol* **39**(4), 407-10 (1995)].

In hyperlipidemic rabbits, administration of ethanolic extract of *M. fragrans* fruits (500mg/kg) for 60 days significantly lowered serum total cholesterol, LDL-cholesterol and triglyceride levels. The total cholesterol/HDL-cholesterol and LDL-c /HDL-c ratios were also decreased in treated hyperlipidemic rabbits. The extract exhibited antiplatelet aggregatory activity. [Ram A, Lauria P, Gupta R, Sharma VN; Hypolipidemic effect of *Myristica fragrans* fruit extract in rabbits, *J Ethnopharmacol* **55**(1), 49-53 (1996)].

Myrtus communis (Myrtle, H. Vilayiti Mehandi)**:** Myrtle extracts rich in polyphenolic compounds, were shown to have a potent antioxidant activity, the hydroalcoholic extract was most potent. Human LDL exposed to copper ions was used to evaluate the antioxidant activity of the myrtle extracts. [Romani A, Coinu R, Carta S, Pinelli P, Galardi C, Vincieri FF, Franconi F; Evaluation of antioxidant effect of different extracts of *Myrtus communis* L., *Free Radical Res* **38**(1), 97-103 (2004)].

Experiments showed that the volatile oil of *M. communis* exerts hypoglycemic as well as mild hypotriglyceridemic activity in diabetic animals. [Sepici A, Gurbuz I, Cevik C, Yesilada E; Hypoglycaemic effects of myrtle oil in normal and alloxan-diabetic rabbits, *J Ethnopharmacol* **93**(2-3), 311-18 (2004)].

N

Nardostachys jatamansi (H. Jatamansi): See *Curcuma longa*: [Dixit *et al.*; *Indian J Physiol Pharmacol* **32**(4), 299-304 (1988)].

Nelumbo nucifera (H. Kamal, S. Padma): Aqueous extracts of leaves of *N. nucifera*, leaves and stems of *Lonicera japonica* and stems of *Akebia quinta* were administered to rats loaded with a high fat diet containing 1.5% cholesterol and 1.0% cholic acid in order to screen the hypocholesterolemic activity of these crude drugs. Significant decreases in serum total cholesterol, free cholesterol and phospholipid were observed in the high fat-loaded groups given these crude drugs. Total cholesterol in the liver did not show any reduction in the groups receiving the extracts of these plant drugs as compared with the high fat-loaded control group. The overall effects in suppressing serum lipids elevation were in the order of *L. japonica* $>$ *A. quinta* $>$ *N. nucifera*. [Onishi E, Yamada K, Yamada T, Kaji K, Inoue H, Seyama Y, Yamashita S; Comparative effects of crude drugs on serum lipids, *Chem Pharm Bull* (Tokyo) **32**(2), 646-50 (1984)].

Nepata hindostana (H. Badrangboya): Administration of alcoholic extract of *N. hindostana* (20mg/kg/d) for 15 days produced marked hypocholesterolemia in pigs. It also exhibited some beneficial effects in experimental myocardial infarction as evidenced by histopathological changes. [Arora RB; Beneficial effects of *Nepata hindostana* in hypercholesterolemia and myocardial infarction, *Hamdard Medicus* **30**(1-2), 159-62 (1987)].

See *Allium sativum* (Garlic): [Arora *et al.*; *Hamdard Medicus* **30** (1-2), 163-74 (1987)]. *Hamdard Medicus* **30**(1-2), 175-84 (1987)].

See *Bombax mori:* [Ahmad et *al.*; *National Symposium on Emerging Trends in Indian*

Medicinal Plants, Lucknow p 89 (8-0/8)10-12 October, 2003].

Nephelium lappaceum (Rambutan): Supplementation of Rambutan ((400-500 g) to the normal diets of male and female subjects (21 each) for a period of 4 weeks exhibited a significant decrease in serum cholesterol and HDL-cholesterol only in female subjects. The cholesterol-lowering effect of rambutan supplementation was most pronounced in the high basal cholesterol group. [Mongkolsirikieat S, Areegitranusorn P, Limratana N, Limpaiboon T, Lulitanond V; Hypocholesterolemic effect of Rambutan (*Nephelium lappaceum*) supplementation in Thai adults, *Nutr Reports International* **39**(4), 797-804 (1989)].

Nigella sativa (Black cumin, H. Kala jeera, S. Krishnajeeraka): Feeding of *Nigella sativa* seed fixed oil (1ml/kg) to rats for 12 weeks caused significant lowering of serum cholesterol, triglycerides and glucose levels as compared to controls. These observations substantiated the traditional use of *Nigella sativa* for the treatment of dyslipidemia and hyperglycemia. [Zaoui A, Cherrah Y, Alaoui K, Mahassine N, Marouch H, Hassar M; Effect of *Nigella sativa* fixed oil on blood homeostasis in rats, *J Ethnopharmacol* **79**(1), 23-26 (2002)].

Oral administration of *N. sativa* fixed oil (2 ml/kg) for twelve weeks to rats, significantly lowered serum cholesterol, triglyceride and glucose levels compared to controls. Treated animals exhibited slowing of body weight gain. The hematocrit and haemoglobin levels were also increased in treated rats. No change in key hepatic enzyme and morphology of heart, liver, kidney and pancreas of treated rats suggested that *Nigella sativa* fixed oil was safe for therapeutic use. [Zaoui A, Cherrah Y, Mahassini N, Alaoui K, Amaronch H, Hassar M; Acute and chronic toxicity of *Nigella sativa* fixed oil, *Phytomedicine* 9(1), 69-74 (2002)].

The effect of a 4-week intragastric gavage with a petroleum ether extract of *Nigella sativa* seeds on blood glucose, insulin and lipids in normal rats was studied. The extract caused a 25% reduction in food intake that translated into a transient weight loss. At the end of 4-week treatment, *N. sativa*-treated rats had lower fasting plasma levels of insulin and triglycerides, and higher HDL-cholesterol as compared to controls. The results of the investigation suggested that the petroleum ether extract of *N. sativa* seeds had a slight anorexic effect, and that it possessed hypolipidemic activity. [Le PM, Benhaddou-Andaloussi A, Elimadi A, Settaf A, Cherrah Y, Haddad PS; The petroleum ether extract of *Nigella sativa* exerts lipid-lowering and insulinsensitizing actions in the rat, *J Ethnopharmacol* **94**(2-3), 251-59 (2004)].

The methanolic extract of black cumin (*N. sativa*) seeds yielded new dolabellane type diterpene alkaloids, nigellamines A3, A4, A5 and C. In primary cultured hepatocytes, nigellamines lowered the triglyceride levels. Such an activity of nigellamine A5 was comparable to clofibrate, a known hypolipidemic agent. [Morikawa T, Xu F, Ninomiya K, Matsuda H, Yoshikawa M; Nigellamines A3, A4, A5 and C new dolabellane type diterpene alkaloids with lipid metabolism promoting activities from the Egyptian medicinal food black cumin, *Chem Pharm Bull* (Tokyo) **52**(4), 494-97 (2004)].

Nymphaea lotus: See *Berberis aristata:* [Kamran & Ahmad; *Int J Pharmacogn* **30**(1), 5-8 (1992)].

O

Ocimum sanctum (H. Tulsi): See *Allium sativum* (Garlic): [Dwivedi S; *Ann Natl Acad Med Sci* (India) 32(3&4), 159-175(1996)].

A significant reduction in fasting blood sugar, uronic acid, total amino acids, total cholesterol, triglyceride, phospholipids and total lipids was observed by feeding leaf powder of the plant at 1% level in normal and diabetic rats for a period of one month. The results of the investigation indicated the hypoglycemic and hypolipidemic effect of *O. sanctum* leaf powder in diabetic rats. [Rai V, Iyer U, Mani UV; Effect of Tulasi (*Ocimum sanctum*) leaf powder supplementation on blood sugar levels, serum lipids and tissue lipids in diabetic rats, *Plant Foods Hum Nutr* **50**(1), 9-16 (1997)].

Feeding of aqueous extract of *Ocimum sanctum* (200mg/kg) mixed with diet to streptozotocin-induced diabetic rats for 8 weeks caused a significant reduction in the serum lipid profile, lipid peroxidation, blood glucose levels and an improvement in glucose tolerance. An increase in the plasma, liver, brain and kidney antioxidant enzymes i.e. superoxide dismutase, catalase and glutathione was also observed following treatment with *O. sanctum* extract. [Halim EMA, Hussain KJ, Rao M; Hypoglycemic, hypolipidemic and antioxidant properties of Tulsi (*Ocimum sanctum* L.) in streptozotocin induced diabetes in rats, *Indian J Clin Biochem* **16**(2), 190-94 (2001)].

See *Commiphora mukul:* [Raut et *al.*; *J Mahatma Gandhi Inst Med Sci* **7**(2), 10-16 (2002)].

Ocimium sanctum extract significantly decreased serum malondialdehyde (MDA) and platelet-rich plasma (PRP) levels in hypercholesterolemic animals. In view of *O.*

sanctum-induced enhanced antioxidant defence and free radical scavenging activity, this drug was considered useful in atherosclerosis and coronary artery disease. [Arora D, Khanna N, Mahajan P, Sharma SB; Antioxidant activity of *Ocimum sanctum* in hypercholesterolemic model, *Indian J Pharmacol* **35**(2), 135 (2003)].

See *Commiphora mukul:* [Mary et al.; *Phytomedicine* **10** (6-7), 474-82 (2003)].

Oenothera biennis (Evening primrose)**:** With an objective of comparing the hypocholesterolemic effect of polyunsaturated fatty acids, male rats were given highcholesterol diets containing either evening primrose oil (linoleic plus γ-linolenic acids) or safflower oil (linoleic acid) at the 10% level. Evening primrose oil with a phytosterol content of 1.47% was found to be more hypocholesterolemic than safflower oil (phytosterols 0.34%), and rats given primrose oil excreted more neutral (cholesterol and its metabolites) but not acidic steroids during the first 2 weeks of the feeding. Even when the phytosterol content of primrose oil and safflower oil was adjusted to be the same (0.67%), the former was still more hypocholesterolemic than the latter but to a lesser extent, although faecal neutral steroid excretion was comparable in these two dietary fat regimens. The results indicate a significant hypocholesterolemic efficacy of γ-linolenic acid present in evening primrose oil. [Sugano M, Ide T, Ishida T, Yoshida K; Hypocholesterolemic effect of *gamma*-linolenic acid as evening primrose oil in rats, *Ann Nutr Metab* **30**(5), 289-99 (1986)].

The hypocholesterolemic efficacy of various polyunsaturated fatty acids was compared in rats, given cholesterol-enriched diets with (0.004%) or without indomethacin, a cyclooxygenase inhibitor. Evening primrose oil (linoleic plus γ-linolenic), safflower oil (linoleic) or soybean oil (linoleic plus α-linolenic) were added to diets at the 10% level. The serum cholesterol level of the evening primrose oil group was consistently lower than the other groups and after 3 weeks, it was significantly different from the safflower oil group without indomethacin and the soybean oil group with indomethacin. In rats, fed with evening primrose oil, the aorta tended to produce more prostacyclin whereas the concentration of plasma thromboxane B2 was much lower than in rats fed safflower or soybean oil. The effects of indomethacin on these eicosanoids were less evident in rats, fed evening primrose oil. Thus γ-linolenic acid appears to cultivate an environment suitable for the prevention of cardiovascualr disease even in the presence of excess cholesterol in the diet. [Sugano M, Ishida T, Ide T, Effects of various polyunsaturated fatty acids on blood cholesterol and eicosanoids in rats, *Agric Biol Chem* **50**(9), 2335-40 (1986)].

The hypocholesterolemic efficacies of various oils (*Oenothera biennis* oil, safflower oil, palm oil and soybean oil) having polyunsaturated fatty acids were compared in rats, given cholesterol-enriched diets. The serum total and very low density lipoprotein + intermediate lipoprotein + low density lipoprotein cholesterol concentrations were consistently lower in rats receiving *O. biennis* oil as 10 and 20% of diet than those in the other groups. The liver weight of the *O. biennis* oil group was significantly lower than that of other groups. The results of this study demonstrate that *O. biennis* oil group inhibit the increasing of serum total cholesterol and VLDL + IDL + LDL-cholesterol concentrations in the presence of excess cholesterol in the diet compared with the other dietary oils. [Fukushima M, Akiba S, Nakano M; Comparative hypocholesterolemic effects of six vegetable oils in cholesterol-fed rat, *Lipids* **31**(4), 415-19 (1996)].

Rats fed on conventional diet were shifted to diets containing 10% vegetable oils with 0.5% cholesterol for 13 weeks. Of the different dietary oils used, oils from cultivated and wild evening primrose (*O. biennis*) were found to be the best in inhibiting the increase of serum total cholesterol and VLDL + intermediate density lipoprotein + LDL-cholesterol concentrations in the presence of excess cholesterol in the diet. [Fukushima M, Matsuda T, Yamagishi K, Nakano M; Comparative hypocholesterolemic effects of six dietary oils in cholesterol-fed rats after long-term feeding: *Lipids* **32**(10), 1069-74 (1997)].

***Oenothera paradoxa*:** The effect of *O. paradoxa* oil on blood serum and liver lipids metabolism in rats, fed with a semisynthetic high fat cholesterol-enriched diet, was investigated. It was found that the addition of cholesterol to the diet decreased the hypocholesterolemic and hypotriglyceridemic effects of *O. paradoxa* oil both in blood serum and liver. [Biernat J, Grajeta H; Effect of high fat cholesterol-enriched diets on hypolipemic action of *Oenothera paradoxa* oil in rats. Part 1: Blood serum and liver lipids, *Nahrung* **41**(1), 46-49 (1997)].

Dietry evening primrose (*O. paradoxa*) cake extract significantly decreased total plasma cholesterol and low density lipoprotein cholesterol without any change in high-density lipoprotein cholesterol in rats, fed with cholesterol-free or cholesterol containing (1%) diet. Plasma and erythrocyte malondialdehyde concentration were also increased in treated rats. [Balasinska B; Hypocholesterolemic effect of dietary evening primrose (*Oenathera paradoxa*) cake extract in rats, *Food Chem* **63**(4), 453-59 (1998)].

Olea europaea (Olive): Administration of olive oil and sunflower oil (0.25 ml/100g/d) to cholesterol-fed rats significantly decreased serum cholesterol and triglyceride levels. Sunflower oil showed an initial enhancement of cholesterol and triglyceride levels followed by lowering of these levels. Olive oil, however, consistantly decreased cholesterol and triglyceride levels throughout the experiment. [Siddique HH, El Hwuegi AS, El-Sagher MR, Ali FM, Sahib FA, El-Zarok AA; Effect of olive and sunflower oil on serum lipids and myocardial triglycerides in rats, *Planta Med* (1), 46-49 (1986)].

A survey of diets of various countries, especially the Mediterranean countries, revealed that the use of olive oil possibly helped in preventing and reducing the incidence of coronary heart disease and hypercholesterolemia. [Keys A; Olive oil and coronary heart disease, *Lancet* **1**(8539), 983-84 (1987)].

Maslinic acid, prepared from wastes from manufacture of olive oil and preserved olives, exhibits hypocholesterolemic, hypoglycemic activities and produces a favourable effect on the blood coagulative and anticoagulative systems in experimental hypercholesterolemia. [Movsumov IS, Manafova MI, Aliev AM; Preparation of maslinic acid and the examination of its effects on some metabolic processes, *Farmatsiya* (Moscow) **39**(1), 54-57 (1990) Article in Russian].

The effects of glycero-alcoholic extracts of shoots and leaves of *O. europaea* and of oleuropein on diet and triton-induced hypercholesterolemia were studied in Wistar rats. The hypocholesterolemic effects of olive extracts can be ascribed to a synergistic action of oleuropein and polyunsaturated fatty acids contained in the drug. [De Pasquale R, Monforte MT, Trozzi A, Raccula A, Tommasini S, Ragusa S; Effects of leaves and shoots of *Olea europaea* L and oleuropein on experimental hypercholesterolemia in rat, *Plantes Medicinaleset Phytotherapie* **25**(2-3), 134-40 (1991)].

Dietary supplementation with virgin olive oil is known to lower plasma cholesterol level. It was demonstrated in animals that olive oil supplementation also suppresses the conversion of 20:3n-6 fatty acids to 20:4n-6 (*delta* 5-desaturation). The results of the investigation indicated that the components in olive oil responsible for suppressing both plasma cholesterol and *delta* 5-desaturation activity are contained mainly in the non-glyceride fraction of the oil and that the hypocholesterolemic activity and the suppression of *delta* 5-desaturation are two independent functions modulated by different components in the virgin olive oil. [Huang YS, Redden P, Lin X, Smith R, Mackinnon S, Horrobin DF; Effect of dietary olive oil: Non-glyceride fraction on plasma cholesterol level and liver phospholipid fatty acid composition, *Nutr Res* **11**(5), 439-48 (1991)].

The effects of supplementing the existing diet with fish oil or olive oil on lipids and cell function in patients with peripheral vascular disease were examined. Thirty two patients with symptomatic and angiographically demonstrated peripheral vascular disease were screened, matched, and randomly allocated to take either 15 g/d fish oil or olive oil for 4 weeks. Fish oil reduced serum triglyceride levels by 26%, but increased total cholesterol levels due to a significant increase in both low density lipoprotein cholesterol (LDL-c) and high density lipoprotein 2-cholesterol (HDL 2-c). Olive oil reduced total cholesterol levels, accountable to a significant decrease in LDL-c levels. Serum thromboxane B-2 levels remained unchanged following fish oil, but were significantly increased by olive oil. Platelet aggregation was significantly reduced after fish oil, but was increased by olive oil. The hypocholesterolemic action of olive oil was confirmed along with new evidence of a possible adverse effect on platelet hyperactivity. [Mori TA, Vandongen R, Mahanian F, Douglas A; Plasma lipid levels and platelet and neutrophil function in patients with vascular disease following fish oil and olive oil supplementation, *Metab Clin Exp* **41**(10), 1059-67 (1992)].

See *Cocos nucifera* (Cocoanut): [Nicolosi *et al.*; *Med Sci Sports Exercise* **29**(11), 1422-28 (1997)].

See *Rosa canina:* [Gonzalez et *al.*; *Rev Esp Fisiol* **53**(2), 199-204 (1997)].

See *Brassica campestris:* [Trautwein et *al.*; *Ann Nutr Metab.* **43**(3), 159-72 (1999)].

The effects of Virgin and Lampante olive oils on lipid metabolism and antioxidant activity were investigated on male Wistar rats adapted to cholesterol-free or 1% cholesterol diets. Hypolipidemic and antioxidant properties of Virgin olive oil was clearly demonstrated by the results of the investigation. Lampante oil were relatively less active. The hypolipidemic and antioxidant properties are more evident when these oils are added to the diets of rats, fed with cholesterol. [Gorinstein S, Leontowicz H, Lojek A, Leontowicz M, Ciz M, Krzeminski R, Gralak M, Czerwinski J, Jastrzebski Z, Trakhtenberg S, Grigelmo Miguel N, Soliva Fortuny R, Martin Belloso O; Olive oils improve lipid metabolism and increase antioxidant potential in rats fed diets containing cholesterol, *J Agric Food Chem* **50**(21), 6102-08 (2002)].

The mechanism of the hypocholesterolemic effect of olive oils (Virgin and lampante) was investigated in Wistar rats. Significant hypocholesterolemic and antioxidant effects were registered in groups of rats fed cholesterol-containing diets supplemented with olive oils. Significant increases in the bile flow, the bile cholesterol and bile acids concentration were also observed. Faecal output and faecal excretion of bile acids and cholesterol were also increased in these rats. The hypocholesterolemic effect of olive oils is genuine and is most likely mediated through increases in bile flow and biliary cholesterol and bile acids concentrations and subsequent increases in their faecal excretion. [Krzeminski R, Gorinstein S, Leontowicz H, Leontowicz M, Gralak M, Czerwinski J, Lojek A, Ciz M, Martin Belloso O, Gligelmo Miguel- N, Trakhtenberg S; Effect of different olive oils on bile excretion in rats fed with cholesterol containing and cholesterol-free diets, *J Agric Food Chem* **51**(19), 5774-79 (2003)].

Olea europaea subsp. ***africana*:** A biossay-directed study of triterpenoids isolated from the leaves of *Olea europaea* from Greece, from wild African olive and from a cultivar of *O. europaea* grown in Cape Town showed that while the isolate of Greek olive leaves contained 0.71% oleanolic acid and that of Cape Town cultivar contained 2.47% oleanolic acid, the isolate of the African wild olive leaves was found to contain 0.27% 1:1 mixture of oleanolic acid and ursolic acid. All three isolates, in a dose of 60 mg/kg bw for 6 weeks treatment, prevented the development of severe hypertension and atherosclerosis and improved the insulin resistance of the experimental animals. [Somova LI, Shode FO, Ramnanan P, Nadar A; Antihypertensive, antiatherosclerotic and antioxidant activity of triterpenoids isolated from *Olea europaea*, subspecies *africana* leaves, *J Ethnopharmacol* **84**(2-3), 299-305 (2003)].

Olea europea var. ***oleaster:*** The decoction of leaves of the plant, prepared at 10% was given orally at the rate of 1.5 ml/100g during 3 months to sand rats, which were fed on hypercaloric diet during 7 months. The plant extract presented a hypocholesterolemic effect (42%) related to decreases in LDL and VLDL-cholesterol. No significant reduction in plasma levels of triglycerides and HDL-cholesterol was, however, observed. [Bennani Kabchi N, Fdhil H, Cherrah Y, El Bouayadi F, Kehel L, Marquie G; Therapeutic effect of *Olea europea* var. *oleaster* leaves on carbohydrate and lipid metabolism in obese and prediabetic sand rats (*Psammomys obesus*), *Ann Pharm Fr* **58**(4), 271-77 (2000) [Article in French].

***Opuntia dillenii*:** See *Saccharum officinarum:* [Tarvady & Dhar; *Biomedicine* **9** (1) 39-42 (1989); *Indian J Exp Biol* **28**(7), 657-60 (1990)].

***Opuntia ficus-indica* var. *saboten*:** In dietary hyperlipidemic rats, the hypolipidemic action of cactus fruits and stem extract was examined. High fat diet-induced changes in various components of lipids and cholesterol were effectively prevented by administration of cactus fruits and stem extracts. The fruit extract was relatively more effective than the stem extract.[Choi J, Lee CK, Lee YC, Moon YI, Park HJ, Han YN; Biological activities of extracts from fruits and stem of prickly pear (*Opuntia ficus-indica var. saboten*) II- effects on dietary induced hyperlipidemia, *Korean J Pharmacogn* **33**(3), 230-37 (2002)].

The antiatherosclerotic effect of fruits and stem extract of cactus (*Opuntia ficus-indica var. saboten*) was investigated in sub-acute alcoholic hyperlipidemic rats. The extract effectively prevented or corrected the alcohol-induced hyperlipidemia. However, the hepatic HMG-Co A reductase and alcohol dehydrogenase activity remained unaffected in treated animals. In view of these findings it was suggested that the extract might promote faecal excretion and delay the absorption of alcohol in these rats. [Choi J, Lee CK, Moon YI, Park HJ, Han YN; Biological activities of extracts from fruits and stem of prickly pear (*Opuntia ficus-indica var. saboten*) III- effects on sub acute alcoholic hyperlipidemia in rats, *Korean J Pharmacogn* **33**(3), 238-44 (2002)].

Opuntia robusta (Prickly Pear): Young cladodes of prickly pear (*Opuntia* spp.) exhibited hypocholesterolemic and hypoglycemic activity. [Mulas M; Medicinal properties and yield possibilities of prickly pear (*Opuntia* spp.) in the Mediterranean environment, *Acta Horticulturae* (331), 79-84 (1993)].

Prickly pear leads to a decrease of total cholesterol (12%), low density lipoproteincholesterol (15%), apolipoprotein B (9%), triglycerides (12%), fibrinogen (11%), blood glucose (11%), insulin (11%) and uric acid (10%), while body weight, high density lipoprotein-cholesterol, and apolipoprotein A-I, remained unchanged. The hypocholesterolemic action of prickly pear may be partly explained by the fibre (pectin) content. [Wolfram RM, Kritz H, Efthimiou Y, Stomatopoulos J, Sinzinger H; Effect of prickly pear (*Opuntia robusta*) on glucose and lipid metabolism in non-diabetics with hyperlipidemia-A pilot study, *Wien Klin Wochenschr* **114**(19-20), 840-6 (2002)].

Prickly pear was found to exert a significant hypolipidemic action via receptor upregulation. [Palumbo B, Efthimiou Y, Stamatopoulos J, Oguogho A, Budinsky A, Palumbo R, Sinzinger H; Prickly pear induces upregulation of liver LDL binding in familial heterozygous hypercholesterolemia; *Nucl Med Rev Cent East Eur* **6**(1), 35-9 (2003)].

Origanum tyttanthum: Oil of *O. tyttanthum* showed hypocholesterolemic and hypolipidemic activity. [Nuraliev Yu N, Zubaidova TM; Hypocholesterolemic and hypolipidemic effects of ether oil of *Origanum tyttanthum* Gontsch, *Khim Farma Zh* **28**(10), 63-64 (1994)].

Oryza sativa (Rice, H. Chawal, S. Dhanya): See *Glycine max* (Soya bean, soybean): [Malinow *et al.*; *Am J Clin Nutr* **29**(8), 905-11 (1976)].

Supplementation with the unsaponifiable matter of rice bran oil to hypercholesterolemic diet-fed to rats, produced lowering of the total serum cholesterol and LDL+VLDL-cholesterol fraction but did not affect significantly the HDL-cholesterol fraction and triglycerides. Liver lipids were also reduced significantly. [Sharma RD, Rukmini C; Hypocholesterolemic activity of unsaponifiable matter of rice bran oil, *Indian J Med Res* **85**(March), 278-81 (1987)].

The hypocholesterolemic activity of oryzanol isolated from rice bran oil was investigated in rats fed one per cent cholesterol in the diet. Feeding oryzanol for 3 weeks did not cause any lowering in serum cholesterol levels of rats fed with cholesterol diet whereas after 5 weeks serum cholesterol levels were significantly reduced. When oryzanol was fed at 0.5% level for 7 weeks, significant decreases were observed in serum total cholesterol as also in free, esterified and low density lipoprotein (LDL)-cholesterol and triglycerides. In the group fed with cholesterol diet, the high density lipoprotein (HDL)-cholesterol level decreased significantly when compared with the control group. Addition of oryzanol to cholesterol diet did not alter the HDL cholesterol level. The increase in the level of low density lipoproteins (LDL) caused by feeding the cholesterol diet was significantly reversed in rats fed oryzanol along with cholesterol and this change was also reflected in a significant enhancement of the percentage of high density lipoproteins (HDL). There was no change in serum phospholipid content. Liver total cholesterol, triglyceride and phospholipids also decreased significantly in rats fed with 0.5% level of oryzanol. [Seetharamaiah GS, Chandrasekhara N; Hypocholesterolemic activity of oryzanol in rats, *Nutr Reports International* **38**(5), 927-36 (1988)].

Chemical, nutritional and toxicological properties of rice bran oil were systematically evaluated. Rice bran oil is similar to groundnut oil, in fatty acid composition, having 36% linoleic acid but its unsaponifiable matter (4.1%) is higher than that of ground nut oil. Nutritional evaluation was carried out in weanling albino rats of the Wistar strain and compared with groundnut oil. Growth, feed efficiency, mineral balance, fat absorption and serum haematology were comparable in both rice bran oil and groundnut oil-fed animals. Toxicological studies of rice bran oil were carried out by the food safety evaluation protocol of WHO/FDA/DGHS in rats for three generations and there were no abnormalities in any of the parameters studied. [Rukmini C,

Chemical, nutritional and toxicological studies of rice bran oil, *Food Chem* **10**(12), 257-68 (1988)].

The serum total, free, esterified and (LDL + VLDL)-cholesterol levels of rats maintained on a 10% refined rice bran oil diet were significantly lower than those on a 10% groundnut oil diet; HDL-cholesterol showed a tendency to be higher. Addition of oryzanol at 0.5% level to the diet containing rice bran oil showed a further significant decrease in serum total cholesterol. Liver lipids of rats fed bran oil were also markedly lower than their groundnut oil-fed counterparts. [Seetharamaiah GS, Chandrasekhara N; Studies on hypocholesterolemic activity of rice bran oil, *Atherosclerosis* **78**(2-3), 219-24 (1989)].

In hamsters, stabilized rice bran and oat bran were equally effective in lowering cholesterol. Cholesterol lowering activity of full fat rice bran was elicited by an Australian clinical study. Other studies also indicated that stabilized par-boiled rice bran lowered cholesterol. It was suggested that active hypocholesterolemic component was present in oil itself. [Haumann BF; Rice bran linked to lower cholesterol (feature), *J Am Oil Chem Soc* **66**(5), 615-18 (1989)].

The hypocholesterolemic effect of γ-oryzanol, a mixture of ferulic acid derivatives present in rice bran oil, was investigated in 67 patients with hyperlipidemia (World Health Organization type IIa: 35 patients, IIb: 19 patients, IV: 13 patients). γ-Oryzanol (300 mg) was administered daily, for three months. In type IIa and IIb patients, plasma cholesterol significantly decreased from the second month. The mean plasma triglyceride levels of all subjects decreased significantly after three months. High density lipoprotein (HDL)-cholesterol was also significantly elevated in the type IIb subjects after three months. The reduction in plasma-cholesterol was attributable to the decrease in low density lipoprotein (LDL)- cholesterol in the type IIa and IIb subjects. Thus a mild but significant hypocholesterolemic effect of γ-oryzanol was observed. [Yoshino G, Kazumi T, Amano M, Tateiwa M, Yamasaki T, Takashima S, Iwai M, Hatanaka H, Baba S; Effects of *gamma* oryzanol on hyperlipidemic subjects, *Curr Ther Res* **45**(4), 543-52 (1989)].

The possible effects of rice bran and wheat bran on rats, fed on a purified diet with or without a marine fish oil, were studied. Rice bran rather than wheat bran significantly lowered plasma and hepatic triacylglycerols and hepatic lipogenesis in rats fed on fish oil. Plasma cholesterol and hepatic cholesterol synthesis were significantly lower in animals fed fish oil with either bran. Liver microsomal free cholesterol was significantly lower in rats fed rice bran alone [Topping DL, Illman RJ, Roach PD, Trimble RP, Kambouris A, Nestel PJ; Modulation of the hypolipidemic effect of fish oils by dietary fibre in rats: Studies with rice and wheat bran, *J Nutr* **120**(4), 325-30 (1990)].

See Plant fibres in Appendix: [Thomas *et al.*; *J Food Sci Technol* **27**(5), 290-93 (1990)].

The hypolipidemic response of rice bran oil was investigated in non-human primates, fed with semi-purified diets containing blends of oils, which included rice bran oil. From the results of the investigation it was suggested that rice bran oil might be an additional vegetable oil, which lowers serum cholesterol levels by a unique mechanism. Further study is, however, warranted for its verification. [Nicolosi RJ, Ausman LM, Hegsted DM; Rice bran oil lowers serum total and low density lipoprotein cholesterol and apo B levels in nonhuman primates, *Atherosclerosis* **88**(2-3), 133-42 (1991)].

The unsaponifiable fraction of rice bran oil lowers cholesterol levels. Feeding phytosterols, cycloartenol, and 24-methylene cycloartanol in amounts present in the oil to hypercholesterolemic rats for 8 weeks indicated that cycloartenol alone reduced cholesterol and triglyceride levels significantly. Endogenous sterol excretion increased in animals given cycloartenol. The accumulation of cycloartenol in the liver was found to inhibit cholesterol esterase activity, which in turn led to reduction in circulating cholesterol levels. [Rukmini C, Raghuram TC; Nutritional and biochemical aspects of the hypolipidemic action of rice bran oil: A review, *J Am Coll Nutr* **10**(6), 593-601 (1991)].

Chicks were fed with full-fat rice bran, defatted rice bran or corn/soy diets, balanced for 18% protein, 14.47% total dietary fibre and 10.78% lipid with 0.5% added cholesterol. Both total cholesterol and triglycerides were significantly lower in chicks fed with full fat rice bran and corn/soy diets. Significant differences were found in HDL values for all three diets; full fat rice bran exhibiting the highest mean value (155 mg/dl) and corn/soy exhibiting the lowest mean value (114 mg/dl). All diets also showed significant differences in LDL values. Full fat rice bran appears to increase HDL and to lower LDL in chicks, but does not always affect total cholesterol, whereas defatted rice bran may increase all three serum lipid components. [Newman RK, Betschart AA, Newman CW, Hofer PJ; Effect of full fat or defatted rice bran on serum cholesterol, *Plant Foods Hum Nutr* **42**(1), 37-43 (1992)].

See Tocotrienols in Appendix: [Pearce *et al.*; *J Med Chem,* **35**(2), 3595-606 (1992)].

A comparison of hypocholesterolemic activities of oryzanol (isolated from rice bran oil), curcumin (yellow pigment from *Curcuma longa*) and ferulic acid was made. Incorporation of 0.5% oryzanol, 0.15% curcumin or 75 mg ferulic acid in 1% cholesterol containing diet and its feeding for 7 weeks significantly decreased serum total cholesterol, LDL-c and VLDL-c alongwith enhancement of HDL-cholesterol. The LDL-c / HDL-c ratio was lowered following administration of all the above mentioned compounds. However, maximum decrease was observed in oryzanol treated animals followed by curcumin and ferulic acid treated ones. [Seetharamaiah GS, Chandrashekhara N; Comparative hypocholesterolemic activities of oryzanol, curcumin and ferulic acid in rats, *J Food Sci Technol* **30**(4), 249-52 (1993)].

The influence of extraction reagents on the properties of soluble dietary fibre was examined in defatted rice bran. The soluble fibres, extracted with solutions of sodium hydroxide (pH 14) and calcium hydroxide (pH 12), suppressed the elevation of serum cholesterol levels. The results of the investigation indicate that calcium hydroxide is appropriate for the extraction of soluble fibre from defatted rice bran because it produces the least color, gives a desirable composition and yield, and retains the hypocholesterolemic activity. [Aoe S, Oda T, Tatsumi K, Yamauchi M, Ayano Y; Extraction of soluble dietary fibres from defatted rice bran, *Cereal Chem* **70**(4), 423-25 (1993)].

See *Eleusine coracana:* [Kurup and Krishnamurthy; *Ind J Exp Biol* **31**(3), 291-93 (1993)].

The fatty acid composition of rice bran oil is very close to that of groundnut oil. The oil has high unsaponifiable matter (4.2%), it is rich in minor constituents such as phytosterols, triterpene alcohols, tocopherols and tocotrienols. Experimental as well as human studies have demonstrated the hypolipidemic effects of rice bran oil. Minor constituents of unsaponifiable fractions of rice bran oil were found to be responsible for its hypolipidemic effect. No toxic effect was noted in animals fed with rice bran oil. Considering the hypolipidemic activity and safety of rice bran oil, its use as an edible oil was suggested. [Raghuram TC, Rukmini C; Nutritional significant of rice bran oil, *Ind J Med Res* **102**(Nov), 241-44 (1995)].

The observation, that blending rice bran oil with safflower oil at a specific proportion magnifies the hypocholesterolemic efficacy, is of particular interest with regard to its utilization. [Sugano M, Tsuji E; Rice bran oil and human health, *Biomed Environ Sci* **9**(2-3), 242-46 (1996)].

Blending rice bran oil with safflower oil (7:3, wt/wt) improves the hypocholesterolemic efficacy and the blend has been found to be superior to the individual oils. Although the mechanism underlying this effect is not apparent at present, the blending may have a practical significance. The blending effect was reproduced in rats fed on cholesterol-enriched diet, and there was a decrease in liver cholesterol. [Sugano M, Tsuji E; Rice bran oil and cholesterol metabolism, *J Nutr* **127**(3), 521S-524S (1997)].

The effect of blends of PUFA-rich vegetable oils with the unconventional and hypocholesterolemic rice bran oil on the serum lipid profile of rats was studied. Rats fed with blends of rice bran oil and safflower oil or rice bran oil and sunflower oil at 70:30 ratio for a period of 28 days showed significantly lower levels of total cholesterol, triglycerides and low density lipoprotein cholesterol and increased high density lipoprotein cholesterol. Liver total cholesterol and triglycerides were also reduced. Faecal excretion of neutral sterols and bile acids was increased with use of blends of rice bran oil. Rice bran oil, which is rich in tocopherols and tocotrienols, may improve the oxidative stability of the blends. Tocotrienols are known to inhibit HMG-COA reductase (rate limiting enzyme in cholesterol biosynthesis), resulting in hypocholesterolemia. [Sunitha T, Manorama R, Rukmini C; Lipid profile of rats fed with blends of rice brain oil in combination with sunflower and safflower oil, *Plant Foods Hum Nutr* (Dordrecht) **51**(3), 219-30 (1997)].

See *Glycine max* (Soya bean, soybean): [Morita *et al.*; *J Nutr* **127**(3), 470-77 (1997)].

The nutritive value and hypocholesterolemic effect of sake cake, prepared by the new sake brewing method using liquefied rice, were examined. Growing rats were fed for 3 and 4 weeks on 33.3% sake cake diets with and without 0.5% cholesterol + 0.15% sodium cholate. There was no significant difference in growth between the sake cake and casein groups. The serum and liver cholesterol levels in the sake cake group were significantly lower than those in the casein group. Sake cake feeding increased faecal excretion of bile salts, cholesterol, and lipid more as compared with casein feeding. [Ashida Y, Saito Y, Kawato A, Suginami K, Imayasu S; Effects of dietary sake cake on cholesterol metabolism in rats, *Nippon Nogeikagaku Kaishi* **71**(2), 137-43 (1997) Article in Japanese].

Sake lees, obtained by brewing liquefied rice, were freed from water and alcohol by lyophilisation. Freeze-dried sake lees powder was not only rich in protein and lysine content but also was effective in lowering the serum triacylglycerol concentration. [Tsutsui N, Yamamoto Y, Iwami K; Protein-nutritive assessment of sake lees obtained by brewing from liquefied rice, *J Nutr Sci Vitaminol* (Tokyo) **44**(1), 177-86 (1998)].

Dietary soluble fiber is known to be beneficial for the treatment of hyperlipidemia. Rice bran contains minimal soluble fiber, but rice bran oil has a hypolipidemic effect. Full-fat rice bran was compared with oat bran and a rice starch placebo in moderately hypercholesterolemic, non-smoking, non-obese adults for a period of 6-weeks. Serum cholesterol decreased significantly in the rice bran and oat bran groups but there was no change in the rice starch group. This change was attributable to the reduction of LDL-c. There was no consistent effect on triglycerides within each group and HDL-c and apoA concentrations did not change. The LDLc/ HDL-c ratio decreased significantly in the rice bran and oat bran groups. Stabilized, full-fat rice bran or oat bran, added to the prudent diet of hyperlipidemic adults, similarly reduced cholesterol and LDL-c and improved lipid ratios in 78% of these individuals. [Gerhardt AL, Gallo NB; Full-fat rice bran and oat bran similarly reduce hypercholesterolemia in humans, *J Nutr* **128**(5), 865-69 (1998)].

Physicochemical properties of γ-oryzanol, its presence in the rice bran oil, its antioxidant and hypocholesterolemic activity, as well as, identification, quantitation and extraction methods have been reviewed. [Scavariello EM, Arellano DB, Gamma-oryzanol: An important component in rice bran oil, *Arch Latinoam Nutr* **48**(1), 7-12 (1998) [Article in Spanish].

Brans from rice, oats, corn, and wheat were cooked in a twin-screw extruder at either high or low energy input, and their cholesterol-lowering effects were compared with those of unprocessed brans when fed to four-week-old male golden Syrian hamsters for three weeks. Peanut oil was added to oat, corn, and wheat bran during the extrusion process to match the oil content of rice bran. Extrusion did not alter the hypocholesterolemic effects of rice, oat, or corn brans. Relative cholesterol-lowering effects of the brans, determined with pooled (extruded and unextruded) bran data, were rice bran > oat bran > corn bran > wheat bran. Rice bran diets resulted in significantly lower levels of total plasma cholesterol and very low density lipoprotein cholesterol compared with all other brans. Total liver cholesterol and liver cholesterol concentrations (mg/g) were significantly lower with high energy extruded rice bran compared with the cellulose control group. Plasma cholesterol and total liver cholesterol values with low energy extruded wheat bran were similar to those with rice bran (unextruded or extruded) diets. Lowered cholesterol with rice bran diets may result, in part, from greater lipid and sterol excretion with these diets. Results with low energy extruded wheat bran suggest that this type of processing may improve the potential for lowering cholesterol with wheat bran products. [Kahlon TS; Edwards RH, Chow FI; Effect of extrusion on hypocholesterolemic properties of rice, oat, corn, and wheat bran diets in hamsters, *Cereal Chem* **75**(6), 897-903 (1998)].

Rice bran oil, which is known to exert hypocholesterolemic activity better than more commonly used vegetable oils, is characterized by a relatively high content of non-fatty acid components (γ-oryzanol and tocotrienols). These compounds might be responsible for its hypocholesterolemic effects. Blending of rice bran oil with safflower oil enhanced its hypocholesterolemic effect, but no enhancement of activity was observed by blending with sunflower oil. [Sugano M, Koba K, Tuji E; Health benefits of rice bran oil, *Anticancer Res* **19**(5A), 3651-57 (1999)].

Two novel tocotrienols (desmethyl tocotrienol and didesmethyl tocotrienol), in addition to known α-, β-, γ- and δ-tocopherols and tocotrienols, were isolated from stabilized and heated rice bran. These tocotrienols significantly lowered serum total and LDL-cholesterol levels and inhibited HMG-CoA reductase activity in chickens. They had much greater *in vitro* antioxidant activities than α-tocopherol and known tocotrienols. [Qureshi AA, Mo H, Packer L, Peterson DM; Isolation and identification of novel tocotrienols from rice bran with hypocholesterolemic, antioxidant, and antitumor properties, *J Agric Food Chem* **48**(8), 3130-40 (2000)].

Hypertriglyceridemic rats, prepared by feeding a high-fructose diet, were given dried Anka powder (2%), a rice product fermented with *Monascus* sp., mixed with basic high-fructose (30%) or basal-diet feed for a period of six months. The concentrations of serum triglycerides, total cholesterol, VLDL-c, and LDL-c had significantly decreased, whereas that of HDL-c had slightly increased in 30% fructose-Anka-fed rats as compared with the 30% fructose-fed rats. On the basis of these findings, it was suggested that Anka might be used to suppress hypertriglyceridemia and hyperlipidemia in rats and possibly in man. [Wang IK, Lin-Shiau SY, Chen PC, Lin JK; Hypotriglyceridemic effect of Anka (a fermented rice product of monascus sp.) in rats, *J Agric Food Chem* **48**(8), 3183-89 (2000)].

Rice bran oil (RBO), when blended with safflower oil (SFO) at the ratio of 7 to 3, has been shown to lower serum cholesterol in humans consuming cholesterol. The mechanism as to how this oil blend exerts its effect is not yet clear. The effect of cholesterol supplementation on the cholesterol-lowering ability of different RBO/SFO blends was studied using 4 weeks old male Sprague Dawley rats. The findings of the investigation suggested that cholesterol supplemented at the level of 0.5% masked the cholesterol-lowering effect of rice bran oil. [Koba K, Liu JW, Bobik E, Sugano M, Huang YS; Cholesterol supplementation attenuates the hypocholesterolemic effect of rice bran oil in rats, *J Nutr Sci Vitaminol* (Tokyo). **46**(2), 58-64 (2000)].

From an investigation it was concluded that black and red rice might be effective in reducing atherosclerotic plaques in the aorta of rabbits, fed with a cholesterol-enriched diet. The effectiveness of black and red rice against atherosclerosis might be related to the high level of serum HDL-c and apolipoprotein A1 (apoA1) [Chen Q, Ling W, Ma J, Mei J; Effects of black and red rice on the formation of aortic plaques and blood lipids in rabbits, Wei Sheng *Yan Jiu* **29**(3), 170-02 (2000) Article in Chinese].

Non-fatty acid components (unsaponifiables) of rice bran oil can contribute significantly to its cholesterol-lowering capability. [Wilson TA, Ausman LM, Lawton CW, Hegsted DM, Nicolosi RJ; Comparative cholesterol lowering properties of vegetable oils: beyond fatty acids *J Am Coll Nutr* **19**(5), 601-7 (2000)].

The antioxidant activities of vitamin E (α-tocopherol, α -tocotrienol, γ-tocopherol, and γ - tocotrienol) and γ-oryzanol components (cycloartenyl ferulate, 24-methylenecycloartanyl ferulate, and campesteryl ferulate) purified from rice bran were investigated in a cholesterol oxidation system. The highest antioxidant activity was found in 24-methylenecycloartanyl ferulate, and all three γ-oryzanol components had activities higher than that of any of the four vitamin E components. Because the quantity of γ-oryzanol is up to 10 times higher than that of vitamin E in rice bran, γ oryzanol may be a more important antioxidant of rice bran in the reduction of cholesterol oxidation than vitamin E. The potential hypocholesterolemic property of rice bran is probably due to the antioxidant function of these components against cholesterol. [Xu Z, Hua N, Godber JS; Antioxidant activity of tocopherols, tocotrienols, and gammaoryzanol components from rice bran against cholesterol oxidation accelerated by 2,2'-azobis(2- methylpropionamidine) dihydrochloride, *J Agric Food Chem* **49**(4), 2077-81 (2001)].

The effects of α-tocopherol, the tocotrienol-rich fraction and didesmethyl tocotrienol of rice bran on the pathogenesis of atherosclerotic lesions were studied in C57BL/6 apolipoprotein (apo)E-deficient (-/-) mice, which are an excellent model because they become hyperlipidemic even when they consume a low fat diet and they develop complex atherosclerotic lesions similar to those of humans. These results of the study demonstrated the superior efficacy of tocotrienols compared with α-tocopherol. The low fat diet supplemented with tocotrienol-rich fraction or didesmethyl tocotrienol fed to apoE-deficient (-/-) mice for 14 weeks decreased atherosclerotic lesion size by 42% and 47%, respectively, whereas α-tocopherol supplementation resulted in only an 11% reduction. Although tocotrienols are known to decrease serum triglycerides, total and LDL-cholesterol levels, this is the first report of a significant reduction in the atherosclerotic lesion size in all three genotypes of apoE mice fed with a novel tocotrienol (didesmethyl tocotrienol) of rice bran. [Qureshi AA, Salser WA, Parmar R, Emeson EE; Novel tocotrienols of rice bran inhibit atherosclerotic lesions in C57BL/6 ApoEdeficient mice, *J Nutr* **131**(10), 2606-18 (2001)].

Feeding of rice bran oil or the unsaponifiable compounds of the oil to exogenously hypercholesterolemic rats resulted in lowering of serum and liver cholesterol concentration and prevented reduction of high density lipoprotein-cholesterol. Dietary rice bran oil or the unsaponifiable compounds led to an elevation of faecal neutral sterol excretion, but no significant change in faecal bile acid excretion or in hepatic abundance of mRNAs for HMGCoA reductase, cholesterol-7α-hydroxylase, and low density lipoprotein receptor. Serum and liver α-tocopherol concentrations were also lowered in rats, fed rice bran oil or the unsaponifiable compounds. [Nagao K, Sato M, Takenaka M, Ando M, Iwamoto M, Imaizumi K; Feeding unsaponifiable compounds from rice bran oil does not alter hepatic mRNA abundance for cholesterol metabolism-related proteins in hypercholesterolemic rats, *Biosci Biotechnol Biochem* **65**(2), 371-77 (2001)].

The effects of long-term feeding of cholestin (*Monascus purpureus*-fermented rice, red yeast rice) on serum lipids and atherosclerosis were studied in cholesterol-fed rabbits. Administration of cholestin (1.35g/kg/d) to rabbits led to significant lowering of serum total cholesterol, compared to controls. Following treatment for 200days, serum LDL, triglyceride and atherogenic index were also significantly decreased. [Wei W, Li C, Wang Y, Su H, Zhu J, K David; Hypolipidemic and antiatherogenic effects of long-term cholestin (*Monascus purpureus*fermented rice, red yeast rice) in cholesterol-fed rabbits, *J Nutr Biochem* **14**(6), 314-18 (2003)].

See *Zea mays:* [Kim *et al.*; *J Nutr Biochem* **14**(3), 166-72 (2003)].

Red yeast rice has been shown to exert moderate cholesterol lowering activity with minimum adverse effects. The presence of agents showing more potent hypolipidemic activity in other types of pigmented rice is considered to be a possibility and might also be explored. [Journoud M, Jones PJH; Red yeast rice: A new hypolipidemic drug, *Life Sci* **74**(22), 2675-83 (2004)].

A dose-dependent hypolipidemic and antioxidant effect of tocotrienol-rich fraction of rice bran oil was investigated on experimentally-induced hyperlipidemic rats. Feeding of atherogenic diet for three weeks resulted in a significant increase in plasma triglycerides, total cholesterol and LDL-cholesterol levels. Reduction of HMG-CoA reductase activity and increase in the formation of thiobarbituric acid reactive substances and conjugated dienes were also observed in these animals. After the induction of hyperlipidemia for three weeks, rats were supplemented with different doses of tocotrienol-rich fraction of rice bran oil for one week. This supplementation decreased the lipid parameters in a dose-dependent manner. The results of the detailed investigation suggest that tocotrienol-rich fraction of rice bran oil supplementation has significant health benefits through the modulation of physiological functions that include various atherogenic lipid profiles and antioxidants in hypercholesterolemia. [Minhajuddin M, Beg ZH, Iqbal J; Hypolipidemic and antioxidant properties of tocotrienol-rich fraction isolated from rice bran oil in experimentally induced hyperlipidemic rats, *Food Chem Toxicol* **43**(5), 747-53 (2005)].

P

***Paeonia lactiflora*:** Paeoniflorin, isolated from the methanol extract of *P. lactiflora*, showed a lipid lowering effect in the experimentally induced hyperlipidemic rats. Paeoniflorin significantly lowered total cholesterol, LDL and triglyceride levels compared with the control group at the dose of 200 and 400 mg/kg, p.o. once a day for 4 weeks. [Yang HO, Ko WK, Kim JY, Ro HS; Paeoniflorin: an antihyperlipidemic agent from *Paeonia lactiflora*, *Fitoterapia* **75**(1), 45-49 (2004)].

***Paeonia moutan*:** CJ90002, a pentagalloylglucose isolated from *P. moutan* (Paeoniaceae) and a potent inhibitor of rat microsomal squalene synthase, inhibited cholesterol biosynthesis *in vitro*. In addition, the intraperitoneal and oral administration of CJ90002 had a significant lowering effect on plasma cholesterol levels in hamsters. [Park JK, Cho HJ, Lim Y, Cho YH, Lee CH; Hypocholestrolemic effect of CJ90002 in hamsters: A potent inhibitor for squalene synthase from *Paeonia moutan*, *J Microbiol Biotechnol* **12**(2), 222-27 (2002)].

***Paeoniae rubra*:** See *Typha angustifolia*: [Park *et al.*; *Phytother Res* **18**(3), 224-29 (2004).].

***Panax ginseng*:** The effect of ginsenosides (Rb$_1$, Rc, Rd, Re and Rg$_1$), isolated form of ginseng, on cholesterol metabolism was investigated. Intraperitoneal administration of each ginsenoside (5mg/kg), particularly ginsenoside Rb$_1$ enhanced the biosynthesis of cholesterol [Sakakibara K, Shibata Y, Higashi T, Sanada S, Shoji J; Effect of ginseng saponins on cholesterol metabolism I: The levels and synthesis of serum and liver cholesterol in rats treated with ginsenosides, *Chem Pharm Bull* (Tokyo) **23**(5), 1009-16 (1975)].

Petroleum ether and water extracts of *P. ginseng* contained most of the active principles responsible for decreasing serum cholesterol and LDL-cholesterol levels in chickens and were more effective than *P. ginseng* root powder. Ginsenosides (saponins) were considered responsible for hypocholesterolemic activity of *Panax ginseng.* [Qureshi AA, Abuirmeilch N, Din ZZ, Ahmad Y, Burger WC, Elson CE; Suppression of cholesterogenesis and reduction of LDL cholesterol by dietary ginseng and its fractions in chicken liver, *Atherosclerosis* **48**(1), 81- 94 (1983)].

In high fat diet-fed rats, administration of red ginseng (*P. ginseng*) saponins (150mg/kg/d) for 4 weeks caused lowering of plasma cholesterol levels without any change in HDL-cholesterol. However, serum triglyceride levels were increased in treated rats. [Moon CK, Kang NY, Yun YP, Lee SH, Lee HA, Kang TL; Effect of red ginseng: Crude saponins on plasma lipid levels in rats fed on a diet high in cholesterol and triglyceride, *Arch Pharm Res* **7**(1), 41- 45 (1984)].

In cholesterol-fed rats, the effect of ginsenoside-Rb-2 (isolated from *Penax ginseng*) on lipid metabolism was studied. Single intraperitoneal injection of ginsenoside to rats led to significant lowering of serum total cholesterol, free cholesterol, LDL-cholesterol and triglyceride levels. A significant increase in HDL-cholesterol level was also noted in these treated rats. Following repeated administration of ginsenoside, high cholesterol diet-induced hyperlipidemic rats also exhibited marked decrease in total and free cholesterol, LDL-cholesterol and triglyceride along with enhancement of HDL-cholesterol levels. However, these effects of ginsenoside were relatively more pronounced following repeated administration as compared to single injection. [Yokozawa T, Kobayashi T, Kawai A, Oura H, Kawashima Y; Hyperlipemic improving effects of ginsenoside-Rb-2 in cholesterol-fed rats, *Chem Pharm Bull* **33**(2), 722-29 (1985)].

Effect of the saponin fraction of *P. ginseng* on LDL uptake by rat and rabbit livers and the disappearance rate of LDL from the blood stream were investigated using [124] LDL to understand the mechanism of hypocholesterolemic action of ginseng saponin fraction. It was realised that LDL uptake by the liver and LDL disappearance rate from the blood were stimulated in saponin administered animals and the decrease of blood cholesterol level was mainly due to the decrease of VLDL and LDL concentration of the blood. [Kang BH, Joo CN; Biochemical studies on ginseng saponin XXVI: The effect of ginseng saponin fraction on low density lipoprotein uptake by rat and rabbit livers, *Korean Biochem J* **19**(2), 168-72 (1986) Article in Korean].

The effect of saponin fraction from *Panax ginseng* and the purified ginsenosides-Rb1, -Rb2, -Re, -Rg1 on LDL receptor biosynthesis in high cholesterol-fed rat was investigated. Supplementation of ginsenoside in the diet of high cholesterol-fed rats significantly lowered the level of serum cholesterol suggesting the hypocholesterolemic action of ginsenosides. Analysis of LDL receptor from various organs such as liver, kidney, adrenal cortex and testes showed that the population of LDL receptors was significantly increased in the above organs suggesting that the hypocholesterolemic action might be brought about by the increase of LDL receptor. [Lee YW, Koo JH, Joo CN; Biosynthesis of low density lipoprotein receptor: Effect of ginsenosides on the inhibition of low density lipoprotein receptor biosynthesis, *Korean Biochem J* **20**(4), 362-67 (1987) Article in Korean].

Liver cholesterol level of high cholesterol diet and ginsenoside administered rats (test group) was found to be considerably lower than that of control group (high cholesterol diet-fed rats). Acyl-coenzyme A: Cholesterol acyltransferase (ACAT) activity of the test group was found stimulated. The effect of ginsenoside on the biosynthesis of bile acid from cholesterol by rat liver homogenate was also investigated *in vitro* and found that ginsenoside as well as several amphiphiles such as sodium dodecyl sulfate stimulated the ACAT activity considerably when present in an adequate amount. The nonspecific enzyme stimulating effect of the ginsenoside might be due to the surface activity of ginsenoside. From the above experimental results, it seemed that hypocholesterolemic activity of ginsenosides might be due to the lowered liver cholesterol level by enhanced ACAT activity as well as rapid bile acid biosynthesis from cholesterol. Low cholesterol level might also prevent the LDL receptor biosynthesis inhibition-induced by high cholesterol diet resulting in a rapid removal of raised plasma LDL level. [Choi JY, Lee YW, Joo CN; Biosynthesis of low density lipoprotein receptor, stimulation of liver cholesterol metabolism by ginsenosides, *Korean Biochem J* **20**(4), 368-72 (1987) Article in Korean].

The effect of the ginseng root powder on avian hepatic cholesterol biosyntheis and serum lipoprotein cholesterol levels were examined. Lohman strain broiler females were fed for 4 weeks a corn-based diet (control) or an experimental diet in which 0.25% Korean ginseng was incorporated (treatment). The HMG-CoA reductase activity was significantly lower in the treatment group than that of the control group. Ginseng treatment effected a lowering of the serum total cholesterol level and of serum low density lipoprotein cholesterol level. The mechanism of the hypocholesterolemic action of ginseng involves the suppression of cholesterol biosynthesis. [Muwalla MM, Abuirmeileh NM; Suppression of avian hepatic cholesterogenesis by dietary ginseng, *J Nutr Biochem* **1**(10), 518-21 (1990)].

The effect of Ginseng (G-115) on serum lipids in hyperlipidemic monkeys was investigated. Serum triglyceride and cholesterol levels were markedly reduced in Rhesus monkeys following treatment with Ginseng (G-115). HDL-c / total cholesterol ratio was also increased in these animals. A reduction in the serum LDL-c and VLDL-c levels suggested possible antiatherogenic activity of Ginseng. [Dixit VP, Jain P, Bhandari K, Purohit AK; Effects of Ginseng (G-115) on serum lipid of hyperlipidemic monkeys (*Macaca mulata.*), *Indian J Pharm Sci* **53**(3), 88-91 (1991)].

See *Glycine max* (Soya bean, soybean): [Lanksy PS; *Acta Horticulturae,* (332), 131-36 (1993)].

See *Allium sativum* (Garlic): [Ismail *et al.*; *Pharmacol Res* **39**(2), 157-66 (1999)].

A technology was developed for complete extraction of a water-soluble polysaccharide complex from the above ground part of ginseng. With this extraction procedure, the output of the target product amounted to as much as 16.8% of the mass of dry raw material compared to only 8.17% obtained by the routine procedure. The hypocholesterolemic effect of the water soluble polysaccharide complex, obtained by this procedure, was comparable with that of the official drug (58.2% reduction in cholesterol levels). [Kudimov Yu N, Kazub VT, Muravyeva DA, Vasilyeva ON, Martirosyan KV; Improving the preparation of a polysaccharide complex from ginseng, *Farmatsiya* (Moscow) (6), 24-26 (2002)].

In high fat diet-induced hyperlipidemic rats, the effect of methanolic extract of adventitious root culture of *Panax ginseng* was investigated. The cultured ginseng roots (CBN3) extract significantly lowered the serum cholesterol and LDL-cholesterol and enhaned HDL-cholesterol levels. HPLC analysis revealed that CBN3 contained more Rb1 and Rd ginsenosides than any other cultured or cultivated ginseng samples. The lipid lowering activity of this cultured ginseng root might be attributed to its high Rb_1 and Rd contents. [Lee EJ, Zhao HL, Lee DW, Jeong CS, Kim JH, Kim YS; Effect of the MeOH extract of adventitious root culture of *Panax ginseng* on hyperlipidemic rats induced by high fat-rich diet, *Korean J Pharmacogn* **34**(2), 179-84 (2003)].

The effects of *Panax ginseng* extract on lipid metabolism in humans were examined by measuring cholesterol, malondialdehyde, superoxide dismutase, and catalase. Serum total cholesterol, triglyceride, low density lipoprotein (LDL) and plasma malondialdehyde levels were decreased and high density lipoprotein (HDL) was increased by administration of ginseng extract for 8 weeks (6 g per day). Administration of *P. ginseng* extract increased superoxide dismutase and catalase activities while decreased malondialdehyde level indicating that antioxidant potential of ginseng extract might induce hypolipidemic effect as one of the action mechanisms. [Kim SH, Park KS; Effects of *Panax ginseng* extract on lipid metabolism in humans, *Pharmacol Res* **48**(5), 511-13 (2003)].

Pandanus odorus (H. Keora, S. Ketak): Plasma glucose and total lipid levels in normal and streptozotocin-induced diabetic rats were determined after oral administration of an aqueous extract of *P. odorus* root. Plasma non-esterified fatty acids were significantly decreased after 1 and 2 hours of single oral administration of the *Pandanus* extract at doses of 0.25 and 0.5 g/kg. Plasma cholesterol and triglyceride levels were also significantly decreased by the extract after once daily oral administration of *Pandanus* extract at a dose of 0.5 g/kg for 7 days. The hypolipidemic effect of an aqueous extract of *P. odorus* in streptozotocin-diabetic rats was confirmed. [Peungvicha P, Thirawarapan SS, Watanabe H; Hypoglycemic and hypolipidemic effects of a water extract of *Pandanus odorus* Ridl. roots in streptozotocin-diabetic rats, *Asia Pacific J Pharmacol* **12**(1-2), 3-8 (1997)].

Papaver somniferum var. ***Sujata*** (H. Afim, S. Ahiphena): A non-narcotic, opium and alkaloid-free variety of opium poppy (Sujata) has been developed. Its seeds possess higher oil content (>50 - 52%) with greater proportion of hypocholesterolemic unsaturated fatty acids, than the major oilseed crops, *viz.* rapeseed and mustard in India. [Sharma JR, Lal RK, Misra HO, Naqvi AA, Patra DD; Combating opium-linked global abuses and supplementing the production of edible seed and seed oil: A novel non-narcotic var. Sujata of opium poppy (*Papaver somniferum* L.), *Curr Sci* (Bangalore) 77(12), 1584-88 (1999)].

Peganum harmala (H. Hurmal): See Polysaccharides in Appendix: [Khushbaktova et al.; *Khim Farm Z* **21**(11), 1348-52 (1987)].

Pentaphylloides fruticosa: Administration of extract from sprouts of *P. fruticosa* at a dose of 300 mg/kg to animals with experimental diabetes mellitus inhibits the processes of lipid peroxidation, offers a protective effect on the functions of the pancreas, liver and kidneys and decreases the level of cholesterol and glucose content in the blood. [Aryayeva MM, Azhunova TA, Nikolaev SM, Aseeva TA, Lesiovskaya EE, Nikolaeva IG; Effect of extraction from sprouts of *Pentaphylloides fruticosa* (L.) O. Schwarz on the course of experimental diabetes mellitus, *Rastitel'nye-Resursy* **35**(1), 91-97 (1999)].

Perilla frutescens (Perilla): See *Carthamus tinctorius:* [Sakai et al.; *Chem Pharm Bull* (Tokyo) **40**(8), 2129-32 (1992)].

High α-linolenate perilla seed oil was hypocholesterolemic but to a lesser degree than highdocosahexaenoate fish oil. [Ishihara A, Ito A, Sakai K, Watanabe S, Kobayashi T, Okuyama H; Dietary high-linoleate safflower oil is not hypocholesterolemic in aged mice after a long-term feeding in comparison with lard, perilla oil and fish oil, *Biol Pharm Bull* **18**(4), 485-90 (1995)].

A comparison of the hypocholesterolemic activity of α-linolenic acid-rich perilla oil was made with that of linoleic acid-rich safflower oil using male Wistar rats, 4 and 33 weeks of age. Serum total cholesterol was lower in the perilla oil diet group of both ages. On the other hand, hepatic cholesterol and phospholipids were significantly higher in the perilla oil group than in the safflower oil group of the adult rats. The perilla oil group showed significantly lower 20:4 n-6 but higher 18:2 n-6 acyl groups in hepatic phosphatidylcholine compared with the safflower oil group of both ages. Hepatic HMG-CoA reductase mRNA was significantly lower in the perilla oil diet group than in the safflower oil diet group, irrespective of age. The results show that α-linolenic acid has a greater hypocholesterolemic activity than linoleic acid in rats irrespective of age and these fatty acids behaved differently in affecting hepatic mRNA expressions of HMG-CoA reductase, LDL receptor, and cholesterol 7α-hydroxylase. [Ihara Watanabe M, Umekawa H, Takahashi T, Furuichi Y; Comparative effects of safflower oil and perilla oil on serum and hepatic lipid levels, fatty acid compositions of serum and hepatic phospholipids, and hepatic mRNA expressions of 3-hydroxy-3-methylglutaryl CoA reductase, LDL receptor, and cholesterol 7α-hydroxylase in young and adult rats, *Food Res International* **33**(10), 893-900 (2000)].

The effects of dietary perilla oil were compared with those of beef tallow, corn oil and fish oil on male Sprague-Dawley rats. Hepatic and plasma triacylglycerol levels were decreased in rats fed-perilla oil and fish oil diets, compared with corn oil and beef tallow diets. The activities of hepatic lipogenic enzymes such as fatty acid synthase, glucose-6-phosphate dehydrogenase, and malic enzyme were suppressed in the fish oil, perilla oil, and corn oil-fed groups. The activity of fatty acid synthase, the key regulatory enzyme in lipogenesis, was positively correlated with hepatic and plasma triacylglycerol levels and reduced significantly in the perilla oil-fed group compared with corn oil-fed group. The suppression of fatty acid synthase plays a significant role in the hypolipidemic effects observed in rats fed α-linolenic acid-rich perilla oil and these effects were associated with the increase of hepatic microsomal eicosapentaenoic acid and docosahexaenoic acid contents. [Kim HK, Choi S, Choi H; Suppression of hepatic fatty acid synthase by feeding α-linolenic acid rich perilla oil lowers plasma triacylglycerol level in rats, *J Nutr Biochem* **15**(8), 485-92 (2004)].

Persea americana (Avocado)**:** The effects of two controlled diets—one rich in oleic acid obtained from avocado and olive oil and the other rich in complex carbohydrates—on fasting and postprandial serum lipids and glycemic control were studied in 12 women with noninsulin- dependent diabetes mellitus (NIDDM). The diet with high monounsaturated fatty acids (avocado as one of its main sources) was associated with a greater decrement in plasma triglycerides. Glycemic control was similar with both diets. The results of the investigation led to conclusion that partial replacement of complex digestible carbohydrates with monounsaturated fatty acids in the diet of patients with NIDDM improves the lipid profile favourably, maintains an adequate glycemic control and offers a good management alternative. [Lerman Garber I, Ichazo Cerro S, Zamora Gonzalez J, Cardoso Saldana G, Posadas Romero C; Effect of a high monounsaturated fat diet enriched with avocado in NIDDM patients, *Diabetes Care* **17**(4), 311- 5 (1994)].

Phaseolus aconitifolius (Moth bean)**:** See *Phaseolus mungo:* [Joshi & Singhal; *Indian J Nutr Dietet* **19**(11), 337-41 (1982)].

Compared to casein, protein concentrates of moth bean and pigeon pea (*Cajanus cajan*) produced significantly lower levels of liver total lipid and cholesterol except that pigeon pea protein concentrate caused only non-significant decrease of total cholesterol in the heart. Protein concentrates of both the legumes significantly lowered serum triglycerides, total lipids as well as total and low density lipoprotein cholesterol levels. However, only moth bean protein produced a significantly higher level of serum high density lipoprotein cholesterol and it was more potent at lowering the elevated hepatic and serum lipids and cholesterol levels, which were attributed to the amino acid profile of this lesser known legume. [Mayilvaganan M, Singh SP, Johari RP; Hypocholesterolemic effect of protein prepared from *Phaseolus aconitifolius* (Jacq.), *Indian J Exp Biol* **42**(9), 904-08 (2004)].

***Phaseolus angularis*:** Incorporation of protein concentrates from *P. angularis*, *P. calcaratus* and *Dolichos lablab* seeds at 12 % level in the diet, fed to golden Syrian hamsters for 30 days significantly lowered serum triglyceride, total cholesterol and low density lipoprotein cholesterol along with hepatic total lipid and cholesterol contents. Serum high density lipoprotein cholesterol levels were increased only in the *P. calcaratus* protein concentrate-fed hamsters. Proteins from *P. calcaratus* and *D. lablab* were comparatively more effective in lowering cholesterol levels than that of *P. angularis*. [Chan CF, Cheung PCK, Wong YS; Hypocholesterolemic effects of protein concentrates from three Chinese indigenous legume seeds, *J Agric Food Chem* **46**(9), 3698-701(1998)].

Phaseolus aureus (Greengram): See *Cicer arietinum* (Bengal gram, chickpea): [Sharma RD; *Lipids* **14**(6), 535-39 (1979)].

See *Cicer arietinum* (Bengal gram, chickpea): [Jaya *et al.*; *Nutr Reports International* **20**(3), 371-82 (1979)].

See *Cicer arietinum* (Bengal gram, chickpea): [Jaya & Venkataraman, *Nutr Reports International* **20**(3), 383-92 (1979)].

See *Cicer arietinum:* [Soni *et al.*; *Indian J Nutr Dietet.* **19**(6), 184-90 (1982)].

The source of dietary protein is known to play an important role in the effectiveness of ascorbate as hypocholesterolemic and hypolipidemic agent. Accordingly, ascorbate was found more effective in lowering the lipid levels in atherogenic diet-fed guinea pigs, when given alongwith greengram dal (*Phaseolus aureus*) as a protein source than casein or egg albumin. Moreover, green gram dal itself has been reported to exert hypolpidemic and hypocholetserolemic activity. [Larroya S, George M, Soni GL, Jethi RK, Rattan Singh; Effect of mega doses of ascorbate with different dietary protein sources on lipid metabolism in guinea pigs fed on atherogenic diet, *Indian J Exp Biol* **18**(12), 1430-32 (1980)].

Feeding of whole seed diet of green gram for 4 weeks to normal and alloxan-induced diabetic guinea pigs led to significant lowering of serum total lipid and triglycerides in both groups of animals. Free and esterified fractions of cholesterol were lowered in diabetic animals following consumption of green gram. However, in normal guinea pigs only esterified fraction was decreased. The total cholesterol/phospholipid ratio was also reduced in green gram-fed diabetic guinea pigs. [Srivastawa A, Joshi L D, Singh SP; Changes in serum lipid in normal and diabetic guinea pigs on feeding *Phaseolus aureus* (green gram), *Indian J Clin Biochem* **4**, 50-57 (1989)].

***Phaseolus calcaratus*:** See *Phaseolus angularis:* [Chan *et al*; *J Agric Food Chem* **46**(9), 3698-701(1998)].

Phaseolus lunatus (Butter beans): See *Vigna subterranea* (Bambara groundnuts): [Dabai *et al.*; *British J Nutr* **75**(4), 557-71 (1996)].

Phaseolus mungo (Black gram, H. Mung, S. Mudga): The hypolipidemic effect of a protein and insoluble polysaccharide fraction, isolated from *P. mungo*, was examined in high fat and high cholesterol diet-fed animals. These isolates decreased the serum, aortic and hepatic cholesterol and phospholipids levels in high fat diet-fed rats. The fatty acid, isolated from the lipid fraction, also elicited mild hypolipidemic activity. [Saraswathi Devi K, Kurup PA; Hypolipidemic activity of *Phaseolus mungo* (Black gram) in rats fed a high-fat-cholesterol diet: Isolation of a protein and polysaccharide fraction, *Atherosclerosis* **15**(2), 223-30 (1972)].

The effect of polysaccharides from black gram on lipid levels, lipoprotein lipase and lipogenesis was studied. The polysaccharides caused lowering of tissue cholesterol, phospholipids and triglycerides in comparision to glucose. The activity of lipogenic enzymes i.e. malic enzyme, malate dehydrogenase, glucose-6-phosphate dehydrogeanse, 6- phosphogluconate dehydrogenase and triosephosphate isomerase was also decreased following administration of polysaccharides isolated from black gram. Hepatic and heart lipoprotein lipase activity did not differ much between polysaccharides and glucose-fed animals. However, the aortic lipase activity was higher in glucose-fed rats compared to polysaccharide fed ones. [Menon PVG, Kurup PA; Hypolipidemic action of the polysaccharides from *Phaseolus mungo* (Black gram): Effect on lipid metabolism, *Ind J Exp Biol* **13**(March), 46-48 (1976)].

See *Cicer arietinum:* [Sharma RD; *Lipids* **14**(6), 535-39 (1979)].

The effects of *P. mungo* on experimental hyperlipidemia and atherosclerosis, produced by feeding rabbit with high cholesterol high fat diet and were studied. *P. mungo* showed preventive and therapeutic effects on hyperlipidemia as well as on vascular atherosclerotic lesions. Since *P. mungo* can significantly reduce the lesions of coronary arteries and is nontoxic, its clinical use for the prevention and treatment of coronary heart disease has been recommended. [Li Z, *et al.*; Preventive and therapeutic effects of *Phaseolus mungo* on experimental hyperlipidemia and atherosclerosis in rabbits, *Zhonghua Xinxueguanbing Zazhi* **9**(3), 228-31 (1981)].

See *Cicer arietinum:* [Soni *et al.*; *Indian J Nutr Dietet* **19**(6), 184-90 (1982)].

Evaluation of hypocholesterolemic and hypoglycemic effects of some pulses (*Phaseolus mungo, P. aconitifolius, P. radiatus, and Cajanus cajan*) in normal rats revealed that all these pulses possessed highly significant hypocholesterolemic activity. This study further indicated that the fraction responsible for hypocholesterolemic effect of *P.mungo, P. aconitifolius and P. radiatus* was insoluble in water while that of *Cajanus cajan* was completely soluble in water. [Joshi LD, Singhal PC; Feeding effect of some pulses on blood sugar and serum cholesterol, *Indian J Nutr Dietet* **19**(11), 337-41 (1982)].

Feeding of black gram fibre (30%) to ethanol-treated animals led to significant lowering of serum, liver, heart and aortic cholesterol contents as compared to controls.

Black gram fibre-fed animals also exhibited significant reduction of serum and liver triglycerides along with an increase in the faecal sterols and bile acids excretion. [Indira M, Kurup PA; Effect of black gram fibre on ethanol-induced hyperlipidemia in rats, *Atherosclerosis* **41**(2-3), 241-46 (1982)].

The hypocholesterolemic activity of *Phaseolus mungo* fibre was studied in rats fed with cholesterol diet with beef or soya bean protein. In soya bean protein fed rats, *P. mungo* fibre significantly decreased serum and aortic cholesterol levels compared to beef-fed group of animals. Similar reduction in the cholesterol levels of heart, liver, and serum LDL + VLDL fractions alongwith an increase in the hepatic bile acid and its faecal excretion was also observed in the soya bean protein-fed rats (in the presence of black gram fibre) compared to beef-fed animals. [Molly Thomas, Leelamma S, Kurup PA; Effect of dietary protein on cholesterol lowering action of black gram fibre, *Ind J Exp Biol* **23**(June), 179-81 (1986)].

The hypocholesterolemic action of neutral detergent fibre from blackgram (*Phaseolus mungo*) in rats may be due to hemicellulose, since removal of hemicellulose resulted in the loss of cholesterol-lowering action. Blackgram neutral detergent fibre showed different binding affinities for different bile acids, with maximum binding observed with chenodeoxycholic acid. Faecal excretion of inorganic cations was greater in rats fed with blackgram neutral detergent fibre than in rats fed a fibre-free diet. Absorption of glucose and cholesterol was lower in rabbits fed with blackgram neutral detergent fibre than in rabbits fed a fibre-free diet. [Indira M, Kurup PA; Effects of neutral detergent fibre from blackgram (*Phaseolus mungo*) in rats and rabbits, *J Nutr* **119**(9), 1246-51 (1989)].

Feeding of whole seed diet of *Phaseolus mungo* to diabetic guinea pigs for 4 weeks significantly lowered the serum total lipids, triglycerides, esterified fraction of cholesterol and blood sugar levels. However, serum phospholipids remained unaltered. Lowering of total cholesterol/phospholipids ratio following consumption of *P. mungo* suggested its antiatherogenic potential. [Sriwastwa A, Joshi LD; Effect of feeding of black gram (*Phaseolus mungo*) on serum lipids of normal and diabetic guinea pigs, *Ind J Med Res* **92B**(Oct.), 383-86 (1990)].

See Plant fibres in Appendix: [Thomas *et al.*; *J Food Sci Technol* **27**(5), 290-93 (1990)].

See *Cocos nucifera:* [Thampi *et al.*; *Indian J Exp Biol* **29**(6), 563-67 (1991)].

See *Zea mays:* [Sharma and Kawatra; *Plant Foods Hum Nutr* **47**(4), 287-92 (1995)].

Phaseolus radiatus (H. Urid, S. Masha)**:** See *Phaseolus mungo:* [Joshi & Singhal; *Indian J Nutr Dietet* **19**(11), 337-41 (1982)].

See *Zea mays* (Corn): [Sharma & Kawatra; *Plant Foods Hum Nutr.* **47**(4), 287-92 (1995)].

Administration of *P. radiati semen* (seeds of *Phaseolus radiatus*) extract to ethanol-fed rats markedly reduced serum and hepatic triglyceride levels. This herbal extract also decreased the blood ethanol concentration in a dose dependant manner. The drug also normalised ethanol-induced decrease of hepatic alcohol dehydrogenase (ADH) and aldehyde dehydrogenase (ALDH) activities. These observations indicated that *P. radiati semen* prevented hepatic triglyceride deposition and stimulated alcohol metabolism by increasing ADH and ALDH activities. [Kim MH, Kwon OH, Park CK; Inhibition of hepatic triglyceride accumulation and stimulation of alcohol metabolism by herbal extract containing *P. radiati semen* in rats fed with alcohol, *Yakhak Hoeji* **40** (1), 78-83(1996)].

Phaseolus vulgaris (Black beans, locust beans, baked beans, H. Rajmah): See Polysaccharides in Appendix: [Tsuji *et al.*; *Annual Report National Inst Nutr* (24), 83-91 (1975)].

Investigation showed that the use of food products with locust bean gum in children and adults is a unique approach to treat familial hypercholesterolemia. Acceptance of locust bean gum food was good, and there were no significant side effects. Locust bean gum in food products appears to be an effective and safe approach to control hyperlipidemia. [Zavoral JH, Hannan P, Stat M, Fields DJ, Hanson MN, Frantz ID, Kuba K, Elmer P, Jacobs DR Jr.; The hypolipidemic effect of locust bean gum food products in familial hypercholesterolemic adults and children, *Am J Clin Nutr* **38**(2), 285-94 (1983)].

Incorporation of cellulose, carboxymethyl cellulose gum, locust bean gum and karaya (*Bassora tragacanth*) gum in basal diet, given to 12 human volunteers, decreased the serum cholesterol without affecting the HDL-cholesterol levels. [Behall KM, Lee KH, Moser PB; Blood lipid and lipoproteins in adult men fed four refined fibres, *Am J Clin Nutr* **39**(2), 209-14 (1984)].

Incorporation of locust bean (*P. vulgaris*) gum in the diet at 2% and 5% levels, significantly reduced the levels of serum cholesterol (13%) and hepatic tissue cholesterol (30%) in rats . Hepatic calcium and zinc contents were also decreased along with an increase in the copper levels in these animals. [Haldar K; Effect of locust bean gum on liver and serum cholesterol and on some trace elements of liver, *J Instt Chem* (India) **59**(Part II), 125-26 (1987)].

See *Cicer arietinum* (Bengal gram): [Sharma RD; *Nutr Res* **7**(4), 351-64 (1987)].

Feeding of whole-bean (*Phaseolus vulgaris*) diet to rats significantly decreased serum cholesterol by 20%, and markedly increased biliary cholesterol output by 200% and hepatic cholesterol esters by 100%. The bean starch diet also decreased serum cholesterol by 20%. In these animals, biliary cholesterol saturation increased by 180%, biliary phospholipid output by 100%, and biliary cholesterol output by 400% hepatic cholesterol esters also increased by 100%. The bean protein and bean lipids had no effect on these parameters. Saponins, which are known to have hypocholesterolemic effects, were only detected in the whole-bean and bean starch diets. When 0.3% bean sapogenins were fed to rats for 3 days, biliary cholesterol output increased by 300%. These experiments indicated that the effects of beans on serum, biliary cholesterol, and phospholipid outputs, and on hepatic cholesterol ester concentration are dependent on the starch fraction of beans, presumably on its sapogenin content. [Amigo L, Marzolo MP, Aguilera JM, Hohlberg A, Cortes M, Nervi F; Influence of different dietary constituents of beans (*Phaseolus vulgaris*) on serum and biliary lipids in the rat, *J Nutr Biochem* **3**(9), 486-90 (1992)].

See *Vigna subterranea* (Bambara groundnuts): [Dabai *et al.*, *British J Nutr* **75**(4), 557-71 (1996)].

Black beans without hulls were found to promote cholesterol output and that whole beans, although lowered blood cholesterol to an extent, kept it in the enterohepatic circulation. The hypocholesterolemic compounds of beans were thought to be located in the inner part of the grain. Further studies were considered necessary to identify these compounds and to elucidate their mechanisms of action. [Rosa CO, Costa NM, Leal PF, Oliveira TT; The cholesterol-lowering effect of black beans (*Phaseolus vulgaris* L.) without hulls in hypercholesterolemic rats, *Arch Latinoam Nutr* **48**(4), 299-305 (1998) [Article in Portuguese].

Oral administration of an aqueous extract of *P.vulgaris* pods (200 mg/kg bw) to streptozotocin-induced diabetic rats for 45 days significantly reduced the elevated blood glucose, serum triglycerides, free fatty acids, phospholipids, total cholesterol, very low density lipoprotein cholesterol, and low density lipoprotein cholesterol. The decreased serum levels of high density lipoprotein cholesterol, antiatherogenic index, plasma insulin, vitamin C, and glutathione in the diabetic rats were also reversed toward normalisation. [Venkateswaran S, Pari L, Saravanan G; Effect of *Phaseolus vulgaris* on circulatory antioxidants and lipids in rats with streptozotocin-induced diabetes, *J Med Food* **5**(2), 97-103 (2002)].

The effects of *Phaseolus vulgaris* on blood glucose, plasma insulin, cholesterol, triglycerides, free fatty acids, phospholipids, and fatty acid composition of total lipids in liver, kidney, and brain of normal and streptozotocin-induced diabetic rats were studied. Oral administration of the aqueous extract of *P. vulgaris* pods (200 mg/kg bw) for 45 days to diabetic rats decreased the concentrations of lipids and fatty acids. It decreased the concentrations of palmitic, stearic, and oleic acids but elevated the concentrations of linolenic and arachidonic acids. The administration of *P. vulgaris* pod extract to normal animals resulted in a significant hypolipidemic effect. The hypolipidemic effects of *P. vulgaris* pod extract both in normal and streptozotocin-induced diabetic rats were thus confirmed. The extract also prevented the fatty acid changes produced during diabetes. The effect of *P. vulgaris* pods extract at 200 mg/kg of body weight was better than that of glibenclamide. [Pari L, Venkateswaran S; Protective role of *Phaseolus vulgaris* on changes in the fatty acid composition in experimental diabetes, *J Med Food* **7**(2), 204-09 (2004)].

***Phellodendron amurense*:** See *Artemisia* species: [Jing *et al.*; *Chin J Integ Trad West Med* **6**(1), 21-23 (1986)].

Phoenix dactylifera (Date palm, H. Khajur, S. Pinda kharjura) Dietary fibres from date waste were examined as a hypolipidemic agent on albino rats. The total lipids, total cholesterol, triglycerides and phospholipids in the liver of rats fed on date waste dietary fibres (100 g/kg) were significantly lower than those of control rats fed on high carbohydrate diet free of fibre. The date waste dietary fibres, cultured with *Endomycopsis fibuligera* for a period of 60 hours, produced decrease in all these parameters. The highest decrease was shown in the phospholipids content (51-56%) during the entire experimental period (8 weeks). [Jwanny EW, Rashad MM, Moharib SA, el Beih NM; Studies on date waste dietary fibres as hypolipidemic agent in rats, *Z Ernahrungswiss* **35**(1), 39-44 (1996)].

Phyllanthus niruri (H. Bhuiamla, S. Bhumiamalaki): Administration of alcoholic extract of *P. niruri* (200 mg/kg) simultaneously with triton, decreased the levels of cholesterol (27%), phospholipid (25%) and triglycerides (24%). *P. niruri* extract (100 mg/kg) also reduced elevated levels of very low density lipoprotein and low density lipoprotein in cholesterol-fed hyperlipidemic rats. [Khanna AK, Ramesh Chander; Lipid lowering activity of *Phyllanthus niruri*, *J Med Arom Plant Sci* **22**(Suppl.1), 29-30 (2000)].

The hypolipidemic activity of *P. niruri* was studied in triton and cholesterol-induced hyperlipidemic rats. Oral feeding of *P. niruri* extract (250mg/kg) to triton-induced hyperlipidemic animals decreased serum lipid levels. In rats fed with cholesterol and the drug (100mg/kg) simultaneously for 30 days produced reduction in the lipids and apoprotein levels of VLDL and LDL. The lipid lowering activity of this drug was attributed to inhibition of hepatic Cholesterol biosynthesis, enhanced excretion of faecal bile acids and increased plasma lecithin: cholesterol acyl transferase activity. [Khanna AK, Rizvi F, Chander R; Lipid lowering activity of *Phyllenthus niruri* in hyperlipidemic rats, *J Ethnopharmacol* **82**(1), 19-22 (2002)].

Picrorhiza kurroa (H. Kutaki, S. Katuka): Antihyperlipidemic effect of "Picroliv", a standardised preparation of *P. kurroa* was studied in normal as well as in triton (WR-1339) and cholesterol-induced hyperlipidemic rats. In triton-induced hyperlipidemic rats, Picroliv (25mg/kg) decreased serum lipids. In normal and cholesterol-fed animals, this drug caused lowering of lipids and β-lipoproteins alongwith an increase in HDL-cholesterol. Lipolytic activity in plasma, liver, heart and adipose tissues was also altered in treated animals. Lipid lowering action of *P. kurroa* is attributed to inhibition of cholesterol biosynthesis in liver, increased faecal bile acid excretion and enhanced plasma lecithin cholesterol acyl transferase activity. [Khanna AK, Chander R, Kapoor NK, Dhawan BN; Hypolipidemic activity of Picroliv in albino rats, *Phytother Res* **8** (7), 403-07 (1994)].

The preventive effects of *Picrorhiza kurroa* on D-galactosamine-induced hepatitis in rats were examined. Oral treatment with an alcoholic extract of *P. kurroa* significantly prevented the D-galactosamine-induced decreases in the levels of protein and glycoprotein and in the activities of superoxide dismutase and catalase. A tendency to prevent the D-galactosamine induced alterations in the levels of cholesterol, phospholipids and lipid peroxides was also observed. The antihepatotoxic potential of *P. kurroa* might be ascribed to its antioxidant and hypolipidemic nature. [Anandan R, Pandima Devi K, Devai T, Govindaraju P; Preventive effects of *Picrorhiza kurroa* on D-galactosamine-induced hepatitis in rats, *J Clin Biochem Nutr* **25**(2), 87-95 (1998)].

***Pinus cembra*:** Oral administration of aqueous alcoholic extract of nuts of *Cembra pine* and four other medicinal plants in elixir form to hyperlipidemic animals, led to significant lowering of serum and liver tissue total cholesterol and triglycerides. The hypolipidemic effect of this extract was comparable to that of Gemifibrozil. In patients of metabolic syndrome (insulin resistance), treatment with the extract for 3 months resulted in lowering of lipids and insulin with an enhancement of HDL-cholesterol. The hypolipidemic activity of this drug was attributed to its general adaptive and antioxidative effects. [Ryzhenkov VE; Hypolipidemic and antioxidative properties of new plant origin drug elixir kedrovit, *Phytomedicine* **7**(Suppl II), 67 (2000)].

Pinus koraiensis (Korean pine): Pinolenic acid (*cis*-5, *cis*-9, *cis*-12- octadecatrienoic acid) is a peculiar trienoic acid of the seed oil of Korean pine. The effects of dietary Korean pine seed oil on various lipid variables were compared in rats with those of flaxseed (*Linum usitatissimum*) oil, safflower (*Carthamus tinctorius*) oil and evening primrose (*Oenothera biennis*) oil. In Sprague-Dawley rats fed on diets containing 100 g fat and 5 g cholesterol/kg, the hypocholesterolemic activity of pinolenic acid was intermediate between α-linolenic and linoleic acids. Analysis of the fatty acid composition of liver phosphatidylcholine indicated that in contrast to α-linolenic acid, pinolenic acid does not interfere with the desaturation of linoleic acid to arachidonic acid. However, the effects on ADP-induced platelet aggregation and aortic prostacyclin production were comparable. [Sugano M, Ikeda I, Wakamatsu K, Oka T; Influence of Korean pine (*Pinus koraiensis*)-seed oil containing *cis*-5, *cis*-9, *cis*-12- octadecatrienoic acid on polyunsaturated fatty acid metabolism, eicosanoid production and blood pressure of rats, *British J Nutr* **72**(5), 775-83 (1994)].

***Pinus messoniana*:** Intragastric perfusion of extract from needles of *P. messoniana* in hyperlipidemic mice (5 gm and 10 gm /kg) and oral administration of the extract to hyperlipidemic rats (8 gm/kg) significantly reduced total cholesterol, low density lipoprotein cholesterol (LDL-c) and enhanced the high density lipoprotein cholesterol (HDL-c) levels. [Hu Jun, Lu Guiynan, Li Wanli; Effect of *Pinus messoniana* needles on lowering lipemia, *J Zhejiang College Traditional Chinese Med* **16**(3), 30-31 (1992)].

Piper longum (H. Piplamul, S. Pippali): Dietary feeding of *"Panchcole"*, a combination of the extracts of *P. longum* root and seeds, *P. officinarum* seeds, *Plumbago zeylanica* bark and *Zingiber officinale* rhizome, significantly inhibited HMG-CoA reductase activity resulting into reduction of serum LDL-cholesterol (88.9%) and triglycerides

(73.6%). "*Panchcole*" extract also decreased cholesterol and phospholipid levels. Atherosclerotic plaque formation in the aorta was prevented in the treated animals. [Sharma I, Verma M, Dixit VP; Hypolipidemic effect of "*Panchcole*" an Ayurvedic remedy in rabbits, *Int J Crude Drug Res* **28**(1), 33-38 (1990)].

Piper nigrum (Black pepper, H. Kalimircha, S. Maricha): The effect of administration of black pepper and its active principle piperine to high fat-fed rats was studied for a period of 10 weeks. Finely powdered drugs were intimately suspended in distilled water. The coarse solution of black pepper at two different doses (250 mg/kg bw and 500 mg/kg bw) and piperine at 20 mg/kg body weight were administered orally by intragastric intubation daily. The plasma and tissue lipid profile showed a remarkable reduction in the levels of total cholesterol, free fatty acids, phospholipids and triglycerides in black pepper as well as in the piperine-treated groups. Supplementation of diets of high fat-fed rats with black pepper or piperine elevated the concentration of high density lipoprotein-cholesterol and reduced the concentrations of low density lipoprotein-cholesterol and very low density lipoprotein-cholesterol in the plasma. Thus dietary intake of black pepper or piperine was found to reduce the risk of atherosclerosis markedly by virtue of its hypolipidemic and antiatherogenic effects. [Vijayakumar RS, Surya D, Senthilkumar R, Nalini N; Hypolipidemic effect of black pepper (*Piper nigrum* Linn.) in rats fed high fat diet, *J Clin Biochem Nutr* **32**, 31-42 (2002)].

Piper officinarum: See *Piper longum*: [Sharma et *al*.; *Int J Crude Drug Res* **28**(1), 33-38 (1990)].

Adminstration of 50% ethanol extract of *P. officinarum* (500mg/kg/d) to hyperlipidemic rabbits showed significant hypolipidemic and antiatherosclerotic activity. The extract also increased the high density lipoprotein cholesterol (HDL-c) along with lowering of atherogenic index. A definite regression of atherosclerotic plaques was also noted in these treated animals. [Sharma I, Gosain D, Dixit VP, Purohit A; *Piper officinarum*: A potent antiatherosclerotic and hypolipidemic agent, *Indian J Pharm Sci* **60**(6), 391-93 (1998)].

Pisum sativum (Marrowfat peas, garden pea, pea, H. Matar, S. Satila): See *Cicer arietinum* [Soni et *al*.; *Indian J Nutr Dietet*. **19**(6), 184-90 (1982)].

See *Vigna subterranea* (Bambara groundnuts): [Dabai et *al*., *British J Nutr* **75**(4), 557-71 (1996)].

The effects of isoproteic and isoenergetic diets containing raw or extruded pea seed meal on nutritional performance and serum lipids, amino acids and enzyme levels were studied in growing rats. Extrusion treatment of peas improved their nutritional quality but did not reduce their hypocholesterolemic properties. [Alonso R, Grant G, Marzo F; Thermal treatment improves nutritional quality of pea seeds (*Pisum sativum* L.) without reducing their hypocholesterolemic properties, *Nutr Res* **21**(7), 1067-77 (2001)].

Aqueous acetone (70%) extract from seed coat of pea was demonstrated to possess strong hypocholesterolemic action. Its antioxidative properties in biological system, especially in animals loaded with dietary cholesterol, are less clear and need further studies. [Troszynska A, Balasinska B; Antioxidant activity of crude tannins of pea (*Pisum sativum* L.) seed coat and their hypocholesterolemic effect in rats, *Polish J Food Nutr Sci* **11**(3), 33-38 (2002)].

The effect of cholesterol-enriched (2.8 g/kg) casein and raw pea seed diets on the cholesterol metabolism of intact and ileorectal anastomosed growing pigs was studied. Plasma total cholesterol was lowered by the raw pea diet through a significant decrease in LDL-cholesterol. This diet also decreased the hepatic concentration of esterified cholesterol and increased HMG CoA reductase activity and LDL receptor synthesis. The biliary total cholesterol and bile acid concentrations were greater in raw pea diet than in casein -fed pigs. The results suggest a hypocholesterolemic effect of the raw pea diet probably due to increased faecal bile acid output and an increased biliary bile acid concentration. [Martins JM, Riottot M, de Abreu MC, Lanca MJ, Viegas-Crespo AM, Almeida JA, Freire JB, Bento OP; Dietary raw peas (*Pisum sativum* L.) reduce plasma total and LDL cholesterol and hepatic esterified cholesterol in intact and ileorectal anastomosed pigs fed with cholesterol-rich diets, *J Nutr* **134**(12), 3305-12 (2004)].

Plantago major (H. Lahuriya): The hypocholesterolemic effect of drugs obtained from *P. major* leaves and composition of polyphenol compounds in them were studied in rats. [Maksyutina NP, Nikitina NI, Lipkan HM, Horin AH, Voitenko IM; Chemical composition and hypocholesterolemic effect of some drugs from *Plantago major* leaves Part 2: Polyphenol compounds, *Farmatsevtychnyi Zhurnal* (Kiev) (4), 56-61 (1978) Article in Ukrainian].

Plantago ovata (Isabgol, Isapgul): See Pectin in Appendix: [Sharma *et al.*; *Indian J Physiol Pharmacol* **24**(2), 136-38 (1980)].

Serum cholesterol and triglyceride levels were decreased following ingestion of Isapgul (10g/d) for 30 days. [Goswami S; Effect of Isapgul on serum lipids, *Ancient Science of Life* **7**(3-4), 164-65 (1988)].

Isabgol husk, a mucilaginous fibre, is an effective hypocholesterolemic agent. Consumption of Isabgol husk was shown to produce significant reductions in plasma fasting total cholesterol, LDL-cholesterol and the ratio of total cholesterol to HDL-cholesterol. However, no change in the level of HDL-cholesterol was observed. [Kawatra A, Kapoor AC, Sehgal S; Hypocholesterolemic effect of Isabgol husk on overweight adults, *Nutr Res* **10**(10), 1177-82 (1990)].

The potential hypolipidemic effects of the seeds from *P. ovata* and the mechanisms associated with the lowering of plasma lipids were tested in male Hartley guinea pigs. Although a dose response was not observed, plasma triglycerides and LDL-cholesterol were lower in the *P. ovata* groups compared with the control. Lecithin cholesterol acyltransferase (LCAT) and cholesterol ester transfer protein (CETP) activities were significantly affected by the *P. ovata* diets. The control group had higher LCAT and CETP activities compared with the *P. ovata* groups. Hepatic total and free cholesterol concentrations were not affected by *P. ovata*. The activity of HMG-CoA reductase, the rate-limiting enzyme of cholesterol synthesis was up-regulated and the activity of cholesterol 7α-hydroxylase, the regulatory enzyme of cholesterol catabolism to bile acids was higher in the *P. ovata* groups. Faecal bile acids were 3 times higher in the *P. ovata* groups than in the control group. The results suggest that *P. ovata* exerts its hypolipidemic effect by affecting bile acid absorption and altering hepatic cholesterol metabolism. [Romero AL, West KL, Zern T, Fernandez ML; The seeds from *Plantago ovata* lower plasma lipids by altering hepatic and bile acid metabolism in guinea pigs, *J Nutr* **132**(6), 1194-98 (2002)].

Plantago psyllium (Psyllium): See *Avena sativa* (Oat): [Anderson JW; *Am J Cardiol* **60**(12), 17G-22G (1987)].

The effect of psyllium husk on plasma total and lipoprotein cholesterol in healthy human subjects was studied and the possible hypocholesterolemic mechanisms have been elucidated. Supplementation of basal diet with psyllium husk (21g/d) reduced total, low-density, and high density cholesterol. Faecal steroid excretion was not affected by psyllium supplementation. The cholesterol lowering mechanism of psyllium may not involve increased bile acid excretion or decreases in nutrient absorption. [Abraham ZD, Mehta T; Three-week psyllium husk supplementation; Effect on plasma cholesterol concentrations, faecal steroid excretion and carbohydrate absorption in men, *Am J Clinical Nutr* **47**(1), 67-74 (1988)].

The hypocholesterolemic effect of psyllium was evaluated in 14 individuals with polygenic hypercholesterolemia. The use of psyllium produced at week 12, a reduction in total cholesterol and LDL-cholesterol with non significant changes in triglycerides and HDL-c. The use of psyllium as a complement of diet in the management of polygenic hypercholesterolemia was recommended. [Lerman Garber I, Lagunas M, Sienra Perez JC, Ahumada Ayala M, Saldana A, Cardoso Saldana G, Posadas Romero C; Hypocholesterolemic effect of *Plantago psyllium, Archivos del Instituto de Cardiologia de Mexico* **60**(6), 535-39 (1990) Article in Spanish].

Sea quails appear to be less sensitive to the hypocholesterolemic action of psyllium than are chickens. [Day CE; Activity of psyllium hydrophilic colloid for reducing serum cholesterol in sea quail fed with a diet supplemented with cholesterol, *Artery* **18**(3), 163-67 (1991)].

African green monkeys were fed for 3.5 years one of three experimental diets: low cholesterol cellulose (LCC), high cholesterol cellulose (HCC), or high cholesterol psyllium (HCP). The LCC and HCP groups had significantly lower plasma cholesterol concentrations (39% lower) at 1 mo than did the HCC group. These responses persisted throughout the study. Plasma cholesterol changes were due to a reduction in intermediate density and low density lipoproteins. Aortic atherosclerosis, evaluated at 3.5 year, was lowest in the LCC group, intermediate in the HCP group, and highest in the HCC group. [McCall MR, Mehta T, Leathers CW, Foster DM; Psyllium husk. I: Effect on plasma lipoproteins, cholesterol metabolism, and atherosclerosis in African green monkeys, *Am J Clin Nutr* **56**(2), 375-84 (1992)].

To study the effect of dietary soluble fibre on serum cholesterol concentration, Sprague- Dawley rats were fed with diets containing 7.5% dietary fibre as cellulose (control), pectin, psyllium or oat bran with or without 0.3% added cholesterol for 3 weeks. Among rats fed with cholesterol, liver total lipid and cholesterol concentrations were significantly lower in groups fed pectin, psyllium and oat bran compared with cellulose-fed controls. When cholesterol was fed, the oat bran-fed group had significantly higher butyrate and the pectin-fed group had significantly higher propionate concentrations in the hepatic portal vein than did cellulose-fed controls. The groups fed psyllium, oat bran and pectin all had significantly higher faecal neutral sterols than did the cellulose-fed group when cholesterol was fed. From the results of this investigation, it was inferred that soluble dietary fibres exert their hypocholesterolemic effect by increasing excretion of faecal neutral sterols. [Arjmandi BH, Ahn J, Nathani S, Reeves RD; Dietary soluble fibre and cholesterol affect serum cholesterol concentration, hepatic portal venous short-chain fatty acid concentrations and faecal sterol excretion in rats, *J Nutr* **122**(2), 246-53 (1992)].

Soluble fibre consistently lowers plasma total and low density lipoprotein cholesterol concentrations in humans and various animal models including the hamster. However, the mechanism of this effect remains incompletely defined. Experiments were performed to determine the activity of dietary psyllium on hepatic 7α-hydroxylase, HMG CoA reductase and LDL receptor expression in the hamster. Although dietary psyllium did not increase hepatic LDL receptor expression in animals fed with the cholesterol-free, very low fat diet, it did increase or at least restore receptor expression that had been downregulated by dietary cholesterol and triglyceride. Thus, 7.5% dietary psyllium produced effects on hepatic 7α-hydroxylase and LDL metabolism that were similar to those of 1% cholestyramine. Induction of hepatic 7α- hydroxylase activity by dietary psyllium may account, in large part, for the hypocholesterolemic effect of this soluble fibre. [Horton JD, Cuthbert JA, Spady DK; Regulation of hepatic 7α-hydroxylase expression by dietary psyllium in the hamster, *J Clin Investigation* **93**(5), 2084-92 (1994)].

The effects of psyllium fibre supplementation to polyunsaturated fatty acid-rich soybean oil and saturated fatty acid-rich coconut oil diets on fat digestibility and faecal fatty acid excretion were investigated in healthy humans. Fat digestibility was significantly lower and faecal fat excretion was significantly higher with soybean oil + psyllium fibre diet than with soybean oil diet. Similar result was observed with coconut oil + psyllium fibre diet and coconut oil diet. Faecal excretion of myristic and lauric acids was not affected by test diets. Increased faecal fat loss, decreased fat digestibility and increased faecal palmitic acid excretion with psyllium supplementation may partly explain the hypocholesterolaemic action of psyllium fibre. [Ganji V, Kies CV, Psyllium husk fibre supplementation to soybean and coconut oil diets of humans: Effect on fat digestibility and faecal fatty acid excretion, *European J Clin Nutr* **48**(8), 595-97 (1994)].

Sources of dietary fibre known to alter cholesterol metabolism and/or bile acid pool size were fed to rats, and activity of the rate-limiting step in bile acid synthesis, cholesterol 7α- hydroxylase, was measured. In the experiment, semipurified diets containing 5% cellulose, psyllium hydrocolloid, pectin or oat bran as dietary fibre sources or 2% cholestyramine were fed to groups of 10 male Wistar rats for 4 weeks. The activity of cholesterol 7α-hydroxylase was highest in the cholestyramine-treated group, followed by groups fed psyllium or pectin, which exhibited more than twice the enzyme activity of groups fed with cellulose or oat bran. The hypocholesterolemic effect of soluble fibres was found to be modulated through increased synthesis and, therefore, pool size of bile acids. [Matheson HB, Colon IS, Story JA; Cholesterol 7α-hydroxylase activity is increased by dietary modification with psyllium hydrocolloid, pectin, cholesterol and cholestyramine in rats, *J Nutr* **125**(3), 454-58 (1995)].

Psyllium, a water-soluble fibre, has been shown to have a cholesterol-lowering effect in studies of adults but in view of variable results reported for the children, a 12-week randomized, single-blind, placebo-controlled, parallel clinical trial was conducted to test the effectiveness of psyllium in lowering total (TC) and low density lipoprotein cholesterol (LDL-c) in 50 healthy 2 to 11 years old children. Greater reduction of total and LDL-cholesterol, and increase in HDL-cholesterol were noted after 12 weeks in children of the psyllium-enriched group compared to the control diet. [Williams CL, Bollella M, Spark A, Puder D; Soluble fibre enhances the hypocholesterolemic effect of the step I diet in childhood, *J Am College Nutr* **14**(3), 251-57 (1995)].

See Plant fibres in Appendix: [Fernandez *et al.*, *J Lipid Res* **36**(10), 2191-202 (1995)].

The effect of psyllium husk fibre (PF) supplementation to the diets of soybean oil (SO) and coconut oil (CO) on serum lipids in normolipidemic humans was studied. SO + PF diet significantly reduced serum cholesterol compared with SO diet, and CO + PF diet significantly reduced serum cholesterol compared with CO diet. Hypocholesterolemic response was greater with SO + PF compared with CO + PF. Reductions in low density lipoprotein cholesterol (LDL-c) and apolipoprotein (apo) B were parallel to reductions of serum cholesterol. SO diet decreased, while CO diet increased serum cholesterol, LDL-c and apo B. Very low density lipoprotein cholesterol, high density lipoprotein cholesterol and apo A-1 were unaffected by psyllium fibre. Psyllium fibre supplementation lowered serum cholesterol regardless of saturation level of dietary fat. [Ganji V, Kies CV; Psyllium husk fibre supplementation to the diets rich in soybean or coconut oil: Hypocholesterolemic effect in healthy humans, *Int J Food Sci Nutr* **47**(2), 103-10 (1996)].

A study was conducted to determine whether the storage conditions and the levels of psyllium in the diet modulate its hypocholesterolemic effects using Sprague-Dawley rats, fed with cholesterol-containing diets for 21 days. Psyllium stored for 8 mo at 5°C (PS5) and 40°C (PS40) were used. The higher storage temperature caused a gradual decrease in molecular weight of the psyllium. Rates of hepatic sterol synthesis were significantly higher in all of the psyllium-fed rats compared with control rats. A similar trend was observed in rates of intestinal sterol synthesis and the difference was significant. Liver total cholesterol and total lipid concentrations were significantly lower in all psyllium-fed rats compared to controls. The findings of this study indicated that the cholesterol-lowering activity of psyllium remains virtually unaltered by storage conditions, despite moderate hydrolysis of PS40. [Arjmandi BH, Sohn E, Juma S, Murthy SR, Daggy BP; Native and partially hydrolyzed psyllium have comparable effects on cholesterol metabolism in rats, *J Nutr* **127**(3), 463-69 (1997)].

See Plant fibres in Appendix: [Ismail *et al.*; *Biochem Arch* **13**(3), 161-70 (1997)].

The effects of cholestyramine and psyllium alone and in combination, on lipoprotein cholesterol and neutral and acidic steroid excretion were studied in hamsters. Psyllium and cholestyramine both showed significant hypocholesterolemic effects but in combination produced additive reductions in lipoprotein and hepatic cholesterol. The combination increased total bile acid excretion by 79% in place of only 26% increase observed with psyllium. Neither of the agents nor the combination affected faecal neutral sterol excretion. The results of the investigation support the use of these agents for lowering of cholesterol. [Daggy BP, O'Connell NC, Jerdack GR, Stinson BA, Setchell KDR; Additive hypocholesterolemic effect of psyllium and cholestyramine in the hamster: Influence on Faecal sterol and bile acid profiles, *J Lipid Res* **38**(3), 491-502 (1997)].

Psyllium, a source of dietary fibre rich in soluble components, results in lower serum cholesterol concentration in several species. Suggested mechanisms for the hypocholesterolemic effect include a greater excretion of faecal bile acids and total steroids and up-regulation of bile acid biosynthesis. Results of the investigation indicate that feeding psyllium to rats increases faecal bile acid and total steroid excretion as well as 7α-hydroxylase activity and 7α-hydroxylase mRNA levels. [Buhman KK; Furumoto EJ, Donkin SS, Story JA; Dietary psyllium increases faecal bile acid excretion, total steroid excretion and bile acid biosynthesis in rats, *J Nutr* **128**(7), 1199-203 (1998)].

Different soluble dietary fibres known to alter cholesterol metabolism were fed to golden Syrian hamsters and their specific impact on lipoproteins, biliary bile acid profile, and faecal sterol excretion was evaluated. Compared to control, psyllium caused a significant reduction in plasma cholesterol, whereas pectin or guar gum had no apparent effect on plasma lipids. Hepatic total and esterified cholesterol were substantially decreased with psyllium, pectin and guar gum but psyllium produced the most pronounced effect. In contrast to pectin and guar gum, psyllium caused a significant increase in the cholate : chenodeoxycholate and the glycine : taurine conjugation ratio. Pectin and guar gum did not alter daily faecal neutral sterol excretion while psyllium caused a 90% increase due to a higher faecal output. Daily faecal bile acid excretion and total faecal bile acid concentration were significantly increased by psyllium, whereas pectin and guar gum revealed only minor effects. The unequal hypocholesterolemic effects of psyllium, pectin, and guar gum on cholesterol and bile acid metabolism in hamsters are possibly related to different physicochemical properties. [Trautwein EA, Rieckhoff D, Kunath Rau A, Erbersdobler HF; Psyllium, not pectin or guar gum, alters lipoprotein and biliary bile acid composition and faecal sterol excretion in the hamster, *Lipids* **33**(6), 573-82 (1998)].

The lipid-lowering effect of psyllium is well established. Enhanced faecal bile acid excretion and stimulation of hepatic bile acid synthesis are discussed as primary mechanisms of this action. Psyllium significantly lowered plasma total cholesterol and triacylglycerol at a magnitude comparable to that induced by cholestyramine in male golden Syrian hamsters fed lithogenic diets. Psyllium did not prevent the hepatic storage of esterified cholesterol but both psyllium and cholestyramine caused distinct alterations in the bile acid profile. Psyllium caused a selective reduction of taurine-conjugated bile acids, especially of taurochenodeoxycholate. As a result, the glycine : taurine conjugation and the cholate : chenodeoxycholate ratios were significantly higher in psyllium-fed hamsters. Psyllium and cholestyramine normalised the lithogenic index and prevented cholesterol gallstone formation compared with controls. The data emphasise the potent lipid-lowering effect of psyllium. Increased faecal bile acid excretion and alterations of the circulating bile acid pool by removal of dihydroxy bile acids (e.g., taurochenodeoxycholate) appear to be main modulators of the hypocholesterolemic action of psyllium by leading to an up-regulation of hepatic bile acid synthesis. [Trautwein EA, Kunath Rau A, Erbersdobler HF; Increased faecal bile acid excretion and changes in the circulating bile acid pool are involved in the hypocholesterolemic and gallstone-preventive actions of psyllium in hamsters, *J Nutr* **129**(4), 896-902 (1999)].

Two groups of female Wistar rats were fed cholesterol-enriched (1% cholesterol and 0.2% cholic acid) semipurified diets containing either 3% cellulose or psyllium for a period of 8 weeks. Cholesterol-enriched diets resulted in a progressive increase in plasma cholesterol levels in both groups during the entire period of the experiment. The rats fed with psyllium, however, had significantly lower plasma cholesterol concentrations than the animals fed with cellulose throughout the experimental period. Most of the plasma cholesterol in both groups at the end of the study was located in the very low density lipoprotein (VLDL) fraction and differences in total plasma cholesterol concentrations were predominantly reflected in differences in VLDL-cholesterol. Liver cholesterol concentrations paralleled the concentrations of plasma cholesterol and were significantly lower in the psyllium-fed rats than in the cellulose-fed rats. Substitution of psyllium for cellulose resulted in an increase in the excretion of faecal bile acids and this increase was predominantly caused by an increased excretion of β-muricholic acid and the bile acids derived from β-muricholic acid. [Terpstra AHM, Lapre JA, de Vries HT, Beynen AC; Hypocholesterolemic effect of dietary psyllium in female rats, *Ann Nutr Metab* **44**(5-6), 223-28 (2000)].

Soluble fibres, including those from psyllium husk, have been shown to augment the cholesterol-lowering effects of a low-fat diet in persons with hypercholesterolemia. A meta analysis was conducted to more precisely define the hypolipidemic effects and safety of psyllium when used adjunctive to a low-fat diet in men and women with hypercholesterolemia. The results of the analysis indicated that psyllium supplementation significantly lowered serum total and LDL-cholesterol concentrations in subjects consuming a low fat diet. Psyllium is well tolerated and safe when used adjunctive to a low fat diet in individuals with mild-to-moderate hypercholesterolemia. [Anderson JW, Allgood LD, Lawrence A, Altringer LA, Jerdack GR, Hengehold DA, Morel JG; Cholesterol-lowering effects of psyllium intake adjunctive to diet therapy in men and women with hypercholesterolemia: Meta analysis of 8 controlled trials, *Am J Clin Nutr* **71**(2), 472-79 (2000)].

See Pectin in Appendix: [Terpstra *et al.*, *Nahrung* **46**(2), 83-86 (2002)].

In patients with mild or moderate hypercholesterolemia, the cholesterol-lowering effect of psyllium husk was investigated. Consumption of 10,15 or 20 g of psyllium husk, twice daily, reduced the raised serum cholesterol levels in a dose dependant manner as compared to their initial value. Almost similar lowering effect of psyllium husk on other lipid components was also noted in these patients. [Jain S, Katarey C; The efficacy of Psyllium husk in hypercholesterolemic patients in Gwalior city, *Nutrition Society of India, 35th Annual Meeting* NIN, Hyderabad p.66, Dec 12-13, 2003].

Psyllium intake decreases plasma LDL-cholesterol (LDL-c) in men and pre and post-menopausal women but its effects on plasma triglycerides are sex related. A significant decrease in plasma triglycerides was observed in men while postmenopausal women experienced an increase in plasma triglycerides concentrations following psyllium supplementation. The mechanisms by which sex and hormonal status influence the effects of psyllium on plasma lipids were explored and it was suggested that the LDL-c lowering induced by psyllium was related to changes in HMG-CoA reductase gene expression in monocytes while the expression of lipoprotein lipase in this system was affected by sex and hormonal status. [Vega Lopez S, Freake HC, Fernandez ML; Sex and hormonal status modulate the effects of psyllium on plasma lipids and monocyte gene expression in humans, J *Nutr* **133**(1), 67-70 (2003)].

The hypolipidemic effects of two solid-state enzymatically- modified psyllium preparations were compared to that of the original psyllium husks in hamsters. The results of the investigation suggest that improving the functional properties of psyllium by solid-state enzymatic procedures does not alter psyllium-mediated hypolipidemic effects. [Allen Kenneth GD, Bristow SJ, Yu L; Hypolipidemic effects of modified psyllium preparations, *J Agric Food Chem* **52**(16), 4998-5003 (2004)].

Plumbago indica: See *Commiphora mukul:* [Mary et al.; *Phytomedicine* **10**(6-7), 474-82 (2003)].

Plumbago zeylanica (H. Chita, S. Chitraka): See *Piper longum* [Sharma et al., *Int J Crude Drug Res* **28**(1), 33-38 (1990)].

Feeding of plumbagin, isolated from roots of *P. zeylanica,* to hyperlipidemic rabbits reduced serum cholesterol (53-86%) and LDL- cholesterol (61-91%). It also lowered cholesterol/ phospholipid ratio (45.8%) and significantly elevated HDL-cholesterol levels. Besides this, plumbagin decreased the cholesterol and triglyceride contents of liver and aorta and regressed the atheromatous plaques in thoracic and abdominal aorta. Faecal cholesterol and phospholipids excretion was also increased in plumbagin-treated animals. [Sharma I, Gusain D, Dixit VP; Hypolipidemic and antiatherosclerotic effects of plumbagin in rabbits, *Indian J Physiol Pharmacol* **35**(1), 10-14 (1991)].

Effect of *P. zeylanica* in hyperlipidemic rabbits and its modification by vitamin E have been discussed. [Dwivedi S; Effect of *Plumbago zeylanica* in hyperlipidemic rabbits and its modification by vitamin E, *Indian J Pharmacol* **29**(2), 138 (1997)].

Polygala senega (Senegae Radix) The hypolipidemic effect of Senegae Radix was investigated in normal and hyperlipidemic mice. The n-butanol fraction of the methanol extract of Senega root (5 mg/kg) significantly reduced the blood triglyceride level of normal mice 7 hours after intraperitoneal administration and also significantly reduced the blood triglyceride level of cholesterol-fed mice under similar conditions. The fraction also decreased the blood triglyceride level in Triton-induced hyperlipidemia. It is suggested that this fraction contains one or more hypolipidemic components including the main triterpenoid glycoside, senegin-II, which significantly reduces the levels of blood triglycerides in normal mice. [Masuda H, Ohsumi K, Kako M, Miura T, Nishiyama Y, Ichimaru M, Moriyasu M, Kato A; Intraperitoneal administration of *Senegae Radix* extract and its main component, senegin-II, affects lipid metabolism in normal and hyperlipidemic mice, *Biol Pharm Bull* **19**(2), 315-17 (1996)].

Polygonatum odoratum (Rhizoma *Polygonatum odorati*)**:** Adminstration of water-soluble extract of *P. odoratum* rhizomes for four weeks to diabetic mice and rats, significantly decreased and prevented hypertriglyceridemia. The extract also lowered fasting blood sugar levels, glycosylated haemoglobin and improved glucose tolerance in diabetic animals. [Chen H, Feng R, Guo Y, Sun L, Jiang J; Hypoglycemic effects of aqueous extract of rhizoma *Polygonatum odorati* in mice and rats, *J Ethnopharmacol* **74**(3), 225-29 (2001)].

***Polygonatum sewezowii*:** See Polysaccharides in Appendix: [Khushbaktova *et al.*; *Khim Farma Zh* **21**(11), 1348-52 (1987)].

***Polygonum cuspidatum*:** The stilbene compounds (resveratrol and piceid), isolated from roots of the plant, prevented deposition of cholesterol and triglycerides in the liver of rats fed with a mixture of cholesterol, corn oil and cholic acid. Administration of piceid caused reduction of serum triglycerides, LDL-cholesterol and atherogenic index of these rats. The stilbenes also decreased the hepatic triglyceride synthesis from ^{14}C-palmitate. [Arichi H, Kimura Y, Okuda H, Baba K, Kozagawa M, Arichi S; Effect of stilbene compounds of the roots of *Polygonum cuspidatum* on lipid metabolism, *Chem Pharm Bull* **30**(5), 1766-70 (1982)].

Polygonum multiflorum: Administration *P. multiflorum* and *Trichiurus chinensis* to normal rats, lowered serum cholesterol levels by 25%. [Mei-chen M, Qing-qi E, Gui-chen L, Wan-Jin X; Screening method for hypocholesterolemic agents, *Acta Pharm Sin* **14**(1), 8-11 ((1979)].

The albino rats treated with *P. multiflorum* roots exhibited a reduction in plasma total cholesterol and high density lipoprotein cholesterol levels. The plasma and liver lipoprotein lipase activity and the ratio of lipoprotein lipase and total lipase activity were increased in treated rats. [Zhang Z, Zhuang QQ, Mei MZ; Effect of some drugs on plasma and liver LPL activities and cholesterol levels in rats, *Acta Pharma Sin* **18**(6), 468-71 (1983)].

Polygonum tinctorium: Administration of *P. tinctorium* to high fat diet-induced hyperlipidemic mice, significantly reduced the serum cholesterol and triglyceride levels. [Inoue SI, Takyama S, Shio S, Iwaki K, Ohashi K, Masaki N, Fukuda S, Kurimato M; Improvement of high fat diet induced hyperlipidemia by *Polygonum tinctorium* Lour, *Natural Medicines* **54**(5), 261-264 (2000)].

***Poncirus trifoliata*:** See *Curcuma zedoaria:* [Liu *et al.*; *Am J Chin Med* **30**(4), 629-36 (2002)].

***Premna tomentosa*:** The hypolipidemic effect of *Premna tomentosa* in acetaminophen induced hepatotoxicity in rats was elucidated. Pretreatment of animals with the plant extract (750 mg/kg, orally) for 15 days significantly inhibited acetaminophen-induced alterations in the levels of cholesterol, triglycerides, free fatty acids, phospholipids, serum lipoproteins, and lipid-metabolising enzymes and resulted in improvement of lipid metabolism. [Devi KP, Sreepriya M, Balakrishna K, Veluchamy G, Devaki T; Assessment of the protective potential of *Premna tomentosa* L. (Verbenaceae) extract on lipid profile and lipid-metabolizing enzymes in acetaminophen-intoxicated rats, *J Altern Complement Med* **10**(3), 540-46 (2004)].

***Prosopis cineraria*:** See *Capparis deciduas:* [Agarwal and Chauhanm; *Plant Foods Hum Nutr* **38**(2), 189-97 (1988)].

Prunella vulgaris (Dharu)**:** The extracts of leaves, stem and rhizomes of *P. vulgaris* exhibited hypocholesterolemic, analgesic and anti-inflammatory activities. [Dhanabal SP, Arun Kumar, Suresh B; Pharmacological and biochemical studies on *Prunella vulgaris, International seminar on recent trends in Pharmaceutical Sciences,* Ootacmund, India, Abstract No E-47, February 18-20, 1995].

Prunus amygdalus (Almonds, H. Badam, S. Badama): In normolipidemic rabbits, the effect of whole seeds, defatted seeds and oil of *P. amygdalus* on lipid profile was investigated. *P. amygdalus,* in all the above mentioned forms, decreased serum total cholesterol, triglycerides, LDL and VLDL- cholesterols alongwith an increase in phospholipids, faecal sterols and HDL- cholesterol. Maximum activity was noted in whole seeds followed by oil and defatted seeds. [Teotia S, Man Singh, Pant MC; Effect of *Prunus amygdalus* seeds on lipid profile, *Indian J Physiol Pharmacol* **41**(4), 483-89 (1997)].

***Prunus bokharensis*:** See *Berberis aristata:* [Kamran & Ahmad; *Int J Pharmacogn* **30**(1), 5- 8 (1992)].

***Prunus davidiana*:** A significant decrease of blood triglyceride and total cholesterol was observed in rats, fed on high fat diets, on administration of the methanolic extract of *P. davidiana* stems for 6 days. The extract also improved the atherogenic index of these rats. In addition to the hypolipemic effect, the methanolic extract was also shown to be effective in reducing an elevated level of glucose in rats with hyperlipemia resulting from high fat feeding. On the other hand, blood triglyceride and total cholesterol in rats, fed with stock diet, were not affected significantly by administration of the methanolic extract of the plant. [Choi JS, Suh SS, Young HS, Park HJ; Hypolipemic and hypoglycemic activities of *Prunus davidiana* in high fat-fed rats, *Arch Pharm Res* **14**(1), 44-7 (1991)].

Methanolic extract of *Prunus davidiana* and its main component prunin, when given intraperitoneally to streptozotocin-induced diabetic rats, produced significant lowering of total blood lipids and sugar levels. It was suggested that the methanolic extract of this plant contained one or more principles including prunin which were responsible for hypolipidemic and hypoglycemic activity in diabetic rats. [Choi JS, Yokozawa T, Oura J; Improvement of hypoglycemia and hyperlipidemia in streptozotocin diabetic rats by a methanolic extract of *Prunus davidiana* stem and its main component prunin, *Planta Med* **57**(3), 208-11 (1991)].

Blood lipid levels in rats with hyperlipidemia resulting from high fat feeding were determined after ip administration of a methanolic extract of *P. davidiana* stems and its flavonoid components, (+)-catechin, prunin and hesperetin 5-O-glucoside. Administration of the extract for 3 days produced a significant decrease of blood triglyceride and total cholesterol, the atherogenic index was also improved. (+)-Catechin was shown to be effective in reducing the elevated level of triglyceride. Prunin and hesperetin 5-O-glucoside did not show such an effect in high fat-fed hypertriglyceridemic rats, but they did exhibit a significant hypocholesterolemic effect.

[Choi JS, Yokozawa T, Oura H; Antihyperlipidemic effect of flavonoides from *Prunus davidiana*, *J Nat Prod*, **54**(1), 218-24 (1991)].

Prunus persica (H. Aru): See *Typha angustifolia*: [Park *et al.*; *Phytother Res* **18**(3), 224-29 (2004).].

Prunus species (Prune, dried plum): Elevated level of cholesterol is quite common among women who have experienced natural or surgical menopause and this has been linked to ovarian hormone deficiency. The efficacy of prune, a good source of dietary fibre and phytochemicals, on lowering cholesterol in an ovariectomized rat model was studied. Ovariectomy of 90 day-old female Sprague-Dawley rats elevated serum total cholesterol by 22% and high dose (25%) of prune diet prevented this increase without affecting high density lipoprotein cholesterol concentrations. Animals fed with high dose of prune diet had lower liver total lipids compared with ovariectomized animals. The findings of this study showed that prune exhibits hypocholesterolemic properties in ovarian hormone deficiency. Dose-response studies should be conducted to establish the effectiveness of prune in prevention of hypercholesterolemia in postmenopausal women who are not on estrogen replacement therapy and seek dietary alternatives. [Lucas EA, Juma S, Stoecker BJ, Arjmandi BH; Prune suppresses ovariectomy-induced hypercholesterolemia in rats, *J Nutr Biochem* **11**(5), 255-59 (2000)].

Psophocarpus tetragonolobus (Winged bean): See *Cicer arietinum* (Bengal gram): [Sharma RD, *Nutr Res* **7**(4), 351-64 (1987)].

Psoralea corrylifolia (H. Babchi, S. Bakuchi)**:** See *Artemisia* species: [Jing *et al.*; *Chin J Integ Trad West Med* **6**(1), 21-23(1986)].

***Psychotria forsteriana*:** Quadrigemine B, quadrigemine A, isopsychotridine C and psychotridine, isolated from *P. forsteriana*, effectively inhibited the ADP, collagen or thrombin-induced aggregation of washed human platelets. [Beretz A, Roth-Georger A, Corre G, Kuballa B, Anton R, Cazenave JP; Polyindolinic alkaloids from *Psychotria forsteriana*: Potent inhibitors of aggregation of human platelets, *Planta Med* (4) 300-03 (1985)].

Pterocarpus marsupium (H. Bijasar. S. Vijayasara)**:** Administration of a decoction of the bark of *P. marsupium* to hypercholesterolemic rabbits significantly lowered the serum cholesterol levels. [Pandey MC, Sharma PV; Hypocholesterolemic effect of bark of *Pterocarpus marsupium* Roxb. (Bijaka): An experimental study, *J Res Indian Med Yoga Homeo* **13**(1), 137-39 (1978)].

The effects of oral administration of ethyl acetate extract of *P. marsupium* heartwood as well of its flavonoid constituents (marsupsin, pterosupin and liquiritigenin) to diet and triton-induced hyperlipidemic rats were studied. Administration of ethyl acetate extract for 14 days caused significant reduction of serum triglyceride, total cholesterol and LDL- and VLDL-cholesterol levels without any significant effect on HDL-cholesterol. Liquiritigenin and pterosupin significantly decreased serum total cholesterol, LDL-cholesterol and atherogenic index, pterosupin being additionally effective in lowering serum triglycerides. [Jahoromi MAF, Ray AB, Chansouria JPN; Antihyperlipidemic effect of flavonoids from *Pterocarpus marsupium*, *J Nat Prod* **56**(7), 989-94 (1993)].

See *Allium sativum* (Garlic): [Dwivedi S; *Ann Natl Acad Med Scs* (India) 32(3&4) 159- 175(1996)].

Pueraria lobata: Total isoflavones from *P. lobata* significantly decreased concentrations of serum total cholesterol and liver triglyceride in ovariectomized rats. [Zheng G, Zhang X, Zheng J, Gong W, Zheng X, Chen A; Hypocholesterolemic effect of total isoflavones from *Pueraria lobata* in ovariectomized rats, *Zhong Yao Cai* **25**(4), 273-75 (2002) [Article in Chinese].

Pueraria thunbergiana: Tectorigenin and kaikasaponin III from the flowers of *P. thunbergiana* showed potent hypoglycemic and hypolipidemic effects in the streptozotocin induced diabetic rats. Intraperitoneal administration of these two compounds (5 and 10 mg/kg, respectively) for seven days to streptozotocin-induced rats significantly reduced the blood glucose, total cholesterol, LDL and VLDL-cholesterol and triglyceride levels when compared with those of control group. Tectorigenin showed *in vitro* antioxidant effects on 1,1-diphenyl-2- pirylhydrazyl radical, xanthine-xanthine oxidase superoxide anion radical, and lipid peroxidation in rat microsomes induced by enzymatic and non-enzymatic methods. Tectorigenin and kaikasaponin III protected the Vero cell line from injury by hydrogen peroxide. From these findings, it seems likely that the antioxidant action of tectorigenin and kaikasaponin III may alleviate the streptozotocin-induced toxicity and contribute to hypoglycemic and hypolipidemic effects. [Lee KT, Sohn Il Cheol, Kim DH, Choi JW, Kwon SH, Park HJ; Hypoglycemic and hypolipidemic effects of tectorigenin and kaikasaponin III in the streptozotocin-induced diabetic rat and their antioxidant activity *in vitro, Arch Pharm Res* (Seoul) **23**(5), 461-66 (2000)].

The effect of kaikasaponin III, obtained from the flower of *P. thunbergiana,* on Phase I and II enzymes and tissue factor activity was investigated to elucidate the pharmacological actions of this immunosuppressive saponin in the diabetic rat. The saponin prolonged the bleeding time and plasma clotting time in streptozotocin-treated rats and increased the tissue factor activity, suggesting that this compound has anti-thrombotic activity in streptozotocin-induced diabetic rats. It also inhibited the formation of malondialdehyde and hydroxy radicals in serum and liver, but promoted superoxide dismutase activity. Low malondialdehyde concentrations and low xanthine oxidase and aldehyde oxidase activities were observed in kaikasaponin III -treated rats, suggesting that such Phase I enzyme activities are the major source of lipid peroxidation. However, the saponin increased Phase II enzyme activities such as superoxide dismutase, glutathione peroxidase, and catalase, suggesting the activation of free radical-scavenging enzymes. From the results of the investigation, it was suggested that kaikasaponin III might exhibit its hypoglycemic and hypolipidemic effects by up-regulating or down-regulating antioxidant mechanisms *via* the changes in Phase I and II enzyme activities. [Choi J, Shin MH, Park KY, Lee KT, Jung HJ, Lee MS, Park HJ; Effect of kaikasaponin III obtained from *Pueraria thunbergiana* flowers on serum and hepatic lipid peroxides and tissue factor activity in the streptozotocin-induced diabetic rat, *J Med Food* **7**(1), 31-37 (2004)].

Punica granatum (Pomegranate, H. Anar, S. Dadim): Inhibition of lipid peroxidation contributes to the attenuation of macrophage cholesterol accumulation, foam cell formation and atherosclerosis. Evidence suggests that nutritional antioxidants such as pomegranate juice can contribute to the reduction of oxidative stress and atherogenesis. Pomegranate juice supplementation to mice with advanced atherosclerosis reduced their macrophage oxidative stress, macrophage cholesterol flux and even attenuated the development of atherosclerosis. Moreover, a tannin-fraction isolated from pomegranate juice had a significant antiatherosclerotic activity. [Kaplan M, Hayek T, Raz A, Coleman R, Dornfeld L, Vaya J, Aviram M; Pomegranate juice supplementation to atherosclerotic mice reduces macrophage lipid peroxidation, cellular cholesterol accumulation and development of atherosclerosis, *J Nutr* **131**(8), 2082-9 (2001)].

Pyrola rotundifolia: The hyperlipidemic patients treated with a Pyrola compound preparation and *P. rotundifolia* alone exhibited a significant reduction in serum cholesterol levels. The Pyrola compound was relatively more effective than the *P. rotundifolia* alone. [Chaohog W, Chuiguang W; Clinical observation on the treatment of 101 hypertensive patients with *Pyrola rotundifolia* preparation, *Chin J Integ Trad West Med* **6**(10), 604-05 (1986)].

Q

***Quercus robur*:** See Proanthocyanidin polymer in Appendix: [Khushbaktova *et al.*; *Khim Farma Zh* **23**(9), 1111-15 (1989)].

***Quillaja saponaria*:** See Saponins and sapogenins in Appendix: [Sidhu & Oakenfull; *Brit J Nutr* **55**(3), 643-50 (1986)].

The relationship between growth depression due to saponins and their cholesterol-lowering effect was investigated under different dietary conditions. Tea and *Quillaja* saponins retarded chick growth rate; the former was more toxic than the latter when cholesterol was not included in the diet. However, the addition of cholesterol alone or together with beef tallow alleviated the growth depression due to saponins partly or completely, the extent of which depended on the dietary saponin levels. Phytosterols and cholestyramine completely prevented the increase in serum cholesterol concentrations due to dietary cholesterol alone or together with beef tallow or sodium cholate. On the other hand, the hypocholesterolemic effect of the two saponins was only observed when cholesterol and beef tallow were incorporated simultaneously into the diet but even in this case, the effect of saponin was inferior to that of phytosterols or cholestyramine. Thus, the growth-depressing effect of saponin was not always accompanied by the hypocholesterolemic effect. [Ueda H, Tanoue K; Growth-depressing and cholesterol lowering effects of Quillaja and tea saponins in chicks as influenced by diet composition, *Animal Sci J* **71**(4), 393-99 (2000)].

See *Yucca schidigera:* [Kim et al.; *Arch Pharm Res* **26**(12), 1042-46 (2003)].

R

Ramulus mori (Sangzhi)**:** Administration of aqueous extract of sangzhi (*R. mori*) to alloxan diabetic rats for 15 days, led to lowering of blood lipid components. This drug also exhibited antidiabetic activity. Hyperglycemia related renal pathological changes were reduced and blood N-acetyl-β-D-glucosaminolase (NAG) activity was reduced following treatment with this plant extract. [Ye F, Shen Z, Qiao F, Zhao D, Xie M; Experimental treatment of complications in alloxan diabetic rats with α-glucosidase inhibitor from the Chinese medicinal herb, *Ramulus mori*, *Acta Pharm Sin* **37**(2), 108-12 (2002)].

Raphanus radicula**:** See Flavonoids in Appendix: [Khushbaktova *et al.*; *Khim Farma Zh* **25**(4), 53-57 (1991)].

Raphanus sativus* var. *niger (Black radish, H. Muli, S. Mulaka)**:** An improvement in all the high fat diet induced histological changes (disruption of epithelial linning, reduction in number of enterocytes and inflammatiom in the mucosa of colon) was observed following administration of granules prepared from the roots of black radish. In treated animals, the mucosal epithelial cells appeared normal without any inflammation. [Sipos P, Hagymasi K, Lugasi A, Felier E, Blazovics A; Effect of black reddish root (*Raphanus sativus* L. var. *niger*) on colon mucosa in rats fed with a fat rich diet, *Phytother Res* **16**(7), 677-79 (2002)].

Administration of black radish juice to lipid rich diet (sunflower oil 20%, cholesterol 2%, cholic acid 0.5%) fed rats, significantly decreased serum cholesterol, triglyceride, malondialdehyde, conjugated diene and liver cholesterol contents. The antioxidant activity of this plant is believed to be responsible for its hypolipidemic effect. [Lugasi A, Blazovics A, Hagymasi K, Labovics VK, Kocsis I, Kery A,

"Beneficial health effect of black radish (*Raphanus sativus* L. var. niger) in *in vitro* and *in vivo* experimental conditions" in *Recent progress in medicinal plants: Phytochemistry and pharmacology*, JN Govil, VK Singh (eds.) Studium press, LLC, Houston, Texas, USA, p.355-373 (2003).

[***Rhapanticum carthamoides***: See Flavonoids in Appendix: [Khushbaktova *et al.*; *Khim Farma Zh* **25**(4), 53-57 (1991)].

Rheum officinale: See *Aloe vera:* [Nada *et al.*; *Fitoterapia* **68**(3), 240-44 (1997)].

Rheum palmatum (Rhubarb): See Proanthocyanidin polymer in Appendix: [Khushbaktova *et al.*; *Khim Farma Zh* **23**(9), 1111-15 (1989)].

Galloyl glucoses and galloyl proanthocynidins, isolated from *R. palmatum*, significantly inhibited rat squalene epoxidase. In view of these observations, the cholesterol-lowering effect of rhubarb may be attributed to inhibition of squalene epoxidase, a rate-limiting enzyme of cholesterol biosynthesis. [Abe I, Seki T, Noguchi H, Kashiwada Y; Galloyl esters from rhubarb are potent inhibitors of squalene epoxidase, a key enzyme in cholesterol biosynthesis, *Planta Med* **66**(8), 753-56 (2000)].

The hypolipidemic and pancreatic lipase inhibitory activity of rhizome of *R. palmatum* was investigated in triton (WR-1339) induced hyperlipidemic mice. Rheum significantly decreased total cholesterol and triglyceride levels. However, in high cholesterol diet-induced hyperlipidemic mice, it did not affect the lipid parameters. *R. palmatum* effectively inhibited the pancreatic lipase activity *in vitro* with IC_{50} value of 6.5 mg/ml. [Yang HK, Kim YS, Bae HS, Cho KH, Shin JE, Kim NJ, Kim DH; *Rhei rhizoma* and chunghyuldan inhibit pancreatic lipase, *Nat Prod Sci* **9**(1), 38-43 (2003)].

Rheum rhaponticum (Rhubarb): A new fibre source was developed by blanching, drying and grinding the fresh stalks of rhubarb, an universal crop. The product was found to contain 74% total dietary fibre (66% insoluble and 8% soluble dietary fibre), on dry weight basis. Preliminary studies involving experimental animals and hypercholesterolemic subjects revealed that this fibre source is potentially hypolipidemic, though the underlying mechanism still remains unknown. However, its potential to complex with bile salts was studied *in vitro* and its ability to bind taurocholate was better than that of cellulose and wheat bran. This ability to bind bile salts might be responsible for its hypocholesterolemic action observed in experimental animals and humans. [Goel V, Cheema SK, Agellon LB, Ooraikul B, McBurney MI, Basu TK; *In vitro* binding of bile salt to rhubarb stalk powder, *Nutr Res* **18**(5), 893-903 (1998)].

Dietary fibre, produced from rhubarb (*R. rhaponticum*) stalks, is potentially hypolipidemic. Animals fed on rhubarb fibre had significantly lower activity of acyl CoA: Cholesterol acyltransferase than the mice maintained on a diet containing cellulose and cholesterol. Feeding of rhubarb fibre accelerated the faecal bile-acid loss and diminished the gall-bladder bile-acid pool in both the normal and the cholesterol-fed mice. The increase in the bile-acid excretion was positively correlated with an increased activity as well as mRNA abundance of cholesterol 7α-hydroxylase. The increased excretion of bile acids and induction of cholesterol 7α- hydroxylase activity may account for the hypocholesterolemic effect of rhubarb fibre. [Goel V, Cheema SK, Agellon LB, Ooraikul B, Basu TK; Dietary rhubarb (*Rheum rhaponticum*) stalk fibre stimulates cholesterol 7α-hydroxylase gene expression and bile acid excretion in cholesterol-fed C57BL/6J mice, *British J Nutr* **81**(1), 65-71 (1999)].

Rosa canina (Rose hip): Male golden Syrian hamsters were fed diets supplemented with 15% (w/w) rose hip, sunflower, olive or cocoanut oils during four weeks and their plasma lipid levels were assessed. In contrast to olive oil and coconut oil (saturated fats), which showed hyperlipidemic effect, rose hip and sunflower oils presented a marked hypolipidemic effect, presumably due to specific action of n-6 linoleic acid. [Gonzalez I, Escobar M, Olivera P; Plasma lipids of golden Syrian hamsters fed with dietary rose hip, sunflower, olive and coconut oils, *Rev Esp Fisiol* **53**(2), 199-204 (1997)].

Rosa indica (H. Gulab): See *Berberis aristata:* [Kamran & Ahmad; *Int J Pharmacogn* **30**(1), 5-8 (1992)].

S

Saccharum officinarum (Sugarcane, H. Ganna, S. Ikshu)**:** Effects of sugar cane wax on serum and liver lipids were studied in male Wistar rats fed with a high level of plant (corn oil) or animal (lard) fat. The addition of 0.5% cane wax to dietary fat caused a significant reduction in the concentration of serum triacylglycerol, while the cholesterol level was significantly decreased only in rats reared on the lard diet. Cane wax did not apparently affect the concentration of liver lipids. Dietary fats and the addition of cane wax to the diet did not affect the faecal excretion of neutral and acidic steroids. The mechanism responsible for the reduction of cholesterol by cane wax may be mediated by changes in cholesterol metabolism in the body, but not faecal steroids. [Fukuda N, Sato M, Oku H, Sho H, Chinen I; Effects of sugar cane wax on serum and liver lipids of rats, *Nippon Nogeikagaku Kaishi* **60**(12), 1023-26 (1986)].

Effect of alkaline extract of bagasse on serum and liver lipid concentration was studied in rats fed with cholesterol and sodium cholate in combination. The alkaline extract was separated into two fractions based on solubility (fraction A and B). Both fractions were found to have potent hypocholesterolemic activity. Fraction B appeared to be more active than fraction A in lowering serum cholesterol concentration. The feeding of the bagasse extract also lowered liver cholesterol concentration. Reduction of serum or liver cholesterol concentration was not always accompanied by increased faecal steroid excretion. [Oku H, Fukuda N, Mori M, Kinjyo M; Motono H, Chinen I; Hypocholesterolemic effect of bagasse alkaline extract in rats fed with atherogenic diet, *Nutr Reports International* **38**(4), 843-52 (1988)].

A herbominiral compound drug (AKRS), prepared from juices of *S. officinarum,*

Opuntia dillenii, Vinca rosea, Bambusa arundinacea, Aristolochia bracteata, Curcuma longa, Cynanchum viminale, Solanum trilobatum, Calotropis gigantea, Cephalandra indica and ferrous sulphate, significantly lowered cholesterol and triglyceride levels in hyperlipidemic rats. The results suggest that this drug prevents assimilation of dietary lipids. [Tarvady S, Dhar SC; Drastic lowering of serum lipid markers by a herbomineral hypolipidemic agent, *Biomedicine* **9**(1), 39-42 (1989)].

The hypocholesterolemic activity of bagasse powder and of products, obtained by three different treatments of bagasse alkaline extract, was studied in rats fed with high cholesterol diets. Treatments of 8% alkaline extracts of bagasse included; acid precipitation and freeze-drying (A), ethanol precipitation and freeze-drying (B-fd) and spray drying (B-sd). Bagasse showed no effect on serum and liver lipids levels. However, high cholesterol diets with bagasse extracts at 3% caused a significant reduction in the concentration of serum cholesterol without influencing food intake and growth. Fraction B-fd was most effective and fractions A and B-sd to a lesser extent, suggesting an activity loss during spray drying. Fraction B-fd also lowered hepatic cholesterol level. No apparent effect was observed on the other lipid classes in serum or liver. Dietary bagasse extracts did not alter the excretion of neutral and acidic steroids, suggesting that the reduction in serum and liver cholesterol levels was not mediated through steroid excretion. [Fukuda N, Oku H, Yoshihara I, Machida M, Chinen I; Effect of bagasse alkaline extract on serum and liver lipids of rats fed high cholesterol diets, *Nippon Nogeikagaku Kaishi* **63**(10), 1599-1606 (1989)].

Cholesterol-lowering activity of enzymatic hydrolysate of bagasse alkaline extract was studied in rats fed with a cholesterol-enriched diet. The bagasse alkaline extract was found to be vulnerable to the enzymic attack of . α-amylase. Thus the alkaline extract was degraded into two fractions: Long-chain fraction (polysaccharides) and short-chain fraction (oligosaccharides). The long-chain fraction was active in lowering the serum cholesterol level while feeding the short-chain fraction resulted in a slightly elevated serum cholesterol level. The feeding by gavage of the long-chain fraction 12 h after the meal was also effective in lowering serum cholesterol concentration. Possible mechanisms responsible for the cholesterol lowering activity of the extract were discussed. [Oku H, Kayano K, Miyagi M, Chinen I; Hypocholesterolemic activity of α-amylase hydrolysate of bagasse alkaline extract in rats fed with atherogenic diet, *J Nutr Sci Vitaminol* **35**(5), 481-94 (1989)].

Administration of AKRS, a herbominiral compound drug containing *Saccharum officinarum, Opuntia dillenii, Vinca rosea, Bambusa arundinacea, Aristolochia bracteata, Curcuma longa, Cynanchum viminale, Solanum trilobatum, Calotropis gigantea, Cephalandra indica* and Ferrous sulphate, to lipid-supplemented diet-fed albino rats for 5 months decreased blood cholesterol and triglycerides [Tarvady S, Dhar SC, Effect of new herbominiral hypolipidemic agent on plasma lipoprotein patterns in rat atherocslerosis, *Indian J Exp Biol* **28**(7), 657-60 (1990)].

D-003, a mixture of long-chain aliphatic acids purified from sugarcane, at 5 and 10 mg/day demonstrated a dose-dependent cholesterol-lowering effects in healthy volunteers characterised by reductions in LDL-c, total cholesterol and atherogenic index, and increases in HDL-c. Effects on triglycerides were modest and uncertain. D-003 inhibited the susceptibility of LDL to lipid peroxidation. Further studies investigating the effect of larger doses and treatment for longer duration are necessary to confirm the reproducibility of the present results in different study populations. [Castano G, Menendez R, Mas R, Ledon N, Fernandez J, Perez J, Gonzalez RM, Lezcay M; Effects of D-003, a new hypocholesterolaemic and antiplatelet compound, on lipid profile and lipid peroxidation in healthy volunteers, *Clin Drug Investigation* **23**(3), 193- 203 (2003)].

Salacia prinoides: Root bark powder of *S. prinoides* significantly decreased serum total cholesterol, triglycerides alongwith enhancement of HDL cholesterol levels in patients of noninsulin dependent diabetes mellitus (NIDDM). Blood glucose levels were also significantly decreased in these treated patients without any side effects [Kowsallya S, Chandrashekar U, Geetha N; Development and evaluation of a hypoglycemic tablet with the herb *Solacia prinoides* (Ekanayakam), *Indian J Nutr Diet* **32**(2), 33-39 (1995)].

Administration of root bark powder of *S. prinoides* (500mg) and a combination of *S. prinoides* and *Strychonos potatorum* (in equal proportions) to 42 patients of non insulin dependant diabetes mellitus for two months exhibited hypocholesterolemic and hypoglycemic activity. [Kowsallya S, Chandrashekar U, Sharmila JB; Development and evaluation of hypoglycemic tablets from selected herbs, *Indian J Nutr Diet* **33**(9), 208-15 (1996)].

Salvadora persica (H. Chhotapilu, S. Brahat Pilu): Administration of a lyophilized decoction of *S. persica* stems to diet-induced hypercholesterolemic rats for 15 and 30 days (by gavage at a dose of 500 mg/kg in an aqueous vehicle in a volume of 0.5 ml/100 g bw) significantly lowered plasma cholesterol and LDL levels. Better activity was observed at 30 days of treatment. [Galati EM, Monforte MT, Forestieri AM, Miceli N, Bader A, Trovato A, Bader A; *Salvadora persica* L.: Hypolipidemic activity on experimental hypercholesterolemia in rat, *Phytomedicine* **6**(3), 181-85 (1999)].

Salvia militiorrhiza: Decoctions of *S. militiorrhiza*, *Polygonum multiforum* and the pollen of *Typha augustifolia* (Jiangzhiling decoction), given at a dose of 100 ml twice daily to hyperlipidemic subjects for 21 days reduced the levels of total triglycerides (92.3%), β-lipoprotein (87.1%) and total cholesterol (93.5 %). [Huang Jinyie, Wang Liechen, Shi Zizhi, Huang xiaojie, Ding Xinjun; Effect of Jiangzhiling decoction on hyperlipidemia *The Practical Journal of Integrating Chinese with Modern Medicine;* **5**(10), 583-84 (1992)].

Saponaria officinalis: See *Glycine max:* [Sautier et *al.*; *Atherosclerosis* **34**(3), 233-241(1979)].

See Saponins and sapogenins in Appendix: [Sidhu & Oakenfull; *Brit J Nutr* **55**(3), 643-50 (1986)].

Sassurea lappa **(H. Kuth, S. Kushtha):** Administration of aqueous extract of *S. lappa* to rabbits (2g/kg) significantly lowered the serum cholesterol and triglyceride levels. [Upadhyay OP, Ojha JK, Bajpayee HS; Experimental study on hypolipidemic activity of kustha (*Sassurea lappa* CS Clarke), *J Res Ayur Siddha* **15**(1-2), 52-63(1994)].

***Satureja khuzestanica*:** Essential oil of *Satureja khuzestanica* (1000 ppm) was administered in drinking water of rats, rendered hyperlipidemic by administration of streptozotocin and lipid diets, for 10 days. The treatment decreased the normal blood lipid peroxidation level and increased total antioxidant power. Significant decreases in fasting blood glucose and triglyceride levels were observed with *S. khuzestanica* essential oil in diabetic and hyperlipidemic rats, respectively. The antioxidant properties of the essential oil are considered responsible for its antidiabetic and triglyceride-lowering effects. [Abdollahi M, Salehnia A, Mortazavi SH, Ebrahimi M, Shafiee A, Fouladian F, Keshavarz K, Sorouri S, Khorasani R, Kazemi A; Antioxidant, antidiabetic, antihyperlipidemic, reproduction stimulatory properties and safety of essential oil of *Satureja khuzestanica* in rat *in vivo*: An oxidopharmacological study, *Med Sci Monit* **9**(9), BR331-35 (2003)].

***Saussurea elegans*:** See Flavonoids in Appendix: [Khushbaktova *et al.*; *Khim Farma Zh* **25**(4), 53-57 (1991)].

***Schizandra chinensis*:** Biochemical studies revealed that oral administration of gomisin A, a lignan component of Schizandra fruits, decreased serum triglyceride and lipid contents of the liver. Gomisin A also showed an antihepatotoxic action. [Takeda S, Maemura S, Sudo K, Kase Y, Arai I, Ohkura Y, Funo S, Fujii Y, Aburada M, Hosoya E; Effects of gomsin A, a lignan component of Schizandra fruits on experimental liver injuries and liver microsomal drug metabolizing enzymes, *Folia Pharmacologica Japonica* **87**(2), 169-88 (1986)].

***Sclerocarya birroea*:** Administration of decoctions of *S. birroea* leaves to diet-induced hypercholesterolemic rats decreased the cholesterol levels. This decoction also elicited hypoglycemic effect and an increase in immunoreactive insulin in normal rats. [Trovato A, Kirjavainen S, Gulati EM, Forestieri AM, Lank I; Effects of *Sclerocarya birroea* Hochst extract on some metabolic activity in the rat, *Phytother Res* **9**(8), 591-93 (1995)].

Secale cereale **(Rye):** See Tocotrienols in Appendix: [Pearce *et al.*; *J Med Chem* **35**(2), 3595-606 (1992)].

The water-soluble fraction extracted from rye bran was separated into a high molecular weight and a low molecular weight fraction. The hypocholesterolemic effects of these fractions were examined in rats, fed on a hypercholesterolemic diet. The elevation of serum and liver cholesterol levels was prevented significantly in the rats fed on a diet containing 3% high molecular fraction of rye bran. However, no such effect was observed in rats fed on low molecular weight fraction of rye bran. The hypotriglyceridemic effects of high molecular weight fraction and rye bran gum preparation were examined in rats fed on a diet containing 20% cocoanut oil, 17.5% glucose and 17.5% fructose. Supplementation of the diet with the high molecular weight fraction or gum at a level of 3%, significantly prevented the elevation of serum and liver triglyceride levels in rats. The results indicate that both the high molecular weight fraction of rye bran and rye bran gum ameliorate hypercholesterolemia and hypertriglyceridemia in rats at the same level. [Tamai Y, Sasaki Y, Fujio T, Ogasawara T, Egashira Y, Ohta T, Sanada H, Ayano Y; The preparation and characterisation of water-soluble functional fraction from rye bran, *J Japanese Soc Food Sci Technol* **41**(4), 265-71 (1994)].

A study was made to determine the hypocholesterolemic effects of whole meal rye and white wheat breads in healthy humans with elevated serum cholesterol concentrations. Rye bread was found effective in reducing serum total and LDL cholesterol concentrations in men. [Leinonen KS, Poutanen KS, Mykkanen HM; Rye bread decreases serum total and LDL-cholesterol in men with moderately elevated serum cholesterol- *J Nutr* **130**(2), 164-70 (2000)].

Semecarpus anacardium (H. Bhilawa, S. Bhallataka): Administration of shell extract of *S. anacardium* nuts to cholesterol-fed rabbits resulted in a significant reduction in serum cholesterol and serum LDL- cholesterol. It also prevented the accumulation of cholesterol/triglycerides in liver, heart muscle and aorta and caused a regression of plaques. In addition to hypocholerolemic activity, shell-extract of *S. anacardium* also prevented cholesterol-induced atheroma. [Sharma A, Mathur R, Dixit VP; Hypocholesterolemic activity of nut shell extract of *Semecarpus anacardium* (Bhilawa) in cholesterol-fed rabbits, *Indian J Exp Biol* **33**(6), 444-48 (1995)].

In DMBA-induced mammary carcinoma bearing rats, antitumor activity of *S. anacardium* nut milk extract was evaluated in terms of plasma lipid levels. The enhanced level of total cholesterol, free cholesterol, ester cholesterol, free fatty acid, phospholipid and triglycerides in tumor bearing rats were reverted back to normal following administration of nut milk of *S. annacardium*. These observations suggest potent hypolipidemic activity in this drug. No side or toxic effects were noted in treated animals. [Sujatha V, Sachidanandan P; Protective effect of nut milk of *Semecarpus anacardium* extract against mammary carcinoma, *J Med Arom Plant Sci* **22**(Suppl. 1), 4 (2000)].

See *Commiphora mukul:* [Mary et al.; *Phytomedicine* **10**(6-7), 474-82 (2003)].

A fraction of *S. anacardium* nuts at a dose of 1mg/100 g body wt, significantly reduced serum cholesterol and increased serum HDL-cholesterol in the rats fed with atherogenic diet. The same fraction also inhibited lipopolysaccharide induced NO production in rat peritoneal macrophages in a dose dependent manner. [Tripathi

YB, Pandey RS; *Semecarpus anacardium* L, nuts inhibit lipopolysaccharide induced NO production in rat macrophages along with its hypolipidemic property, *Indian J Exp Biol* **42**(4), 432-36 (2004)].

Serratula coronata: Ecdysterone was found to be the major component in both *Serratula coronata* and *S. inermis*. The minor components from *S. coronata* were identified as α- ecdysone, polypodine B, integristerone, pterosterone and acetonides of ecdysterone and ajugasterone C. The minor components from *S. inermis* were identified as viticosterone E, 2- desoxyecdysterone, polypodine B, integristerone and 26-hydroxyecdysterone. The ecdysteroids from these plant species showed a variety of biological activities including antioxidant, antiradical and hypocholesterolemic activities in a variety of model systems *in vitro* and *in vivo*. [Kholodova Yu D; Phytoecdysteroids; Biological effects, application in agriculture and complementary medicine, *Ukrainskii Biokhim Zhurnal* **73**(3), 21-29 (2001)].

Serratula inermis: See *Serratula coronata:* [Kholodova Yu D; *Ukrainskii Biokhim Zhurnal* **73**(3), 21-29 (2001)].

Sesamum indicum (Sesame, H. Til, S. Tila): See *Zingiber officinale:* [Singhal and Joshi; *J Sci Res Plants Med* **4**(3), 32-34 (1983)].

Hypocholesterolemic effect of sesame lignan has been studied in humans. [Hirata F, Fujita K, Ishikura Y, Hosoda K, Ishikawa T, Nakamura H; Hypocholesterolemic effect of sesame lignan in humans, *Atherosclerosis* **122**(1), 135-36 (1996)].

The effect of globulin fraction with a lysine: Arginine ratio 0.67, isolated from sesame seeds, on cholesterol metabolism was studied in rats fed with cholesterol-free and cholesterol containing diet and compared with casein having a lysine: Arginine ratio 2.0. Rats, fed sesame seed globulin, showed significantly lower concentrations of cholesterol in the serum and aorta. The decrease in serum was manifested in both HDL and LDL + VLDL fractions. There was increased cholesterogenesis in the liver as was evident from increased incorporation of labeled acetate into cholesterol and increased activity of HMG-CoA reductase. Increased hepatic diversion of cholesterol to bile acid synthesis and increased faecal excretion of bile acids and sterols were also observed in rats fed with sesame seed globulins. The study suggests that low lysine: arginine ratio of a protein exerts hypocholesterolemic effects. [Rajamohan T, Kurup PA; Lysine: arginine ratio of a protein influences cholesterol metabolism: Part 1. Studies on sesame protein having low lysine-arginine ratio, *Indian J Exp Biol* **35**(11), 1218-23 (1997)].

See *Emblica officinalis:* [Anila & Vijayalakshmi; *Phytother Res* **14**(8), 592-95 (2000)].

Silphium perfoliatum: Silphioside, a triterpenic glycoside fraction containing 6 individual compounds, was isolated from the above ground part of *S. perfoliatum*. Silphioside, given orally to albino mice in doses of 10, 50, and 100 mg/kg, showed noticeable hypocholesterolemic and hypotriglyceridemic effects, both in normal and hyperlipidemic rats. [Syrov VN, Khushbaktova ZA, Davidyants ES; Triterpene glycosides of *Silphium perfoliatum* L.; Hypolipidemic activity of silphioside, *Khim Farma Zh* **26**(7-8), 66-69 (1992) [Article in Russian].

Silybum marianum: Silymarin (a standardised mixture of antioxidant flavonolignans from *S. marianum*)-phospholipid complex (SA) exhibited hypolipidemic activity in high fat diet-fed mongrel rabbits. SA also inhibited atherosclerototic plaque formation in aortic intima of these animals [Drozdzik M, Juzwiak S, Wojcieki J, Barcew-Wiszniewska B, Rozewicka L, Mscisz A, Gorecki P; Effect of silymarin phospholipid complex on the development of experimental atherosclerosis in rabbits, *Herba Pol* **41**(3), 132-38 (1995)].

Silymarin, a standardized mixture of antioxidant flavonolignans from *S. marianum*, or its major constituent silybin, were given as dietary supplements, and their influences on serum cholesterol levels were compared to those of probucol, an antioxidant hypocholesterolemic drug. Anticholesterolemic effect of silymarin was parallel to that of probucol, and dose-dependent at dietary drug concentrations of 0.1, 0.5, 1.0% (w/w). However, in contradistinction to probucol, silymarin caused an increase in high density lipoprotein (HDL)-cholesterol and a decrease in liver cholesterol content, changes considered to be of benefit. In addition to its anticholesterolemic effect, silymarin partially prevented the high cholesterol diet-induced decrease in liver reduced glutathione, an endogenous antioxidant. Silybin was not as effective as silymarin. [Krecman V, Skottova N, Walterova D, Ulrichova J, Simanek V; Silymarin inhibits the development of diet-induced hypercholesterolemia in rats, *Planta Med* **64**(2), 138- 42 (1998)].

Oral administration of silymarin, a mixture of flavonolignans extracted from the seeds of *Silybum marianum*, is known to exhibit a hypocholesterolemic effect in rats fed with high cholesterol diet enriched with fat. Similar adminstration of silymarin to rats fed standard laboratory diet, however, failed to show a decrease of serum cholesterol but showed only a mild increase in HDL-cholesterol. Parenterally injected silymarin failed to reduce serum cholesterol both in rats-fed with high cholesterol diet and standard laboratory diet. The results suggest that silymarin could act either due to the fat-mediated improved bioavailability and/or by inhibiting of resorption of dietary cholesterol. [Skottova N, Krecman V, Walterova D, Ulrichova J, Kosina P, Simanek V; Effect of silymarin on serum cholesterol levels in rats, *Acta Universitatis Palackianae Olomucensis Facultatis Medicae* **141**, 87-89 (1998)].

Simmondsia chinensis (Jojoba): In rabbits, effect of jojoba (*S. chinensis*) seed oil on cholesterol and lipoprotein level was studied. Incorporation of jojoba oil (2%) in an atherogenic diet (1% cholesterol) significantly lowered the blood cholesterol and lipoprotein levels. However, at a similar dietary level (2%) safflower oil did not influence the cholesterol levels. [Clarke JA, Yermanos DM; Effect of ingestion of jajoba oil on blood cholesterol levels and lipoprotein patterns in New Zealand white rabbits, *Biochem Biophys Res Commun* **102**(4), 1409-415 (1981)].

Solanum indicum (H. Birhatta, S. Vanbirintaki): In rabbits, feeding of chloroform extract of aerial parts of *S. indicum* elicited significant hypocholesterolemic activity. However, such hypocholesterolemic activity was found to be absent in petroleum ether, alcoholic and water extracts of this plant [Kalhoro MA, Kapadia Z, Badar Y, Ul Hassain SN; Preliminary screening of hypocholesterolemic activity in *Solanum indicum*, *J Faculty of Pharmacy, Gazi Univ* **14**(1), 11-16 (1997)].

Solanum lycocarpum (Wolf Apple): A preparation from the green fruits of *S. lycocarpum* is widely employed in Brazil for management of diabetes and obesity and to decrease cholesterol levels. Phytochemical analysis of this phytomedicine as well as of the fruits of the plant showed polysaccharides as the main component. Attempts have been made to rationalise its use as a hypoglycemic and hypocholesterolemic agent. [Dall'Agnol R, Lino von Poser G; The use of complex polysaccharides in the management of metabolic diseases: The case of *Solanum lycocarpum* fruits, *J Ethnopharmacol* **71**(1-2), 337-41 (2000)].

Solanum melongena (Brinjal, Eggplant, H. Baigan, S. Bhantaki): Flavonoids, extracted from the fruits of *S. melongena,* showed significant hypolipidemic action in normal and cholesterol-fed rats when administered orally at a dose of 1 mg/100 g bw/d. The flavonoids also enhanced HMG-CoA reductase activity and reduced activities of glucose-6-phosphate dehydrogenase and malate dehydrogenase. A significant increase in the concentrations of hepatic and faecal bile acids and faecal neutral sterols was also observed indicating a higher rate of degradation of cholesterol. [Sudheesh S, Presannakumar G, Vijayakumar S, Vijayalakshmi NR; Hypolipidemic effect of flavonoids from *Solanum melongena, Plant Foods Hum Nutr* **51**(4), 321-30 (1997)].

Eggplant (*S. melongena*) is consumed extensively in Brazil and it is believed that infusion of a powdered preparation of the fruit possesses serum cholesterol reducing activity. The results of an investigation, taken up to verify this activity, suggesed that *S. melongena* infusion had a modest and transitory effect, which was not different from that obtained with standard orientation for dyslipidemic patients (diet and physical activities). [Guimaraes PR, Galvao AM, Batista CM, Azevedo GS, Oliveira RD, Lamounier RP, Freire N, Barros AM, Sakurai E, Oliveira JP, Vieira EC, Alvarez-Leite JI; Eggplant (*Solanum melongena*) infusion has a modest and transitory effect on hypercholesterolemic subjects, *Braz J Med Biol Res* **33**(9), 1027-36 (2000)].

The effect of eggplant on cholesterol metabolism and atherogenesis in LDLR(-/-) mice was evaluated. Eggplant extract had high histamine and other amine levels that could enhance LDL oxidation and its endocytosis. Eggplant did not decrease plasma cholesterol nor prevent the development of atherosclerosis in LDLR(-/-) mice. Surprisingly, eggplant increased oxidative stress, representing a risk factor for atherosclerosis. These results did not support the use of eggplant extract as hypocholesterolemic agent. [Botelho FV, Eneas LR, Cesar GC, Bizzotto CS, Tavares

E, Oliveira FA, Gloria MB, Silvestre MP, Arantes RM, Alvarez-Leite JI; Effects of eggplant (*Solanum melongena*) on the atherogenesis and oxidative stress in LDL receptor knock out mice (LDLR(-/-)), *Food Chem Toxicol* **42**(8), 1259-67 (2004)].

The hypolipidemic potential of dried powdered fruits of eggplant, which has been commercialised in Brazil to treat human hyperlipidemia, was investigated in a double-blind placebo-controlled study. From the results of the investigation it was concluded that *Solanum melongena,* at least in the form commercialised in Brazil (dried powdered fruits), requires further clinical trials before being recommended to treat hyperlipidemia. [Silva GE, Takahashi MH, Eik Filho W, Albino CC, Tasim GE, Serri Lde A, Assef AH, Cortez DA, Bazotte RB; Absence of hypolipidemic effect of *Solanum melongena* L. (eggplant) on hyperlipidemic patients, *Arq Bras Endocrinol Metabol* **48**(3),368-73 (2004) Article in Portuguese].

Solanum nigrum (H, Makoi, S. Kakamachi): Administration of 50% alcoholic extract of *S. nigrum* (50mg/100g bw) to albino rats significantly lowered lipid levels. It also prevented the development of fatty liver changes in alcohol-fed rats. [Agrawal SS, Gulati R; Hepatoprotective studies on *Solanum nigrum* Linn. against country-made liquor induced hepatotoxicity in albino rats fed on controlled caloric diet, *Acta Clinica Scientia* **5**(I&II), **6**(I&II), 18-21 (1996)].

***Solanum trilobatum*:** See *Saccharum officinarum:* [Tarvady & Dhar; *Biomedicine* **9** (1) 39- 42 (1989); *Indian J Exp Biol* **28**(7), 657-60 (1990)].

Solanum tuberosum (Potato, H. Aloo): Male rats were fed diets containing 1% cholesterol and 0.2% cholic acid with either 6% cellulose or potato peels as the fibre source. After 4 weeks, rats fed with potato peels showed a 40% decrease in plasma cholesterol content and a reduction of 30% in hepatic fat cholesterol levels as compared to rats fed with cellulose. The data indicate that potato peels might be considered as a source of dietary fibres for human consumption. [Lazarov K, Werman MJ; Hypocholesterolaemic effect of potato peel as a dietary fibre source, *Medical Sci Res* **24**(9), 581-82 (1996)].

See *Glycine max* (Soya bean, soybean): [Morita *et al*; *J Nutr* **127**(3), 470-77 (1997)].

***Sophora japonica*:** See Flavonoids in Appendix: [Khushbaktova *et al.*; *Khim Farma Zh* **25**(4), 53-57 (1991)].

Spinacia oleracea (Spinach, H. Palak, S. Palankya) Spinach extract showed potent dose dependent hypolipidemic activity in high lipid diet-induced hyperlipidemic rats. Spinach extract also reduced hepatic lipid fraction contents in these animals. [Wojcieki J, Samochowiec L, Cynerski Z, Dominiezak K; Effect of spinach extract on serum and liver lipids in rats fed on high lipid diet, *Herba Pol* **26**(1), 5-10 (1980)].

Radish and spinach leaf protein isolates, prepared from chilled aqueous sodium hydroxide (0.2%) extracts of their leaves, were compared with casein for their effects on serum cholesterol level in rats fed with a cholesterol-enriched diet for 14 days.

Each protein isolate was incorporated into the cholesterol-enriched diet to provide a 15% protein level. Radish leaf protein was extremely inferior to spinach leaf protein and casein for body weight gain of rats but addition of methionine to radish leaf protein made it comparable to spinach leaf protein and casein. The serum cholesterol level in rats fed with spinach leaf protein alone or in combination with methionine diets was significantly lower as compared to that of the casein-fed rats. The amounts of excreted cholesterol and bile acids were also significantly higher in rats fed with spinach leaf protein diets than that of the casein-fed rats. The hypocholesterolemic action of spinach leaf protein may partly be due to the inhibition of intestinal absorption of both cholesterol and bile acids. [Satoh T, Goto M, Igarashi K; Effects of protein from radish and spinach leaves on serum lipids levels in rats, *J Nutr Sci Vitaminol* **39**(6), 627-33 (1993)].

The serum total cholesterol, triacylglycerol and phospholipid concentrations in the rats fed with spinach leaf protein concentrate diet containing 2% corn oil were significantly lower than those of the rats fed a corresponding casein diet. The concentrations of serum threonine, serine, glutamine, glycine, cystine, and isoleucine were significantly higher in the rats fed with the spinach leaf protein concentrate diet containing 2% corn oil compared with those of the control rats, but when the dietary fat was raised to 10%, only glycine showed a higher serum concentration. These results indicate that the spinach leaf protein concentrate has a stronger cholesterol lowering effect at a lower dietary fat level (2%), and the activity is partly due to the inhibition of intestinal absorption of cholesterol and bile acid, and partly due to an increase in the concentration of some of the serum amino acids. [Satoh A, Hitomi M, Igarashi K; Effects of spinach leaf protein concentrate on the serum cholesterol and amino acid concentrations in rats fed with a cholesterol-free diet, *J Nutr Sci Vitaminol* **41**(5), 563-73 (1995)].

Strychnos potatorum (H. Nirmali, S. Kataka): See *Salacia prinoides:* [Kowsalya *et al*, *Indian J Nut Diet* **33**(9), 208-15 (1996)].

Syzygium aromaticum (Syn. *Eugenia aromatica,* Cloves, H. Laung, S. Lavanga): Enhancement of lipid peroxidation in high fat diet-induced hyperlipidemic rats was evidenced by an increase in the liver and kidney levels of thiobarbituric acid reactive substances (TABRS), diene conjugate (CD), reduced glutathione (GSH) and lipid parameters. The alterations in above parameters reversed back towards normalcy following administration of cloves to these animals. The activity of antioxidant enzymes like superoxide dismutase, catalase, glutathione peroxidase and glutathione-S-transferase was also enhanced in clove treated hyperlipidemic rats. It was suggested that antioxidant activity of cloves might protect the animals against hyperlipidemia-induced damage. [Shyamala MP, Venukumar MR, Latha MS; Antioxidant potential of *Syzygium aromaticum* (Gaertn.) Linn. (Cloves) in rats fed with high fat diet, *Indian J Pharmacol* **35**(2), 99-103 (2003)].

T

Tamarindus indica (Tamarind, H. Imli, S. Tintrine): See *Brassica nigra* (Mustard): [Sambaiah & Srinivasan; *J Food Sci Technol* **28**(1), 35-38 (1991)].

Terminalia arjuna (H. Arjun, S. Arjuna): Administration of *T. arjuna* and cholestyramine to experimentally-induced hypercholesterolemic rabbits, caused a significant reduction of serum total cholesterol and low density lipoprotein cholesterol levels. *T. arjuna* also prevented cholesterol-rich diet induced increase of serum triglyceride and VLDL-c levels. Total cholesterol /HDL-c ratio was also decreased in treated group of animals. All these changes were relatively more marked in *T. arjuna* treated rabbits than cholestyramine treated ones. [Tewari AK, Gode JD, Dubey GP; A comparative study between *Terminalia arjuna* and cholestyramine effect on serum lipids and lipoproteins in hypercholesterolemic rabbits, *Indian Drugs* **26**(12), 664-(1989)].

The effect of *T. arjuna* bark powder on anginal pain, rhythm disturbances and certain known coronary risk factors was evaluated in patients of Ischemic heart disease. The bark powder of the plant decreased blood sugar, cholesterol, catecholamines and cortisol levels in these patients. It also alleviated anginal pain and reduced body weight and blood pressure. [Dwivedi S, Chansouria JPN, Somani PN, Udupa KN; Effect of *Terminalia arjuna* on Ischemic heart disease, *Alternative Medicine* **3**(2), 115-22 (1989)].

Administration of *T. arjuna* alongwith high cholesterol diet, prevented diet induced enhancement of total cholesterol and triglyceride levels without any change in HDL-c as compared to hypercholesterolemic rabbits. *T. arjuna* treatment of hypercholesterolemic animals significantly decreased elevated levels of cholesterol and triglycerides with an increase of HDL-cholesterol. [Tewari AK, Gode JD, Dubey GP; Effect of *Terminalia arjuna* on lipid profile of rabbits fed hypercholesterolemic diet, *Int J Crude Drug Res* **28**(1), 43-47 (1990)].

Administration of extracts of *T. arjuna, Inula recemosa* and latex of *Commiphora mukul* to 40 heart patients for four months showed hypolipidemic and cardioprotective activity. Six out of 10 patients of angina also exhibited improvement in ECG pattern following treatment with above drugs. [Banerjee S, Bandyopadhyay SK, Muckherjee PK, Muckherjee NK, Chauwdhuri, Muckherjee A; Clinical studies on hypolipidemic and cardioprotective effect of some indigenous drugs, *Proceedings of 25th Indian Pharmacological Society Conference*, Muzaffarpur, Bihar, India, Dec. 5-8, p.80 (1992)].

In triton-induced hyperlipidemic rats, bark powder of *T. arjuna* (100mg/kg) significantly lowered serum lipids. Feeding of this drug (100mg/kg) simultaneously with cholesterol (25 mg/kg) to the animals for 30 days also lowered lipids and β-lipoprotein -cholesterol. Lipolytic activity in plasma, liver, heart and adipose tissues was altered in hyperlipidemic rats after treatment with *T. arjuna* bark powder. Lipid lowering activity of this bark powder was attributed to enhanced faecal bile acids excretion, inhibition of hepatic cholesterol biosynthesis and increased plasma lecithin cholesterol acyl transferase activity along with receptor mediated breakdown of low density lipoprotein [Khanna AK, Ramesh Chander, Kapoor NK; *Terminalia arjuna*: An Ayurvedic cardiotonic, regulates lipid metabolism in hyperlipidemic rats, *Phytother Res* **10**(8), 663-665 (1996)].

See *Allium satium:* [Dwivedi S; *Ann Natl Acad Med Scs* (India) 32(3&4) 159-75 (1996)].

Administration of 50% ethanolic extract of *T. arjuna* bark (100 and 500 mg/kg) to diet induced hyperlipidemic rabbits for 60 days, significantly lowered total serum cholesterol, LDL-cholesterol, triglycerides and LDL/HDL ratio. This drug did not adversely affect hepatic and renal functions. [Ram A, Lauria P, Gupta R, Kumar P, Sharma VN; Hypocholesterolemic effect of *Terminalia arjuna* tree bark, *J Ethnopharmacol* **55**(3), 165-69 (1997)].

Administration of *T. arjuna* bark powder (500mg/kg) to hypercholesterolemic rabbits for 90 days significantly raised HDL-cholesterol along with lowering of LDL-cholesterol. This drug was well tolerated. [Shaila HP, Udupa SL, Udupa AL, Nair NS; Effect of *Terminalia arjuna* on experimental hyperlipidemia in rabbits, *Int J Pharmacogn* **35**(2), 126-29 (1997)].

Serum cholesterol, phospholipids and triglyceride levels were significantly decreased following treatment of cholesterol-fed rabbits with the bark powder of *T. arjuna* (500mg/kg). Pretreatment with this bark powder reduced the heart tissue cholesterol, triglycerides and aortic phospholipids contents in comparison to control group. *T. arjuna* pretreated rabbits showed normal aorta without any atherosclerotic changes.

These observations suggested that this drug prevented deposition of cholesterol in aorta of these animals [Shaila HP, Udupa SL, Udupa AL; Hypolipidemic effect of *Terminalia arjuna* in cholesterol-fed rabbits, *Fitoterapia* **68**(5), 405-09 (1997)].

See *Allium sativum:* [Sharma & Dwivedi; *Indian Drugs* **34**(5), 242-51 (1997)].

Of the three indigenous drugs *Terminalia arjuna*, *T. belerica* and *T. chebula* that were investigated on experimental atherosclerosis, *T. arjuna* was found to be the most potent hypolipidemic agent and it induced partial inhibition of rabbit atheroma. [Shaila HP, Udupa SL, Udupa AL; Hypolipidemic activity of three indigenous drugs in experimentally induced atherosclerosis, *Int J Cardiol* **67**(2), 119-24 (1998)].

Administration of *T. arjuna* bark powder, *Acorus calamus* and "Mruga-shrunga bhasma" to cholesterol-fed rats, significantly lowered serum cholesterol, triglyceride, LDL-cholesterol and VLDL-cholesterol levels. This formulation also increased monocyte population, which is directly related to atheromatous plaque formation. [Dubewar VM; Effect of Arjuna, Vacha and Mruga-shrunga bhasma in atherosclerosis (Dhamani pratichaya) animal experiment, *Phytomedicine* **7** (Suppl II), 116 (2000)].

See *Bombax mori:* [Ahmad et *al.*; *National Symposium on Emerging Trends in Indian Medicinal Plants,* Lucknow p 89 (8-0/8)10-12 October, 2003].

See *Commiphora mukul:* [Mary et *al.*, *Phytomedicine* **10** (6-7), 474-82 (2003)].

Terminalia belerica (H. Bahera, S. Bahira): See *Terminalia chebula* (Haritaki): [Thakur *et al.*, *Int J Cardiol* **21**(2), 167-75 (1988)].

See *Terminalia arjuna* (H. Arjun): [Shaila *et al.*; *Int J Cardiol.* **67**(2), 119-24 (1998)].

See *Terminalia chebula* [Nalini *et al.*; *Plant Foods Human Nutr* **53**(4), 343-49 (1999)].

See *Allium sativum* (Garlic): [Chander et *al.*; *Ethnobotany* **14**(1-2), 123-28 (2001)].

Terminalia chebula (H. Harir, S. Haritaki): See *Emblica officinalis:* [Mishra et *al.*; *Nagarjun* **26**(5), 105-07 (1983)].

In different groups of cholesterol-induced hypercholesterolemic and atherosclerotic rabbits, administration of *T. chebula*, *T. belerica* and *E. officinalis* significantly reduced serum cholesterol levels as compared to untreated hypercholesterolemic animals. Aortic sudanophilia was significantly less in all the treated hypercholesterolemic rabbits. Likewise, the hepatic and aortic cholesterol contents were also significantly decreased in all treated animals. Of all the three drugs, maximum hypocholesterolemic activity was noted in *T. chebula*-treated rabbits. However, these drugs did not affect serum triglyceride, euglobulin lysis time and platelet adhesiveness. [Thakur CP, Thakur B, Singh S, Sinha PK, Sinha SK; The Ayurvedic medicines Haritaki, Amla and Bahera reduce cholesterol induced atherosclerosis in rabbits, *Int J Cardiol* **21**(2), 167-75 (1988)].

In triton-induced hyperlipidemic rats, ethyl acetate soluble fraction of alcoholic extract of *T. chebula* reduced serum lipid. Administration of extract to normal rats for 30 days also decreased the levels of low density lipoprotein lipids and increased the high density lipoprotein cholesterol (HDL-c) levels. Hepatic triglyceride lipase activity was also decreased in these treated rats. The mechanism by which *T. chebula* exerts hypolipidemic activity involves inhibition of cholesterol biosynthesis, increased faecal excretion of bile acid and enhanced plasma lecithin: cholesterol acyl transferase activity. [Khanna AK, Chander R, Kapoor NK, Singh C, Srivastava AK; Hypolipidemic activity of *Terminalia chebula* in rats, *Fitoterapia* **64**(4), 351-56 (1993)].

Administration of a compound herbal preparation containing *Terminalia chebula*, *Acorus calamus*, *Pluchea lanceolata*, *Piper longum*, *Zingiber officinale*, *Hedychium spicatum* and *Inula racemosa* to 20 patients of stable angina for 2 months significantly lowered the serum cholesterol and triglyceride levels. Severity and frequency of chest pain was also considerably reduced in these patients. [Awasthi AK, Kothari K, Sharma RK; Role of Haritakyad vati in management of stable angina, *Aryavaidyam* **9**(4), 214-19 (1996)].

See *Terminalia arjuna:* [Shaila *et al.*; *Int J Cardiol.* **67**(2), 119-24 (1998)].

Administration of dried powder of *Terminalia chebula*, *T. belerica* and *Emblica officinalis* fruits to different groups of diet-induced hypercholesterolemic rats led to lowering of total cholesterol, LDL-cholesterol and triglyceride levels. HDL-cholesterol did not change in rats given *T. chebula* and *T. belerica* fruit powder but increased in *E. officinalis* treated rats. Bile acid excretion was significantly increased in rats consuming the mixture of these three fruits. [Nalini D, Kapoor R; Effect of plant fruits; Indian gall nut, bedda nut and gooseberry on hypercholesterolemic rats, *Plant Foods Human Nutr* **53**(4), 343-49 (1999)].

Administration of *T. chebula* fruit powder in the dose of 2 g twice daily with lukewarm water for 6 weeks significantly decreased serum cholesterol, trigycerides, total lipids, low density lipoprotein and very low density lipoprotein levels. High density lipoprotein cholesterol (HDL-c) was significantly increased in these subjects. However, this drug did not affect body weight and adipose tissue thickness at the level of triceps, nape of neck and abdomen. [Sood R, Sharma AK; Effect of Bala Haritaki on hypercholesterolemia, *J Res Ayur Siddha* **21**(1-2), 11-18 (2000)].

T. chebula powder lowered serum total cholesterol, triglycerides , LDL and VLDL-cholesterol levels in heart patients with sedentary life style.[Amrithaveni M,Vijayalakshmi P, Niklia MN; Lipid profile of the heart patients and healthy volunteers and the effect of supplementation of kadukai (*Terminalia chebula*) on hypercholesterolemic patients, *Indian J Nutr Diet* **38**(3), 83-88 (2001)].

See *Allium sativum* (Garlic): [Chander *et al.*; *Ethnobotany* **14**(1-2), 123-28 (2001)].

Administration of alcoholic extract of immature and mature fruits and ethyl acetate fraction of immature fruits of *T. chebula* to atherogenic diet-induced hyperlipidemic rats, caused significant reduction of total cholesterol, triglycerides and total lipoprotein levels. Blood HDL-cholesterol levels were increased in these treated animals. In normocholesterolemic rats also, the ethanol extract of the drug lowered the total cholesterol and triglyceride levels alongwith enhancement of HDL-cholesterol. The ethyl acetate fraction of immature fruits was most effective in lowering lipids. [Ahirwar B, Singhai AK, Dixit VK; Effect of *Terminalia chebula* fruits on lipid profile of rats, *J Nat Remedies* **3**(1), 31-35 (2002)].

Teucrium polium: Intraperitoneal administration of aqueous extract of *T. polium* aerial parts at doses from 50 to 150 mg/kg for 10 days reduced significantly the serum levels of cholesterol and triglycerides in hyperlipidemic rats. [Rasekh HR, Khoshnood-Mansourkhani MJ, Kamalinejad M; Hypolipidemic effects of *Teucrium polium* in rats, *Fitoterapia* **72**(8), 937-39 (2001)].

Thermopsis alterniflora: See Flavonoids in Appendix: [Khushbaktova *et al.*; *Khim Farma Zh* **25**(4), 53-57 (1991)].

Thermopsis dolichocarpa: See Flavonoids in Appendix: [Khushbaktova *et al.*; *Khim Farma Zh* **25**(4), 53-57 (1991)].

Tilia cordata: See *Brassica campestris:* [Samochowiee and Wojcicki; *Herba Pol* **27**(4), 333- 39 (1981)].

Tinospora cordifolia (H. Giloya, S. Guduchi): Administration of aqueous extract of *T. cordifolia* roots (2.5 and 5 g/kg bw) for 6 weeks significantly lowered serum and tissue cholesterol, phospholipids and free fatty acids in alloxan-induced diabetic rats. Maximum hypolipidemic activity was noted in animals treated with 5g/kg dose. The results were comparable to glibenclamide. [Prince PSM, Menon VP, Gunasekaran G; Hypolipidemic action of *Tinospora cordifolia* roots in alloxan diabetic rats. *J Ethnopharmacol* **64**(1), 53-57 (1999)].

See *Commiphora mukul:* [Mary *et al.*; *Phytomedicine* **10**(6-7), 474-82 (2003)].

Trachyspermum ammi (Syn.*Carum copticum*, H. Ajwan, S. Ajmoda): See *Zingibar officinale:* [Singh VK, Singh S, Singh DK; Pharmacological effects of spices: Recent progress in medicinal plants: Phytochemistry and pharmacology, JN Govil, VK Singh (eds.) Studium press, LLC, Houston, Texas, USA p 321-353(2003)].

Trichilia connaroids: The hexane, chloroform and methanol extracts of *T. connaroids* were examined for hypocholesterolemic activity. In normal rats, hexane and methanol extracts of this plant enhanced the levels of high density lipoprotein cholesterol without affecting the cholesterol and triglyceride levels. In triton-induced hyperlipidemic animals, chloroform and methanol extracts caused significant lowering of cholesterol levels as compared to controls. [Purnima AL, Mathuram V; Hypocholesterolemic and antihypercholesterolemic activity of extracts of *Trichilia connaroids* on rats, *Indian J Pharm Sci* **66,** 537-39 (2004)].

***Trichiurus chinensis*:** See *Polygonum multiflorum*: [Mei chen et *al.*; *Acta Pharm Sin* **14**(1), 8-11 ((1979)].

Trichosanthes dioica (H. Parwal, S. Patola)**:** Effect of raw deseeded fruit powder of *T. dioica* on blood lipid and sugar levels was investigated in normal albino rats. Feeding of fruit powder of *T. dioica* to normal albino rats significantly decreased the blood chholesterol, triglycerides and sugar levels. On the other hand, the serum HDL-cholesterol and phospholipid levels were significantly increased in treated rats. [Sharma G, Pant MC; Effect of raw deseeded fruit powder of *Trichosanthes dioica* (Roxb) on blood sugar, serum cholesterol, high density lipoprotein, phospholipids and triglyceride levels in normal albino rats, *Indian J Physiol Pharmacol* **32**, 160-63 (1988)].

Whole fruit and pulp of *T. dioica* was shown to exert significant cholesterol, LDL-cholesterol, triglycerides and phospholipid lowering effect in normal and mild diabetic subjects. The high density lipoprotein cholesterol (HDL-c) was significantly increased in these subjects. [Sharma G, Sarkar A, Pachori SB, Pant MC; Biochemical evaluation of raw *Trichosanthes dioica* whole fruit and pulp in normal and mild diabetic human volunteers in relation to lipid profile, *Indian Drugs* **27**(1), 24-28 (1989)].

Trifolium alexandrinum (Egyptian clover)**:** The effect of supplementing Egyptian clover or alfalfa (*Medicago sativa*) to an atherogenic diet was investigated in rats by determining the levels of cholesterol and triglycerides in serum and liver and the excretion of bile acids during an experimental period of 20 days. Feeding of clover seed and alfalfa-supplemented diets resulted in a significant ($P<0.01$) reduction in total cholesterol levels of serum and liver. Consumption of alfalfa seed also showed a significant decline in the levels of serum triglycerides as compared to control. [Geetanjali K, Kapoor R; Effect of supplementation of Egyptian clover seeds (*Trifolium alaxandrinum*) on serum and liver lipids of hypercholesterolemic rats, *J Food Sci Technol* **36**(2), 106-08 (1999)].

Trifolium pratense (Red clover)**:** The anti-atherosclerotic and hypocholesterolemic effects of flavonoids and their glycosides, isolated from red clover, were studied in animal models of atherosclerosis. The effect of the total flavonoids somewhat exceeded the action of the standard hypocholesterolemic preparation, cetamiphen. Delayed development of experimental hypercholesterolemia and hyper β-lipoproteinemia by synthetic isoflavones was structure dependent. Development of experimental hypercholesterolemia and hyper β-lipoproteinemia was greatly retarded and time required for normalisation of blood and aortic wall cholesterol content and aortic. β-lipoproteins in sick animals was greatly reduced following administration of 7,3',4'-trimethoxy isoflavone, the action of which was similar to the total flavonoids isolated from clover. [Vasilenko YU K, Dorofeenko GN, Kazakov AL, Lisevitskaya LI, Leonteva TP, Mezheritskii VV, Parfenteva EP, Shinkarenco AL; The effect of flavonoids of red clover and some of their synthetic analogues on the indices of lipid metabolism in animals with experimental atherosclerosis, *Izvestiya Severo Kavkazskogo Nauchnogo Tsentra Vysshei Shkoly Estestvennye Nauki* **6**(4), 99-101 (1978) Article in Russian].

The effect of native and defatted leaf protein concentrate (LPC) from red clover on plasma cholesterol level in rats was studied. The native LPC contained oleic acid as its main fatty acid and the fat present in the native LPC had no hypocholesterolemic effect. LPC was hypocholesterolemic compared with casein in diets not containing added soya bean oil. [Szymczyk B, Gwiazda S, Hanczakowski P; The effect of leaf protein concentrate from red clover on plasma cholesterol level in rats, *J Sci Food Agric* **67**(3), 299-301 (1995)].

Trigonella foenum-graecum (Fenugreek, H. & S Methi)**:** The hypochlesterolemic effects of fenugreek seeds on normal and diabetic hypercholesterolemic dogs were studied. The defatted portion of fenugreek seeds elicited significant cholesterol and sugar lowering effects in normal dogs. Administration of this fraction to diabetic hypercholesterolemic dogs for 8 days caused reduction of blood cholesterol and glucose levels. [Valette G, Sauvaire Y, Baccon JC, Ribes G; Hypocholesterolemic effect of fenugreek seeds in dogs, *Atherosclerosis* **50**(1), 105-11 (1984)].

The influence of fenugreek (*T. foenum graecum*) and ginger (*Zingiber officinale*) on the secretion and composition of bile was investigated in rats. The intragastric administration of fenugreek or dietary feeding of ginger and fenugreek caused an increase in bile flow with a concomitant decrease in bile solids. Feeding these two spices in the diet significantly increased the total bile acid output. The excess bile salt excretion is mainly due to the increased production of taurodeoxycholic acid and taurocholic acid. The results indicate that fenugreek and ginger stimulate the bile forming function of the liver as also the conversion of cholesterol to bile salts. [Bhat BG, Sambaiah K, ChandrasekharaN; The effect of feeding fenugreek (*Trigonella foenum-graecum*) and ginger (*Zingiber officinale*) on bile composition in the albino rat, *Nutr Reports International* 32(5), 1145-52 (1985)].

Fenugreek and its fractions when added to a diet caused hypocholesterolemia in rats. Fenugreek significantly prevented the rise in serum cholesterol in rats, fed on a hypercholesterolemic diet. Among the fenugreek fractions, the defatted fractions, gum isolate and the crude saponins showed hypocholesterolemic activity. Supplementation of hypercholesterolemia-inducing diet with fenugreek for 4 weeks significantly reduced the elevated cholesterol levels but not the triglyceride levels. [Sharma RD; An evaluation of hypocholesterolemic factor of fenugreek seeds (*Trigonella foenum-graecum*), *Nutr Reports International* **33**(4), 669-78 (1986)].

Feeding of 1g dried green leaves (boiled in water) of fenugreek with normal diet for 8 weeks to experimental animals, led to an increase in the excretion of faecal total lipids and sterols. Subsequently the serum total cholesterol and triglycerides levels were also decreased in these animals. [Chaturvedi V, Pant MC; Effect of feeding fenugreek (*Trigonella foenum-graecum*) leaves on faecal excretion of total lipids and sterols in normal albino rabbits, *Curr Sci* **57**(2), 81-82 (1988)].

Ingestion of diet containing 100g of debitterized fenugreek powder for 20 days led to significant reduction in seum total cholesterol, LDL and VLDL-cholesterol and triglycerides levels in hyperlipemic subjects. Though the HDL- cholesterol remained unaltered but its ratio with total choletesterol, LDL-cholesterol and VLDL- cholesterol was significantly increased. [Sharma RD, Raghuram TC, Rao VD; Hypolipidemic effect of fenugreek seeds –A clinical study, *Phytother Res* **5**(3), 145-47 (1991)].

Faeces of alloxan diabetic dogs fed with fenugreek subfractions were analyzed, and diosgenin, smilagenin and gitogenin were identified and measured using capillary gas chromatography/mass spectrometry. The results indicated that saponins were hydrolysed, in part (about 57%), into sapogenins in the digestive tract. The saponins are probably implicated, alone or together with diosgenin, in the observed hypocholesterolemic effect of fenugreek seeds in diabetic dogs. [Sauvaire Y, Ribes G, Baccou JC, Loubatieeres Mariani MM; Implication of steroid saponins and sapogenins in the hypocholesterolemic effect of fenugreek, *Lipids* **26**(3), 191-97 (1991)].

The effects on lipid metabolism of a hypoglycemic principle isolated from fenugreek, was investigated in cholesterol-induced hypercholesterolemic rabbits. The fenugreek principle in the dose of 50mg/kg/d for 4 weeks effectively prevented increase in serum cholesterol, triglycerides, LDL-c, VLDL-c and total cholesterol/HDL-c ratio in cholesterol-fed rabbits. [Puri D, Prabhu M, Murthy PS; Hypocholesterolemic effect of the hypoglycemic principle of fenugreek (*Trigonella foenum-graecum*) seeds, *Indian J Clin Biochem* **9**(1), 13-16 (1994)].

See *Glycine max* (Soya bean, soybean): [Lanksy PS; *Acta Horticulturae* (332), 131-36 (1993)].

See *Cyamopsis tetragonoloba* (Cluster bean, Guar): [Bharadwaj *et al.*; *J Indian Med Assoc* **92**(3), 80-81 (1994)].

In non-insulin dependent diabetic subjects, the lipid lowering activity of *Trigonella foenum graecum* seeds was investigated. Consumption of diet containing 25 g fenugreek seed powder led to a significant reduction of serum total cholesterol, LDL and VLDL-cholesterol and triglyceride levels. [Sharma RD, Sarkar A, Hazra DK, Mishra B, Singh JB, Maheshwari BB, Sharma SK; Hypolipidemic effect of fenugreek seeds: A chronic study in non insulin dependent diabetic patients, *Phytother Res* **10**(4), 332-34 (1996)].

See *Allium sativum* (Garlic): [Dwivedi S; *Ann Natl Acad Med Scs* (India) 32(3&4) 159- 175(1996)].

In non-insulin dependant diabetics, sprouted fenugreek seeds (30g/day) caused mild hypocholesterolemic and hypoglycemic effect [Chandra V, Aruna K, Glycemic and hypocholesterolemic effect of sprouted fenugreek on diabetic subjects, *Indian J Nutr*

Diet **34**(10), 246-251 (1997)].

See *Aloe vera:* [Nada *et al.*; *Fitoterapia* **68**(3), 240-44 (1997)].

See *Allium sativum:* [Sharma & Dwivedi; *Indian Drugs* **34**(5), 242-51 (1997)].

Effect of *T. foenum-graecum* (fenugreek) powder on hypercholesterolemia and hyperglycemia was examined in diabetic patients. Administration of fenugreek powder (9g/day) for 3 months to 15 cases of type II diabetes mellitus significantly decreased serum cholesterol, triglycerides and blood sugar levels. These observations suggested effective use of fenugreek powder in controlling triglyceride and blood sugar levels in diabetic patients. [Kuppu RK, Srivastva A, Krishnaswami CV, Vijay Kumar G, Chellamariappan M, Asha Bai PV, Buchi Babu O; Hypoglycemic and hypotriglyceridemic effects of methika churna (Fenugreek), *Antiseptic* **95**(3), 78-79 (1998)].

Fenugreek seeds (*T. foenum-graecum*) have been shown to influence lipid profile in hypercholesterolemic patients. Experimental studies also demonstrated that fenugreek seeds significantly lower serum total cholesterol, triglycerides, VLDL-, LDL- cholesterol and phospholipids levels . It also controls hepatic cholesterol and triglyceride levels. [Chakravotty S, Mitra M; Anticholesterolemic effect of fenugreek, *National conference on recent trends in spices and medicinal plants research,* Calcutta, WB, India, Abst. B-50, April 2-4, 1998].

The effect of consumption of germinated fenugreek seed powder at two different levels, *i.e.*, 12.5 g and 18.0 g on the blood lipid profiles of twenty hypercholesterolemic adults of both sexes in the age range of 50-65 years was studied. Consumption of 18.0 g of the germinated seed resulted in a significant reduction in total cholesterol and LDL levels. No significant changes were found in HDL, VLDL and triglyceride levels in all the subjects. [Sowmya P, Rajyalakshmi P; Hypocholesterolemic effect of germinated fenugreek seeds in human subjects, *Plant Foods Hum Nutr* **53**(4), 359-65 (1999)].

Fenugreek seeds were powdered and extracted sequentially with hexane and alcohol to remove its lipid content and the saponins, respectively. This powder, given orally before food at 25 and 50 gm twice a day, significantly decreased serum cholesterol, triglycerides and VLDL levels and thus showed promise of being used as a hypolipidemic agent in hypercholesterolemic patients. [Prasanna M; Hypolipidemic effect of Fenugreek: A clinical study, *Indian J Pharmacol* **32**(1), 34-36 (2000)].

Fenugreek seeds, commonly used as food supplement, have been reported to exert antihyperlipidemic and antihyperglycemic activity in rats. Antihypercholesterolemic effect of whole powered seeds of fenugreek in normal and diet-induced hypercholesterolemic rabbits has been discussed. It is suggested that fenugreek-containing diet may be useful in cases of hyperlipidemia in humans. [Kumar H, Bhandari U; Attenuation of experimental hypercholesterolemia by Fenugreek seeds,

Hamdard Medicus **44**(1), 8-10 (2001)].

Composition, nutritional value, physiological properties and uses of fenugreek have been summarised. Consumption of the seed results in a hypocholesterolemic effect presumably due to the presence of steroidal saponins. [Billaud C, Adrian J; Fenugreek; Composition, nutritional value and physiological properties, *Sciences des Aliments* **21**(1), 3-26 (2001) Article in French].

The effects of oral administration of a unique fibre cocktail of fenugreek seed powder, guar gum and wheat bran (Fibrenat) on some aspects of lipid metabolism and cholesterol homeostasis in rats were examined. Rats were administered Fibrenat along with the atherogenic diet containing 1.5 % cholesterol and 0.1 % cholic acid. Amounts of hepatic lipids, hepatic and faecal bile acids and activity of hepatic triglyceride lipase (HTGL) were determined. Fibrenat intake significantly increased apo B, E receptor expression in rat liver. The activity of HTGL increased by approximately 1.5 fold in fibrenat-fed rats as compared to those fed with the atherogenic diet alone. A marked hypocholesterolemic effect was observed. Cholesterol homeostasis was achieved in fibrenat-fed rats. A plausible mechanism has been proposed. [Venkatesan N, Devaraj SN, Devaraj H; Increased binding of LDL and VLDL to apo B,E receptors of hepatic plasma membrane of rats treated with Fibrenat, *Eur J Nutr* **42**(5), 262-71 (2003)].

See *Zingibar officinale:* [Singh VK, Singh S, Singh DK; Pharmacological effects of spices. Recent progress in medicinal plants: Phytochemistry and Pharmacology, JN Govil, VK Singh (eds.) Studium press, LLC, Houston, Texas, USA, p 321-353 (2003)].

Preliminary animal and human trials suggest possible hypoglycemic and antihyperlipidemic properties of fenugreek seed powder. [Basch E, Ulbricht C, Kuo G, Szapary P, Smith M, Therapeutic applications of fenugreek, *Altern Med Rev* **8**(1), 20-27 (2003)].

Administration of crude extracts of seed powder of fenugreek, simultaneously with high fat diet to hamsters for 10 days, produced lowering of lipid levels. However, the chloroform and water extracts showed more pronounced lipid-lowering activity compared to other fractions. [Saxena R, Shwetat AP, Narinder T, Khanna AK, Bhatia G, Chander R, Rastogi AK; Antihyperlipidemic activity of *Trigonella foenum graecum* in high fat-fed hamsters, *National Seminar on New Millennium Strategies for Quality, Safety and GMP of herbal drugs / products,* NBRI, Lucknow, India p 157, Nov 11-13, 2003].

Triticum aestivum (Wheat, H. Gehun, S. Godhuma): See *Glycine max* (Soya bean, soybean): [Malinow *et al.*; *Am J Clin Nutr* **29**(8), 905-11 (1976)].

See Pectin in Appendix: [Sharma *et al.*; *Indian J Physiol Pharmacol* **24**(2), 136-38 (1980)].

Weanling rats, fed with a hypercholesterolemic diet containing 10% protein derived from wheat gluten as the sole protein source for 3 weeks, were compared to other rats fed with a 10% casein-control diet. Rats fed gluten showed a higher uptake of cholesterol by the adrenals, and enhanced excretion of neutral sterols and bile acids. The increased faecal excretion of cholesterol and bile acids induced by the gluten diet represents the main mechanism of the hypocholesterolemic effect of this diet. [Einav P, Mokady S, Cogan U; Effect of wheat gluten on cholesterol metabolism in growing rats, *Nutr Reports International* **24**(5), 1001-08 (1981)].

See Plant fibres in Appendix: [Chen and Anderson; *Am J Clin Nutr* **34**(6), 1077-82 (1981)].

See *Cyamopsis tetragonoloba* (Cluster bean, Guar): [Vahouny GV; *Fed Proc* **41**(11), 2801- 6 (1982)].

See *Glycine max* (Soya bean, soybean): [Mokady and Liener *Ann. Nutr Metab* **26**(2), 138-44 (1982)].

It was ascertained from an investigation with patients with a history of myocardial infarction that inclusion of wheat bran in an amount of 70-80 g into the antiatheroclerotic diet does not exert any hypolipidemic action. [Meshcheriakova VA, Samsonov MA, Frolova IA, Plotnikova OA, Pokrovskaia GR; Effect of wheat bran included in an anti-atherosclerotic diet on the lipid metabolic indices of ischemic heart disease patients, *Vopr Pitan* (3), 9-13 (1985) [Article in Russian].

Anticholesterolemic activity of the processed and purified wheat bran was investigated. Wheat bran was dispersed in water, treated with calcium hydroxide solution, neutralized with oxalic acid and then filtered. Further, the filtrate was purified by activated carbon, concentrated and dried. This dried and purified hemicellulose, exhibited potent hypocholesterolemic activity in rats. [Japan Maize Products Co. Ltd; *Anticholesterolemics from wheat bran.* Patent/ Japan Kokai Tokkyo, Koho JP **58**, 41,841(Cl.A61K35/78) 1988 6pp].

See *Oryza sativa* (Rice): [Topping *et al.*; *J Nutr* **120**(4), 325-30 (1990)].

Wheat germ intake (30g daily) by hypercholesterolemic subjects for 4 weeks significantly decreased plasma cholesterol, VLDL- cholesterol and apoprotein B and A-1 levels. However, LDL- and HDL-cholesterol levels did not change much in these subjects. In hypertriglyceridemic patients, significant reduction in plasma triglycerides and VLDL-triglycerides was also noted following consumption of wheat germ. Previous studies also demonstrated similar results in albino rats. It was suggested that wheat germ might be useful in the dietary management of hyperlipidemia. [Cara L, Borel P, Armand M, Senft M, Lafont H, Portugal H, Pauli AM, Boulze D, Lacombe C, Lairon D; Plasma lipid lowering effects of wheat germ in hypercholesterolemic subjects. *Plant Foods Hum Nutr* **41**(2), 135-50 (1991)].

Several foods rich in water-soluble fibre have documented hypocholesterolemic effects. The cholesterol-lowering effects of high-soluble fibre intake from refined, wheat-based bakery products was studied on 10 hypercholesterolemic subjects. The results of the investigation confirmed that a small increase in soluble-fibre intake of approximately 6 g/d modestly decreases atherogenic serum cholesterol concentrations, regardless of fibre source. [Anderson JW, Riddell-Lawrence S, Floor TL, Dillon DW, Oeltgen PR; Bakery products lower serum cholesterol concentrations in hypercholesterolemic men, *Am J Clin Nutr* **54**(5), 836-40 (1991)].

See *Avena sativa* (Oat): [Bre mer *et al.*; *Australian and New Zealand J Med* **21**(4), 422-26 (1991)].

Addition of a lipopolysaccharide (LPSw) from wheat flour in drinking water caused lowering of serum cholesterol in WHHL (Watanabe heritable hyperlipidemic) rabbits. Following withdrawl of LPSw from drinking water, the serum cholesterol levels remained decreased upto 30-40 days and thereafter increased gradually. The serum apolipoprotein B (a constituent of low density lipoprotein) was also reduced in treated animals. On the contrary, the apolipoperotein A-1 (a constituent of high density lipoprotein) and HDL levels did not change following feeding of LPSw. The atherosclerosis risk factor was also decreased by feeding of LPSw. [Okutomi T, Nishizawa T, Inawaga J, Takano T, Morikawa A, Soma JI, Mizuno D; Homeostasis as regulated by activated macrophage. VII. Supression of serum cholesterol levels by LPSw (a lipopolysaccharide from wheat flour) in WHHL (Watanabe heritable hyperlipidemic) rabbits, *Chem Pharm Bull* **40**(5), 1268-270 (1992)].

See *Hordeum vulgare* (Barley): [Martinez *et al.*; *J Nutr* **122**(5), 1070-76 (1992)].

See Tocotrienols in Appendix: [Pearce *et al.*; *J Med Chem,* **35**(2), 3595-606 (1992)].

Plasma cholesterol concentrations were significantly lower in rats fed with a cholesterol-free diet containing white wheat flour than those fed the diet with whole wheat or wheat bran. Effects of white wheat flour on steroid metabolism and cecal volatile fatty acid resemble those of oat bran and support the observation that wheat flour might be hypocholesterolemic in humans. [Illman RJ, Storer GB, Topping DL; White wheat flour lowers plasma cholesterol and increases cecal steroids relative to whole wheat flour, wheat bran and wheat pollard in rats, *J Nutr* **123**(6), 1094-100 (1993).

See *Hordeum vulgare* (Barley): [Wang & Klopfenstein; *Cereal Chem* **70**(6), 712-15 (1993)].

Serum cholesterol levels were significantly higher in animals fed with the diet containing wheat water solubles, a by-product of a gluten-starch washing plant, in comparison to those fed oat bran. Freeze-dried wheat water solubles have no potential as a dietary hypocholesterolemic agent. [Maziya Dixon BB, Klopfenstein CF, Walker CE; Freeze-dried wheat water solubles from a starch-gluten washing stream: Functionality in angel food cakes and nutritional properties compared with oat bran, *Cereal Chem* **71**(3), 287-91 (1994)].

In alloxan-induced diabetic and hypercholesterolemic rats, the hypolipidemic and hypoglycemic activity of pasta made from whole durum wheat, whole durum wheat supplemented with 7% or 12% defatted soy flour or 12% soy flour plus 0.3% methionine was studied. High fibre, high protein pasta made solely from durum wheat, supplemented with soy flour and soy flour plus methionine significantly lowered plasma cholesterol, lipid fractions and blood glucose levels in these animals. However, maximum hypocholesterolemic and hypoglycemic effect was noted in animals with pasta made from durum wheat flour supplemented with 12% soy flour plus 0.3% methionine. [Taha SA, Wasif MM; Hypoglycemic effect and protein nutritive quality of soy and methionine-supplemented whole durum pasta products, *Nahrung* **40**(5), 281-87 (1996)].

See *Oryza sativa* (Rice): [Kahlon *et al.*; *Cereal Chem* **75**(6), 897-903 (1998)].

Effect of whole-wheat flour and its milling fractions on plasma and liver lipids was investigated in albino rats. Wheat flour and white wheat flour both decreased cholesterol level. However, whole-wheat flour significantly decreased cholesterolemia. All cereal diets caused a significant reduction of liver lipid contents but such an effect was relatively more marked in case of whole wheat flour. It was suggested that total wheat grain was more effective in lowering the cholesterol and triglyceride levels and splitting of wheat grain may affect its hypocholesterolemic activity. [Adam A, Lopez HW, Tressol JC, Leuillet M, Demigne C, Ramesy C; Impact of whole wheat flour and its milling fractions on the cecal fermentation and plasma and liver lipids in rats, *J Agric Food Chem* **50**(22), 6557-62 (2002)].

See *Trigonella foenum-graecum*: [Venkatesan *et al.*; *Eur J Nutr* **42**(5), 262-71 (2003)].

Typha angustata: In experimental animals, *T. angustata* significantly decreased serum cholesterol and triglyceride levels alongwith enhancement of HDL-cholesterol. The drug was free from toxic side effects. [Zhang B *et al.*; Clinical and experimental research of *Typha angustata* on hyperlipidemia, *Chin J Integ Trad West Med* **5**(3), 145-47 (1985)].

Typha angustifolia: Silsosangami, a traditional Korean medicine consisting of the pollens of *Typha angustifolia*, roots of *Paeoniae rubra*, rhizomes of *Cnidium monnier*, seeds of *Prunus persica*, flowers of *Carthamus tinctorius*, tubers of *Curcuma longa* and the faeces of *Trogopterus xanthipes* (flying squirrel) has been reported to have a hypolipidemic effect in human subjects. The inhibitory effects of this Korean medicine on thrombosis in rats, induced by endotoxin treatment and the anti-thrombic properties of this drug with respect to blood parameters were investigated. The results of the investigation indicate that protective effects of the drug on ischemic infarction might be related to its inhibitory effects on disseminated intravascular coagulation, platelet coagulation and thrombotic action. [Park WH, Ahn JC, Kim HM, Lee YC, Kim CH; Effects of a Korean herbal formulation, Silsosangami, consisting of seven medicinal herbs, on endotoxin-induced experimental thrombosis in rats, *Phytother Res* **18**(3), 224-29 (2004).].

U

***Uncaria sinensis*:** The migration and matrix metalloproteinases (MMPs) production of vascular smooth muscle cells may play a key role in the development of atherosclerosis. Results of an investigation showed that the Korean traditional herbal formulation, Cho-Deung- San, composed of 11 herbal ingredients could be used as potential antiatherosclerotic agent and that the hooks and stems of *Uncaria sinensis* provide the major component of the herbal formulation for antimigration in tumor necrosis factor-*alpha* (TNF- α) treated human aortic smooth muscle cells. [Ha KT, Lee TK, Kwak KH, Kim JK, Kim DI, Choi DY, Kim CH; Inhibitory effect of Cho-Deung-San on human aortic smooth muscle cell migration induced by TNF- α through inhibition of matrix metalloproteinase-2 and -9 activity, *Vascul Pharmacol* **41**(3), 83-90 (2004)].

***Ungernia ferganica*:** See Polysaccharides in Appendix; [Khushbaktova *et al.*; *Khim Farma Zh* **21**(11), 1348-52 (1987)].

Administration of a mannan, isolated from the bulbs of *U. ferganica*, elicited potent hypolipidemic activity in normal as well as in experimentally induced hyperlipidemic animals. [Rakhinov DA, Malikova M.K, Khushbaktova ZA, Syrov VN; Plant polysaccharides. XVI. Mannan from *Ungernia ferganica* and its biological activity, *Chem Nat Prod* **32**(5), 680-82 (1996)].

***Ungernia sewerzowii*:** See Polysaccharides in Appendix: [Khushbaktova *et al.*; *Khim Farma Zh* **21**(11), 1348-52 (1987)].

V

***Vaccinium myrtillus*:** In genetically hyperlipidemic rats, oral administration of extract of *V. myrtillus* leaves significantly lowered plasma triglycerides and cholesterol levels without affecting free fatty acid contents. In normolipidemic rats, this drug failed to elicit significant effect on plasma triglycerides and free fatty acid levels. *V. myrtillus* leaves, a known hypoglycemic agent, may also be useful in dyslipidemia. [Cignarella A, Bertozzi D, Pinna C, Puglisi L; Hypolipidemic activity of *Vaccinium myrtillus* leaves on a new model of genetically hyperlipidemic rats, *Planta Med* **58**(Suppl.1), A 581-A582 (1992)].

***Vexibia alopecuroides*:** See Flavonoids in Appendix: [Khushbaktova *et al.*; *Khim Farma Zh* **25**(4), 53-57 (1991)].

Vicia faba (Field beans, Fava beans, Broad beans, H. Bakla): The ability of a faba bean protein concentrate, deprived of all the compounds soluble in hot ethanol, in lowering the level of serum cholesterol was investigated. Male adult rats were fed with a high-fat high-cholesterol diet, or the same diet in which 50% of the protein was substituted by a faba bean protein concentrate, either untreated or extracted with hot ethanol. Untreated faba bean protein concentrate diet always exhibited a significant hypocholesterolemic effect. The lipoprotein fraction in which the cholesterol was more affected was the very low density lipoprotein and then, in order, the intermediate density lipoprotein and low density lipoprotein. Ethanol extracted faba bean protein concentrate diet failed to lower the serum cholesterol. Feeding both untreated and ethanol extracted faba bean protein concentrate increased faecal excretion of cholic acid, deoxycholic acid and cholesterol. The fraction soluble in hot ethanol was thus proved to be responsible for the hypocholesterolemic effect of the faba bean protein concentrate. [Mengheri E, Scarino ML, Vignolini F, Spadoni MA; Effect of a hot ethanol extracted faba bean protein concentrate on rat serum cholesterol distribution, *Nutr Reports International* **26**(5), 751-58 (1982)].

The hypocholesterolemic effect of dietary vegetable proteins was studied by comparing eggwhite protein and fava bean protein concentrate in one normal and seven hypercholesterolemic persons. Fava bean diet did not show a significant effect on lowering serum total and LDL-cholesterol. [Contaldo F, Di Biase G, Giacco A, Pacioni D, Moro CO, Grasso L, Mancini M, Fidanza F; Evaluation of the hypocholesterolemic effect of vegetable proteins, *Prev Med* **12**(1), 138-43 (1983)].

The biochemical studies on blood serum and liver homogenate of rats, activity of the enzymes GOT, GPT, G-6PDh (glucose 6-phosphate dehydrogenase) and quantity of serum cholesterol revealed that a diet with protein concentrate of broad beans showed a tendency to hypocholesterolemic action . [Parlapanova M, Baikova D, Stoyanov Z; Protein concentrate of broad beans as a component of low energy diet, *Khigiena-i Zdraveopazvane* **29**(2), 65-70 (1986) Article in Bulgarian].

The hypocholesterolemic effect of field bean flour was studied on young volunteers with borderline-high or high serum cholesterol values. All subjects (groups A-D) consumed the same basic diet. Additionally, volunteers in the control group (A) consumed 90 g control flour/d whereas those in the three bean groups received either 90 g cooked field bean flour (groups B and C) or 90 g raw field bean flour (group D) daily. After 30 days, serum glucose, insulin, triacylglycerol, total cholesterol, LDL-cholesterol, and very low density lipoprotein (VLDL)-cholesterol values were significantly lower than initial values in all subjects who consumed diets containing field bean flour. Legume intake also resulted in a significant increase in glucagon and high density lipoprotein cholesterol. Neither cortisol nor thyroid hormone values changed significantly. The results suggest that the hypocholesterolemic effect of field bean intake depends at least partly on a concomitant increase in glucagon and decrease in insulin values. The more marked reduction in triacylglycerol and VLDL-cholesterol concentrations in subjects who consumed raw field beans indicates a co-participation of their thermolabile components. [Fruhbeck G, Monreal I, Santidrian S; Hormonal implications of the hypocholesterolemic effect of intake of field beans (*Vicia faba* L.) by young men with hypercholesterolemia, *Am J Clin Nutr.* **66**(6), 1452-60 (1997)].

Vicia truncatula: Butanol extract of the above ground part of *V. truncatula* showed the presence of diosmetin glycosides. The compounds possessed hypolipidemic and capillary-strengthening properties when tested in albino rats. [Andreeva OA, Bandyukova VA, Leonteva TP, Rekkanut SA; Flavonoids from *Vicia truncatula* Fisch. Ex Bieb and their pharmacological properties, *Rastitel'nye Resursy* **23**(1), 96-100 (1987)].

Vigna sinensis (Cowpea): Hypocholesterolemic effect of whole cowpea flour, defatted cowpea flour and hexane extracted fat was investigated in atherogenic diet fed with albino rats. All the three preparations of cowpea markedly lowered the serum and liver cholesterol levels. These preparations also significantly enhanced the faecal bile acid excretion as compared to control. [Mahadevappa VG, Raina PL; Hypocholesterolemic effect of cowpea in rats fed with atherogenic diet, *Ind J Med Res* **78**(Dec), 819-23 (1983)].

Effects of *V. sinensis* seed extract on the cholesterol levels was studied in experimentally induced hypercholesterolemic rats. Aqueous extract of the seeds and the residual seed meal of *V. sinensis* significantly lowered the serum cholesterol levels. [Joshi LD, Singhal PC, Gupta RK, Singh JB; Cholesterolemic action of *Vigna sinensis* (Cow pea), *Indian Heart J* **36**(1), 44-45 (1984)].

Vigna subterranea (Bambara groundnuts): A comparative study of the effects on blood lipids and faecal steroids of five legume species (*Vigna subterranea, Phaseolus vulgaris, Pisum sativum, Lens culinaris* and *Phaseolus lunatus*) was made. Sprague-Dawley rats were fed on hypercholesterolaemic semi-purified diets supplemented with cholesterol (1%) and cholic acid (0.5%). The effects of substitution (33%) of semi-purified diets by different legumes were studied at weeks 4 and 8. The diets incorporating the five different legume species produced very different cholesterolemic effects. Diets incorporating *Phaseolus vulgaris* and *P. lunatus* were more potent at lowering raised plasma cholesterol levels than diets containing *Pisum sativum* and *Lens culinaris*. Inclusion of the Bambara groundnut (*Vigna subterranean*) into the semi-purified diet resulted in an exaggeration of hypercholesterolaemia. Differences in cholesterol-lowering capacity of the various legume diets in this experiment could not be related to concentrations of faecal bile acids or neutral sterols. However, there was evidence that the inclusion of legumes in the diets reduced the faecal excretion of secondary bile acids. [Dabai FD, Walker AF, Sambrook IE, Welch VA, Owen RW, Abeyasekera S; Comparative effects on blood lipids and faecal steroids of five legume species incorporated into a semipurified, hypercholesterolaemic rat diet, *Brit J Nutr* **75**(4), 557-71 (1996)].

Vinca rosea (H. Sadabahar): See *Saccharum officinarum* [Tarvady & Dhar, *Biomedicine.* **9**(1) 39-42 (1989); *Indian J Exp Biol* **28**(7), 657-60 (1990)].

Vitex leucoxylon: Ethanol extract of *V. leucoxylon* leaves lowered serum total cholesterol level. [Makwana HG; Ravishankar B; Shukla VJ; Nair RB; Vijayan NP; Sasikala CK; Saraswathy VN; Bhatt SV; General pharmacology of *Vitex leucoxylon* Linn leaves, *Indian J Physiol Pharmacol* **38**(2), 95-100 (1994)].

Vitis vinifera (Grapes, H. Angur, S. Draksha)**:** The effects of dietary apple and grape pomace on serum cholesterol level were compared to those of pectin and cellulose in rats fed with cholesterol-enriched diets. Pomace from these fruits, particularly that from grape, exhibited a potent hypocholesterolemic activity compared to cellulose, although the efficacy was lower than that of pectin. The results indicate a usefulness of grape pomace as well as apple pomace as a dietary fibre, which is capable of regulating serum cholesterol level. [Sugano M, Nakano Morita M, Yoshida K, Imai J; Influence of dietary apple and grape pomace on serum cholesterol level of the rat, *J Jpn Soc Food Sci Technol* (*Nippon Shokuhin Kogyo Gakkaishi*) **35**(4), 242-45 (1988) Article in Japanese].

The effect of grape seed tannins (monomeric or polymeric form) on plasma cholesterol in rats was studied. Feeding of diets containing 1% cholesterol to Sprague Dawley rats showed an increase in total and low density lipoprotein plasma cholesterol and a decrease in plasma highdensity lipoprotein. These changes were prevented by the addition of 2% polymeric grape tannins in the diet but not by monomeric tannins. The tannin polymers also largely inhibited the observed increases in liver weight, liver lipids and total liver cholesterol in high cholesterol-fed rats. [Tebib K, Bitri L, Besancon P, Rouanet JM; Polymeric grape seed tannins prevent plasma cholesterol changes in high-cholesterol-fed rats, *Food Chem* **49**(4), 403-06 (1994)].

The antiatherosclerotic effect of proanthocyanidin-rich extracts from grape seeds in cholesterol-fed rabbits was studied. Proanthocyanidin-rich extracts (0.1% and 1% in diets w/w) did not appreciably affect the changes in serum lipid profile but the level of cholesteryl ester hydroperoxides (ChE-OOH) induced by 2,2'-azobis(2-amidinopropane-dihydrochloride) were lower in the plasma of rabbits fed proanthocyanidin-rich extract plus cholesterol than in the plasma of rabbits fed with cholesterol alone. Aortic malondialdehyde content decreased in rabbits fed with proanthocyanidin-rich extract and severe atherosclerosis in the aorta significantly reduced. From the results of the investigation, it was suggested that proanthocyanidins, the major polyphenols in red wine, might trap reactive oxygen species in plasma and interstitial fluid of the arterial wall and thus inhibit oxidation of LDL and show antiatherosclerotic activity. [Yamakoshi J, Kataoka S, Koga T, Ariga T; Proanthocyanidin-rich extract from grape seeds attenuates the development of aortic atherosclerosis in cholesterol-fed rabbits, *Atherosclerosis* **142**(1), 139-49 (1999)].

The effect of dietary cellulose (5 or 15%) and dried powdered grape pomace (15%) on the development of hypercholesterolemia and colon carcinoma was studied in male Wistar rats. Hypercholesterolemia was induced by the diet supplemented with 0.3% of cholesterol and 0.55% of bile salts while colon carcinoma was induced by treatment with dimethylhydrazine (20 mg/kg sc 12 doses in one-week intervals). Fibre content in grape pomace was 67 g/100 g of dry matter 10.3% of which was water-soluble. Fourteen weeks after the application of dimethylhydrazine, serum cholesterol level decreased by 38-48% in animals fed with grape pomace diet when compared to cellulose diets. Increased amount of cellulose in the diet showed no hypocholesterolemic effect. Decrease of serum cholesterol in grape pomace fed to animals could be attributed mainly to low density and very low density lipoproteins. A significant reduction (by almost 40%) was also observed for cholesterol levels in aorta and triacylglycerol levels in serum. Compared to cellulose diets, grape pomace diet reduced conjugated diene content in plasma, erythrocytes and liver by 30-60% and it significantly increased catalase activity in erythrocytes and colon. When compared to 15% cellulose diet, an increase in superoxide dismutase activity was observed in liver while glutathione peroxidase activities in liver and colon were reduced. [Bobek P, Galbavy S; Effect of grape pomace on alimentary hypercholesterolemia and chemically induced colon carcinogenesis in rats, *Biologia* (Bratislava) **54**(6), 725-31 (1999)].

The beneficial effects of red wine and other alcoholic beverages in inhibiting atherosclerosis were studied in a hamster model. Beverages tested included red wine, dealcoholized red wine, and red grape juice. Ethanol and all beverages caused a significant reduction in atherosclerosis. The combination of ethanol in red wine had the largest effect in decreasing atherosclerosis by both hypolipemic and antioxidant mechanisms. Red wine's beneficial effects can be attributed entirely to the polyphenols. Grape juice had a significant benefit at a much lower dose of polyphenols than the wines. Grape juice.was calculated to be much more effective than red wine or dealcoholised red wine at the same polyphenol dose in inhibiting atherosclerosis and improving lipids and antioxidant parameters. This data suggest that polyphenolic beverages from grapes are beneficial in inhibiting atherosclerosis by several mechanisms. Grape juice or non-alcoholic red wine is an excellent alternative to red wine in this model of atherosclerosis. [Vinson JA, Teufel K, Wu N; Red wine, dealcoholized red wine, and especially grape juice, inhibit atherosclerosis in a hamster model, *Atherosclerosis* **156**(1), 67-72 (2001)].

The effect of resveratrol, a polyphenolic compound present in grapes and other plants, on proteinuria, hypoalbuminemia and hyperlipidemia was studied in rats with glomerulonephritis. Resveratrol suppressed significantly hyperlipidemia incident to nephritis, the hypotriglyceridemic action being more prominent than the hypocholesterolemic one. The results of the investigation suggested resveratrol to be a potent anti-glomerulonephritic food factor capable of suppressing proteinuria, hypoalbuminemia and hyperlipidemia at the same time. [Nihei T, Miura Y, Yagasaki K; Inhibitory effect of resveratrol on proteinuria, hypoalbuminemia and hyperlipidemia in nephritic rats, *Life Sci* **68**(25), 2845-52 (2001)].

Resveratrol is an antioxidant present in grapes and wines. With an objective to study whether dietary resveratrol could inhibit the proliferation and metastasis of tumors and hyperlipidemia, experiments were conducted on Donryu rats, subcutaneously implanted with an ascites hepatoma cell line of AH109A. By feeding resveratrol (10 or 50 ppm) in the diet to hepatoma-bearing rats for 20 days, solid tumor growth and metastasis tended to be suppressed dose-dependently. Resveratrol (50 ppm) significantly suppressed the serum lipid peroxide level, indicating its antioxidative properties or those of its metabolite(s) *in vivo*. Resveratrol dose-dependently suppressed both the serum triglyceride and very low density lipoprotein + low-density lipoprotein

(VLDL + LDL)-cholesterol levels. The hypocholesterolemic action of resveratrol is attributed, at least in part, to an increased excretion of neutral sterols and bile acids into faeces. [Miura D, Miura Y, Yagasaki K; Hypolipidemic action of dietary resveratrol, a phytoalexin in grapes and red wine, in hepatoma-bearing rats, *Life Sci* **73**(11), 1393-400 (2003)].

See *Brassica campestris* (Rapeseed)**:** [Gorinstein *et al.*; *Nutr Res* **23**(3), 317-30 (2003)].

See *Citrus* species: [Kim *et al.*; *Nutr Res* **23**(12), 1671-83 (2003)].

Antiatherosclerotic effect of commercially available phenolics-rich extracts from grape seeds was studied in cholesterol-fed hamsters and the possible operating mechanisms were investigated. These extracts, fed at a moderate dose (equivalent to two glasses of red wine) per meal, reduced plasma cholesterol but did not affect plasma antioxidant capacity of hamsters. The extracts prevented the development of aortic atherosclerosis by 68%. Phenolic extracts from grape seeds were proved to be beneficial in inhibiting atherosclerosis by indirect mechanism(s). [Auger C, Gerain P, Laurent-Bichon F, Portet K, Bornet A, Caporiccio B, Cros G, Teissedre PL, Rouanet JM; Phenolics from commercialized grape extracts prevent early atherosclerotic lesions in hamsters by mechanisms other than antioxidant effect, *J Agric Food Chem* **52**(16), 5297-302 (2004)].

W

Withania coagulans (H. Doddapaneer)**:** The hypolipidemic activity of the aqueous extract of dried fruits of *W. coagulans* was investigated in triton and high fat diet-induced hyperlipidemic albino rats. Administration of the extract of *W. coagulans* (1g/kg, po) to triton-induced hyperlipidemic rats caused a lowering of serum cholesterol (15%) as compared to untreated animals. Similarly, high fat diet-fed rats exhibited significant decrease in the serum cholesterol and lipoprotein levels following treatment with *W. coagulans* extract. This drug also reduced hepatic cholesterol and lipid peroxidation in comparison to controls. [Hemalatha S, Wahi AK, Singh PN, Chansouria JPN, Hypolipidemic activity of aqueous extract of *Withania coagulans* Dunal in high fat diet model, *55th Indian Pharmaceutical Congress* 19-21 December, 2003, Chennai].

Withania somnifera (H. & S. Aswagandha)**:** Six patients of mild NIDDM (Non-insulin dependent diabetes mellitus) and six mild hypercholesterolemic subjects were treated with the powder of roots of *W. somnifera* for 30 days. Decrease in blood glucose was comparable to that of an oral hypoglycemic drug. Significant increase in urine sodium, urine volume and significant decrease in serum cholesterol, triglycerides, LDL and VLDL-cholesterol-were observed indicating that root of *W. somnifera* is a potential source of hypoglycemic, diuretic and hypocholesterolemic agents. [Andallu B, Radhika B, Hypoglycemic, diuretic and hypocholesterolemic effect of winter cherry (*Withania somnifera*, Dunal) root, *Indian J Exp Biol* **38**(6), 607-09 (2000)].

See *Commiphora mukul:* [Mary et al.; *Phytomedicine* **10**(6-7), 474-82 (2003)].

Y

***Yucca schidigera*:** The effects of a blend of partially purified *Yucca schidigera* and *Quillaja saponaria* extracts on cholesterol levels in the human's blood and gastrointestinal functions were studied. Ultrafiltration and sequential diafiltration increased the amounts of steroidal saponin in aqueous yucca extract and terpenoid saponin in aqueous quillaja extract from 9.3% and 21.4% to 17.2% and 61.8%, respectively. Taking 0.9 mg of the blend (6:4, v/v) of the resulting filtrates a day for 4 weeks resulted in the decreases in total and LDL-cholesterol levels in blood plasma of hypercholesterolemic patients with improvement in gastrointestinal functions of patients. [Kim SW, Park SK, Kang SI, Kang HC, Oh HJ, Bae CY, Bae DH; Hypocholesterolemic property of *Yucca schidigera* and *Quillaja saponaria* extracts in human body, *Arch Pharm Res* **26**(12), 1042-46 (2003)].

***Yucca* species:** The extract of Yucca exhibited antihypercholesterolemic, antiarthritic, antihypertensive and antiviral activity. It was nontoxic when administered orally. [Liberty L, *Yucca* –a monograph, *Lawrence Review of Natural Products* p 1-2 March (1994)].

Z

Zea mays (Corn, H. Makai, S. Yavanala): See *Glycine max* (Soya bean, soybean): [Richard *et al.*; *Atherosclerosis* **37**(4), 513-20 (1980)].

See Plant fibres in Appendix: [Chen & Anderson; *Am J Clin Nutr* **34**(6), 1077-82 (1981)].

The validity of the hypothesis that the hypocholesterolemic activity of corn oil and other unsaturated vegetable oils (sunflower seed and soybean oils) is related to effects of their nontriglyceride components on intestinal lipid absorption was examined. The results indicate that, at the level present in these three oils, the non-triglyceride components do not significantly influence chylomicron lipid composition or size, or the rate of intestinal secretion of lipid components. [Green MH, Green JB; Effects of native and fractionated vegetable oils on lipid absorption in the rat, *Nutr Res* **8**(11), 1265-76 (1988)].

The mechanisms, by which poorly digestible raw amylomaize (corn that has an amylose content of around 50% or greater) starch lowers the serum cholesterol level in rats, were studied by feeding experiments as well as by *in vitro* measurements for the interaction of the starch with bile salts. The animals fed with amylomaize starch showed significantly lower serum cholesterol level than those on sucrose or normal corn starch. Raw potato starch, another poorly digestible starch, was also found to exhibit remarkable hypocholesterolemic effect compared to sucrose. In *in vitro* study, amylomaize starch was proved to adsorb more taurocholate and to inhibit more efficiently the absorption of 14C-cholate by everted ileum sacs than normal corn starch. These findings indicate that amylomaize starch presumably exerts its hypocholesterolemic action by depressing the intestinal reabsorption of bile salts through adsorbing them on undigested starch granules staying in the lower bowel. [Ohta F, Hirayama K, Kai K, Watanabe Y, Ayano Y; Hypocholesterolemic action of poorly digestible raw amylomaize starch in rats fed a cholesterol-free diet, *Tech Bull Faculty of Horticulture Chiba Univ* (41), 35-44 (1988)].

The effect of different types of fats on heart lipid peroxidatiom and blood lipid parameters was studied in albino rats. The animals were fed with either a low fat diet (2.2% lard plus 2.2% corn oil), corn oil diet (17%), salmon oil diet (12.5%) supplemented with 4.5% corn oil or lard diet (15%) supplemented with 2% corn oil for 8 weeks. All these diets also contained 1 % cholesterol. Corn oil-diet significantly lowered the blood triglyceride levels. However, salmon oil diet-fed rats exhibited more pronounced lowering of blood cholesterol, triglycerides and phospholipid levels compared to low fat diet-fed animals. Heart lipid contents were not affected by dietary manipulations. [Nalbome G, Leonard J, Termine E, Portugal H, Lechene P, Paul AM, Lafont H; Effects of fish oil , corn oil and lard diets on lipid peroxidation status and glutathione peroxidase activities in rat heart, *Lipids* **24**(3), 179-86 (1989)].

The industrial procedure for the preparation of dietary fiber materials from corn pericarp was developed by wet milling process. Refined corn bran and soluble corn fiber, prepared by this procedure, were tested for their hypocholesterolemic activity in diet-induced hypercholestreolemic rats and compared with that of corn bran and wheat bran. Refined corn bran was effective in preventing elevation of serum cholesterol levels and it was superior to wheat bran and also to corn bran. Soluble corn fibre and corn bran hemicellulose preparation showed a significant effect on preventing the elevation of serum cholesterol and also on depressing the increase in liver cholesterol content of rats compared with cellulose powder refined corn bran and soluble corn fiber, natural fiber supplement from corn, can play a role in achieving health benefits. [Takeuchi M, Sugawara M, Takesho T, Egashira Y, Sañaa H, Ayano Y; Development of corn dietary fibre materials with physiological functions, *J Jpn Soc Food Sci Technol* (*Nippon Shokuhin Kogyo Gakkaishi*) **38**(11), 981-89 (1991) Article in Japanese].

Hydrogenation of corn oil was found to impair its hypolipidemic effect. Replacing corn oil with a typical corn oil-margarine (by hydrogenation) resulted in a 10-fold increase in dietary *trans* fatty acid intake as well as increases in saturated fatty acids (21%) and mono-unsaturated fatty acids (14%) intake and a 12% decrease in polyunsaturated fatty acids intake. These changes resulted in higher plasma concentrations of total cholesterol, LDL-c, and LDL apoB and a less favourable total cholesterol to HDL-c ratio. Substitution of the corn-oil margarine for corn oil was associated with a less favourable lipid profile with regard to coronary heart disease risk. It was, therefore, recommended that hydrogenation be minimised during the processing of foods for use in cholesterol-lowering diets. [Lichtenstein AH, Ausman LM, Carrasco W, Jenner JL, Ordovas JM, Schaefer EJ; Hydrogenation impairs the hypolipidemic effect of corn oil in humans: Hydrogenation, *trans* fatty acids, and plasma lipids, *Arterioscler Thromb* **13**(2), 154-61 (1993)].

A significant hypocholesterolemic effect of the resistant cornstarch diet was observed only during the postabsorptive period. Hepatic fatty acid synthesis is tightly controlled by carbohydrate availability, but the possibility that volatile fatty acids exert specific effects on lipogenesis could not be ruled out. [Morand C, Levrat MA, Besson C, Demigne C, Remesy C; Effects of a diet rich in resistant starch on hepatic lipid metabolism in the rat, *J Nutr Biochem* **5**(3), 138-44 (1994)].

Isoproteinous diet having one percent cholesterol and ten percent dietary fibre from corn bran and black gram (*Phaseolus radiatus*) seed coat was fed to four groups of albino rats for six weeks. Consumption of both the grain husks lowered total lipids, cholesterol and triglycerides but significantly increased HDL-cholesterol. However, these grain husks did not significantly affect serum phospholipids. Corn bran was observed to be more hypolipidemic than black gram seedcoat. [Sharma M, Kawatra A; Effect of dietary fibre from cereal brans and legume seedcoats on serum lipids in rats, *Plant Foods Hum Nutr* **47**(4), 287-92 (1995)].

The prevention of cholelithiasis by dietary manipulation was investigated in hamsters receiving a fat-free lithogenic diet or the same diet with replacement of sucrose by 12, 36, 48, or 72.5% of autoclaved amylomaize starch for seven weeks. While all hamsters receiving lithogenic diet had cholesterol gallstones, none in the groups receiving 48 and 72.5% amylomaize starch had gallstones. Plasma cholesterol concentrations and hepatic cholesterogenesis of these two groups were also significantly reduced compared to the group receiving lithogenic diet without amylomaize starch. The transformation of cholesterol to bile acids significantly increased in the group receiving 72.5% of autoclaved amylomaize starch. Thus, the autoclaved amylomaize starch, which could be used in human nutrition, was found to prevent cholelithiasis and reduce cholesterolemia. [Khallou J, Riottot M, Parquet M, Verneau C, Lutton C; Antilithiasic and hypocholesterolemic effects of diets containing autoclaved amylomaize starch in hamster, *Dig Dis Sci* **40**(12), 2540-48 (1995)].

The hypolipidemic properties of lime-treated cornhusk containing 69% of fibre (5.0% as soluble fibre) were evaluated in guinea pigs. Lime-treated cornhusk significantly lowered plasma LDL-cholesterol by 25% and VLDL-cholesterol by 37%, although a dose effect was not observed in this parameter. Plasma triacylglycerol concentrations and HDL-cholesterol levels were not affected. The results of the detailed investigation indicate that lower plasma VLDL and LDL-cholesterol concentrations, induced by lime-treated corn husk intake, are associated with decreases in microsomal cholesterol that alter the regulatory enzymes of cholesterol homeostasis and upregulate LDL receptors. [Vidal Quintanar-RL, Hernandez L, Conde K, Vergara jimenez M, Fernandez ML; Lime-treated corn husks lower plasma LDL cholesterol in guinea pigs by altering hepatic cholesterol metabolism, *J Nutr Biochem* **8**(8), 479-86 (1997)].

See *Cocos nucifera* (Cocoanut): [Nicolosi *et al.*; *Med Sci Sports Exerc* **29**(11), 1422-28 (1997)].

See *Oryza sativa* (Rice): [Kahlon *et al.*; *Cereal Chem* **75**(6), 897-903 (1998)].

The mechanisms for the hypocholesterolemic activity of cornhusk oil were tested on male Hartley guinea pigs. The data from this study suggest that cornhusk oil exhibits its hypocholesterolemic effect by decreasing cholesterol absorption and increasing bile acid output. These alterations in the intestinal lumen alter hepatic cholesterol metabolism and may affect the synthesis and catabolism of lipoproteins. [Ramjiganesh T, Roy S, Nicolosi RJ, Young T, McIntyre JC, Fernandez ML; Corn husk oil lowers plasma LDL cholesterol concentrations by decreasing cholesterol absorption and altering hepatic cholesterol metabolism in guinea pigs, *J Nutr Biochem* **11**(7-8), 358-66 (2000)].

The mechanisms involved in the hypocholesterolemic effects of corn fibre oil were studied using male Hartley guinea pigs. The results of the study suggest that corn fibre oil, as a result of decreased bile acid absorption, increased mRNA abundance and activity of cholesterol 7α- hydroxylase. Because hepatic cholesterol is the substrate for cholesterol 7α-hydroxylase, a lowering of cholesterol concentrations in the total and microsomal pools was observed. As a response to the depleted microsomal free cholesterol pool, the LDL receptor was upregulated, drawing more cholesterol from plasma, thus leading to the observed decrease in plasma LDL cholesterol concentrations. [Ramjiganesh T, Roy S, Freake HC, McIntyre JC, Fernandez ML; Corn fibre oil lowers plasma cholesterol by altering hepatic cholesterol metabolism and upregulating LDL receptors in guinea pigs, *J Nutr* **132**(3), 335-40 (2002)].

A comparison of the hypocholesterolemic effect of high amylose cornstarch was made with normal cornstarch on sham-operated and cecectomized rats. In both types of rats, those fed the former diet had a significantly lower plasma total cholesterol concentration and a significantly larger intestinal bile acid pool than those fed the latter diet. In cecectomized rats, those fed with the high amylose cornstarch diet had significantly lower plasma HDL and LDL-cholesterol concentrations, a significantly greater faecal bile acid excretion and a significantly lower hepatic HMG-CoA reductase mRNA concentration than those fed the normal cornstarch diet. In intact rats, biliary bile acid flux into the small intestine was significantly greater in those fed with the high amylose cornstarch diet than in those fed the normal cornstarch diet. Thus, the hypocholesterolemic effect of high amylose cornstarch appears to be mediated by accelerated faecal excretion of bile acids and increases in the intestinal pool and biliary flux of bile acids, and not by cecal fermentation products. [Kishida T, Nogami H, Ogawa H, Ebihara K; The hypocholesterolemic effect of high amylose cornstarch in rats is mediated by an enlarged bile acid pool and increased faecal bile acid excretion, not by cecal fermented products, *J Nutr* **132**(9), 2519-24 (2002)].

Sprague-Dawley streptozotocin-induced diabetic rats were fed diet containing resistant starch from corn or rice. No significant effect of resistant starch feeding on blood glucose and insulin was found. Nonetheless, resistant starch from corn and rice significantly lowered plasma total lipid and cholesterol concentrations compared to the diabetic control. The total liver cholesterol lowering effect was observed with resistant starch from rice. [Kim WK, Chung MK, Kang NE, Kim MH, Park OJ; Effect of resistant starch from corn or rice on glucose control, colonic events, and blood lipid concentrations in streptozotocin-induced diabetic rats, *J Nutr Biochem* **14**(3), 166-72 (2003)].

See *Cyamopsis tetragonoloba* (Cluster bean, Guar gum): [Castro *et al.*; *Food Chem* **80**(3), 323-30 (2003)].

Zingiber officinale (H. Adrak, S. Ardraka)**:** Effect of *Z. officinalis* and *Sesamum indicum* on serum cholesterol and blood sugar was investigated. Adminstartion of 30 % *Z. officinalis* and *S. indicum* to albino rats significantly decreased serum cholesterol levels. However, blood sugar levels were increased following treatment with above plant drugs. [Singhal PC, Joshi LD; Glycemic and cholesterolemic role of ginger and til, *J Sci Res Plants Med* **4**(3), 32-34 (1983)].

Administration of *Z. officinalis* to cholesterol-fed rats significantly prevented increase of the blood cholesterol levels. Ginger also caused lowering of serum and hepatic cholesterol levels in hypercholesterolemic rats. [Giri J, Sakthi Devi TK, Meerarani S; Effect of Ginger on serum cholesterol levels, *Indian J Nutr Diet* **21**(12), 433-36 (1984)].

See *Piper longum:* [Sharma *et al.*; *Int J Crude Drug Res* **28**(1), 33-38 (1990)].

See *Curcuma longa* (Turmeric): [Srinivasan & Sambaiah; *Int J Vitamin Nutr Res* **61**(4), 364-69 (1991)].

In triton (WR-1339)-induced hypercholesterolemic mouse, oral administration of (*E*)- 8β, 17-epoxylabd-12-ene-15,16-diol, isolated from ginger, decreased the cholesterol biosynthesis in rat liver homogenate. General pharmacological screening did not reveal any remarkable activity other than inhibitory effect of the phytochemical on cholesterol biosynthesis. [Tanabe M, Chen YD, Saito KI, Kano Y; Cholesterol biosynthesis inhibitory component from *Zingiber officinalis*, *Chem Pharm Bull* **41**(4), 710-13 (1993)].

Adminstration of ethanolic extract of *Z. officinale* (200mg/kg) to atherogenic diet-fed rabbits for 10 weeks significantly reduced hyperlipidemia. The ginger extract also brought down the levels of serum cholesterol, triglycerides and phospholipids along with an increase in the HDL-cholesterol levels and coagulation time compared to untreated hyperlipidemic rabbits. The results were comparable to gemfibrozil, a lipid- and cholesterol-modifying medicine. [Bhandari U, Grover JK, Sharma JN; Effect of *Zingibar officinale* (ginger) on lipid metabolism in albino rabbits, *International Seminar on Recent Trends in Pharmaceutical Sciences, Ootacomund,* Abstr. **A41**, Feb 18-20, (1995)].

In cholesterol-fed rabbits, ethanolic extract of ginger (*Z. officinale*) in a dose of 200mg /kg po for 10 weeks significantly reduced serum and tissue cholesterol, serum triglyceride, lipoproteins, and phospholipid levels. The results were comparable to gemfibrozil. According to gross grading, the ginger extract-treated rabbits showed comparatively less marked atherosclerotic changes than the hypercholesterolemic animals [Bhandari U, Sharma JN, Zafar R; The protective action of ethanolic ginger (*Zingibar officinale*) extract in cholesterol fed rabbits, *J Ethnopharmacol* **61**(2), 167-171 (1998)].

The effect of administration of ginger (*Z. officinale*) on high fat fed-rats was studied for a period of 10 weeks. Ginger, as a coarse solution with distilled water, was administered orally by intragastric intubation daily, at two different doses, 35 mg and 70 mg/kg body weight. There was a significant decrease in the levels of cholesterol, phospholipids, and free fatty acids in the liver, intestine, kidney, aorta and serum of the ginger-treated rats. Levels of serum triglyceride were also significantly reduced in the ginger-treated groups. Supplementation of diets of the control and high fat-fed rats with ginger increased the concentration of HDL and decreased the concentration of LDL and VLDL in the serum as compared with control and high fat-fed animals not receiving the supplement. Thus, dietary intake of ginger was found to reduce the risk of atherosclerosis markedly by virtue of its hypolipidemic and antiatherogenic effects. [Murugaiah JS, Namasivayam N, Menon VP; Effect of ginger (*Zingiber officinale* R.) on lipids in rats fed with atherogenic diet, *J Clin Biochem Nutr* **27**(2), 79-87 (1999)].

The effect of rhizome of *Z. officinalis* (dry ginger) on blood lipid and sugar levels was examined in 20 cases of mild hypercholesterolemia and 20 patients of NIDDM. Dried rhizomes of ginger significantly lowered the serum total cholesterol, triglycerides, LDL- and VLDL-cholesterol levels along with significant enhancement of HDL-cholesterol in hypercholesterolemic subjects. Atherogenic index was also decreased in these treated patients. A significant lowering of blood and urinary sugar levels was also noted in the treated diabetic cases. [Andulla B, Radhika B; Evaluation of rhizomes of *Zingiber officinalis* for hypoglycemic and hypolipidemic activity. *Ethnobotany* **13**(1-2), 150-54 (2001)].

See *Commiphora mukul:* [Raut et al.; *J Mahatma Gandhi Inst Med Sci* **7**(2), 10-16 (2002)].

Chemical investigations done so far on *Zingiber officinale, Trachyspermum ammi, Trigonella foenum-graecum, Allium sativum, Allium cepa, Eugenia aromatica*, and *Curcuma longa* and their pharmacological activity like hypocholesterolemic, antiplatelet, antioxidant etc, have been reviewed. [Singh VK, Singh S, Singh DK; Pharmacological effects of spices. Recent progress in medicinal plants: Phytochemistry and pharmacology, JN Govil, VK Singh (eds.) Studium press, LLC, Houston, Texas, USA, p 321-353 (2003)].

The antiatherosclerotic effect of air-dried ginger powder (0.1g/kg bw for 75 days) was studied in cholesterol-induced atherosclerotic rabbits. Ginger administration significantly inhibited the cholesterol-induced atheroma in aorta and coronary arteries of these rabbits. The treated animals also exhibited decreased lipid peroxidation and enhancement of fibrinolytic activity. However, no significant change in blood lipid levels was noted in these animals. The antiatherosclerotic activity of ginger was ascribed to its free radical scavenging, prostaglandin inhibitory and fibrinolysis enhancing properties. [Verma SK, Singh M, Jain P, Bordia A; Protective effect of ginger, *Zingiber officinale* Rosc on experimental atherosclerosis in rabbits, *Indian J Exp Biol* **42**(7), 736-38 (2004)].

Zygophyllum coccineum (Kammun Quaramany): A single dose of alloxan (120 mg/kg bw) showed 2-fold increase in the plasma glucose level of rats, relative to the mean value of control group. Furthermore, the levels of total lipid, triglyceride, cholesterol, LDL and VLDL were significantly increased in the plasma and the liver tissues of diabetic rats compared to the control group, whereas HDL level was significantly decreased. The plasma levels of all the above parameters were normalised after treatment of the diabetic rats with aqueous suspension of the herb (1.5 ml /100 g bw, equivalent to 75 mg/100 g bw) for a period of four weeks. The plants Halfa barr (*Cymbopogon proximus*) and Termis (*Lupinus termis*) showed similar activity. [Newairy AS, Mansour HA, Yousef MI, Sheweita SA; Alterations of lipid profile in plasma and liver of diabetic rats: Effect of hypoglycemic herbs, *J Environ Sci Health* **B**. **37**(5), 475-84 (2002)].

Zygophyllum cornutum: *Zygophyllum cornutum* elicited hypocholesterolemic and hypolipidemic activity. The major flavonoid constituent of this plant was found to be quercetin 3β-D-glucpyranose-3'-methyl ether. [Aclinou P, Abdessemed K, Massiot G, Le Men-Oliver L; Plants of Aures III; Structure of a flavanoid of *Zygophyllum cornutum*, *Plantes Medicinales et Phytototherapie* **22**(4), 212-18 (1988)].

Zizyphus mistol: Nutritional evaluation was carried out on growing and reproducing mice fed with a semisynthetic diet containing *Z. mistol* seed oil, having a high percentage of unsaturated fatty acids, as the only added fat. After 20 weeks on mistol diet a hypocholesterolemic and hypolipemic effect was achieved. *Z.mistol* oil seed could be a valuable source of edible fat mainly as a rich vegetable source of α-linolenic acid. [Eynard AE, Munoz S, Lamarque A, Silva R, Guzman CA; Lipidic composition and nutritional evaluation of the (Rhamnaceae) *Zizyphus mistol* oil seed as the sole source of fat for mice, *Comunicaciones Biologicas* **10**(3), 213-24 (1992)].

APPENDIX

In addition to reports of hypolipidemic and antiatherosclerotic activity of plants reported above, similar activity is also known to be elicited by phytochemicals (flavonoids, lignans, sterols, triterpenes, saponins etc.), not specific to a particular plant, and these are presented in this Appendix. The roles played by amino acids, dietary fats and fatty acids, proteins and peptides, polysaccharides, dietary fibres, gums and many other similar compounds in regulating dyslipidemia, are also recorded in the Appendix.

AMINO ACIDS: The effect of lysine- and threonine-supplemented wheat gluten (gluten is the viscid, tenacious substance which gives adhesiveness to dough) on cholesterol metabolism was studied using male weaning rats. Animals were fed on cholesterol-free diets containing 100 or 200g gluten/kg diet with or without amino acid supplementation, and compared with animals given 50, 100 and 200 g casein/kg diets, for 3 weeks. A hypocholesterolemic effect was observed with the wheat gluten-fed rats, compared with the animals given 100 and 200g casein/kg diets. The hypocholesterolemic effect was accompanied by increased turnover of cholesterol as expressed by enhanced cholesterol biosynthesis and increased faecal excretion of cholesterol and bile acids. This effect was not abolished by lysine and threonine supplementation. A mechanism, related to impairment of cholesterol transport from the liver, was most likely responsible for the hypocholesterolemia found in these protein-malnourished animals. The effect on cholesterol metabolism produced by dietary wheat gluten was independent of the low quality of the protein and of its specific deficiency in lysine and threonine. [Bassat M, Mokady S; The effect of amino acid supplemented wheat gluten on cholesterol metabolism in the rat, *Brit J Nutr* **53**(1), 25-30 (1985)].

The lysine:arginine ratio of a protein shows significant effect on the metabolism of cholesterol in rats fed with cholesterol diet. A lysine:arginine ratio of 1.0 significantly lowered cholesterol in the serum, liver and aorta and increased hepatic cholesterogenesis as well as degradation of cholesterol to bile acid when compared to a lysine:arginine ratio of 2.0. Activity of lipoprotein lipase in the extrahepatic tissues and that of plasma lecithin cholesterol acyltransferase were also higher with lys:arg ratio of 1.0. [Rajamohan T, Kurup PA; Lysine to arginine ratio of protein and its effect on cholesterol metabolism, *Indian J Biochem Biophys* **23**(5), 294-96 (1986)].

Taurine is a non-essential sulfur-containing amino acid. The effect of oral administration of taurine (3.2 g/d, 2 wk) on the metabolism of lipids and bile acids was studied in healthy humans. The results suggested that taurine administration alone did not influence the serum lipid level although taurine-conjugated bile acids were increased. The taurine intake increased serum low density lipoprotein cholesterol and biliary cholesterol levels when excessive cholesterol was administered simultaneously.[Tanno N, Oikawa S, Koizumi M, Fuji Y, Hori S, Suzuki N, Sakuma E, Kotake H, Namai K, Toyota T; Effect of taurine administration on serum lipid and biliary lipid composition in man, *Tohoku J Exp Med* **159**(2),: 91-100 (1989)].

Soy protein induces a low postprandial insulin/glucagon ratio in both hypercholesterolemic and normocholesterolemic subjects. Casein induces a high postprandial insulin/glucagon ratio among hypercholesterolemic subjects. Amino acids such as arginine and glycine are associated with a decrease, while lysine and branched-chain amino acids are associated with increased serum cholesterol levels. The data are consistent with the hypothesis that the control of cholesterol by insulin and glucagon is regulated by dietary and plasma amino acids. [Sanchez A, Hubbard RW; Plasma amino acids and the insulin-glucagon ratio as an explanation for the dietary protein modulation of atheroscleroses, *Medical Hypotheses* **36**(1), 27-32 (1991)].

Effects of low casein diets supplemented with either cystine alone, cystine plus glycine, or cystine plus threonine on hyperlipidemia and proteinuria were studied in rats with nephrotoxic serum nephritis. The results suggest that cystine-threonine supplemented low casein diets have beneficial effects on hyperlipidemia and proteinuria with neither growth retardation nor fatty liver induction in nephritis. They also suggest that the hypocholesterolemic effect of the 8% casein supplemented with cystine and threonine diet in nephritic rats may be, at least in part, attributed to an increased excretion of steroids. [Fujisawa K, Yagasaki K, Funabiki R; Reduction of hyperlipidemia and proteinuria without growth retardation in nephritic rats by amino acids-fortified low casein diets, *J Nutr Biochem* **5**(1), 21-27 (1994)].

A methionine-threonine-supplemented 8.5% casein diet, when compared with a basal 20% casein diet, improved hypoalbuminemia as well as hyperlipidemia and proteinuria without noticeable growth retardation and fatty liver induction in nephritic rats. Faecal bile acid excretion and microsomal cholesterol 7α-hydroxylase activity were enhanced by feeding amino acid supplemented casein diet. The results suggest that the hypocholesterolemic action of methionine-threonine-supplemented 8.5% casein diet may be, at least in part, due to increased faecal bile acid excretion accompanied by elevated microsomal cholesterol 7α-hydroxylase activity. [Fujisawa K, Yagasaki K, Miura Y, Funabiki R; Improvement of hyperlipidemia and proteinuria without noticeable growth retardation by feeding a methionine and threonine supplemented low casein diet to nephritic rats, *Biosci Biotechnol Biochem* **59**(10), 1896-900 (1995)].

The effect of dietary lysine and arginine on growth performance and tissue cholesterol levels in chicks, fed the wheat gluten diet containing 20% crude protein was studied. The best growth performance was achieved by 0.5% supplementary lysine and both deficient and excess levels of lysine elevated serum cholesterol level in chicks fed with the cholesterol-supplemented diet. Supplementation of arginine along with lysine reduced the serum cholesterol level in cholesterol-fed chicks. Supplementation of 1% to 3% excess lysine increased serum cholesterol levels with concomitant growth retardation. This deleterious effect was completely alleviated by 3% excess arginine. The extent of hyper-and hypo-cholesterolemic effect respectively, of lysine and arginine in excess, was not proportional to their supplementary levels in the diet, so that the dietary ratio of lysine to arginine was not a determinant factor regulating serum cholesterol level. [Ueda H, Imanishi T, Fukumi R, Kumai S; Effect of dietary lysine and arginine addition on growth performance and serum cholesterol level in chicks, *Animal Sci Technol* **66**(5), 412-21 (1995)].

The effects of the amino acids methionine and cystine on the cholesterol concentrations in the serum and liver of chicks, fed diets containing 1% cholesterol, were studied. From the results of the investigation, it was inferred that methionine and cystine were not positively involved in the control of serum cholesterol concentrations in chicks. [Ueda H, Fukui W; Effects of methionine and cystine on the cholesterol concentrations in the serum and liver of cholesterol-fed chicks, *Animal Sci Technol* **67**(6), 533-40 (1996)].

The effects of dietary taurine supplementation on plasma and hepatic lipid levels and phospholipid profiles were evaluated in rats fed with a high-cholesterol diet. Taurine supplementation to high-cholesterol diet significantly lowered hepatic cholesterol and triglyceride concentrations compared to those fed high cholesterol diet alone. Rats fed with high-cholesterol diet had significantly higher phosphatidylcholine/phosphatidylethanolamine ratio in the liver homogenates than those fed cholesterol-free diet but taurine supplementation to high-cholesterol diet significantly lowered this ratio. The results suggest the hypocholesterolemic and hypotriglyceridemic effects of dietary taurine supplementation in rats fed with a high cholesterol diet. [Park T, Lee K, Um Y; Dietary taurine supplementation reduces plasma and liver cholesterol and triglyceride concentrations in rats fed a highcholesterol diet, *Nutr Res* **18**(9), 1559-71 (1998)].

The effect of dietary taurine on hypercholesterolemia, induced by a high-cholesterol diet in streptozotocin -induced diabetic rats, was investigated. The concentrations of serum and liver cholesterol were markedly elevated in streptozotocin -diabetic rats fed on the cholesterol-containing diet, and dietary taurine significantly reduced this elevated level of cholesterol in the serum and liver. The gene expression of cholesterol 7α-hydroxylase, which is the rate-limiting enzyme for cholesterol degradation, was induced by the supplementation of taurine to the high cholesterol diet. It is suggested that enhancement of cholesterol degradation might be one of the reasons for this hypocholesterolemic action by taurine. [Mochizuki H, Takido J, Oda H; Yokogoshi H; Improving effect of dietary taurine on marked hypercholesterolemia induced by a high cholesterol diet in streptozotocin-induced diabetic rats, *Biosci Biotechnol Biochem* **63**(11), 1984-87 (1999)].

The effects of dietary supplementation of taurine or glycine, the two amino acids involved in bile acid conjugation in the liver, on plasma and hepatic lipid concentrations were evaluated in rats fed with a cholesterol-free diet. Three groups of male rats were fed a cholesterol-free diet (CFD), a taurine-supplemented diet (CFD + 1.5% taurine) or a glycine-supplemented diet (CFD + 1.5% glycine) for 5 weeks. No significant difference in organ weights and cumulative body weight gain was observed between groups at the end of the experimental period. Plasma triglyceride level was significantly lower in rats of taurine supplemented group compared to those fed the CFD. Both taurine and glycine supplementation significantly lowered the plasma levels of total cholesterol and LDL-plus VLDL-cholesterol. Liver cholesterol concentration was not significantly influenced by the dietary supplementation of taurine or glycine, which, however, significantly lowered hepatic triglyceride concentrations, and elevated hepatic free fatty acid levels. The results suggest the possible roles of dietary taurine or glycine as hypocholesterolemic and/or hypotriglyceridemic agents. [Park T, Oh J, Lee K; Dietary taurine or glycine supplementation reduces plasma and liver cholesterol and triglyceride concentrations in rats fed with a cholesterol-free diet, *Nutr Res* **19**(12), 1777-89 (1999)].

The effect of taurine on hypercholesterolemia induced by feeding a high cholesterol diet (10g/kg) to rats was examined. The hypocholesterolemic effects of taurine observed in the hypercholesterolemic rats fed with the high-cholesterol diet were mainly due to the enhancement of cholesterol degradation and the excretion of bile acid. [Yokogoshi H, Mochizuki H, Nanami K, Hida Y, Miyachi F, Oda H; Dietary taurine enhances cholesterol degradation and reduces serum and liver cholesterol concentrations in rats fed a high-cholesterol diet, *J Nutr* **129**(9), 1705-12 (1999)].

Carnitine, a derivative of the amino acid lysine, plays an important role in the mitochondrial uptake of long-chain fatty acids in mammals. It has recently been shown that this compound has a marked hypocholesterolemic effect when used in conjunction with lipid-rich diets. The effects of L-carnitine on the fatty acid composition of plasma lipoproteins in rabbits fed with different diets were examined. The results of the investigation suggested that the hypocholesterolemic effects of L-carnitine could be associated with increased systemic breakdown of cholesteryl esters, a probable increase in reverse cholesterol transport and the stabilization of a phospholipid-based structure of VLDL + LDL particles. [Diaz M, Lopez F, Hernandez F, Urbina JA; L-Carnitine effects on chemical composition of plasma lipoproteins of rabbits fed with normal and high cholesterol diets, *Lipids* **35**(6), 627- 32 (2000)].

The effect of taurine on plasma cholesterol and liver lipid levels, and on the level of faecal bile acid excretion, was examined in ovariectomized 10-month-old retired breeder female rats. The findings of the investigation indicate that taurine can effectively prevent the ovarian hormone deficiency-associated increase in plasma cholesterol, and that an increased level of faecal bile acid excretion is one of the factors involved in the hypocholesterolemic effect of taurine. [Kishida T, Ebihara K;

Ovarian hormone deficiency-induced hypercholesterolemia is reversed by taurine, *Nutr Res* **20**(8), 1173-82 (2000)].

The effects of taurine feeding on plasma cholesterol concentrations and faecal bile acid excretion were examined in young and aged male and female rats. In female rats, plasma cholesterol concentrations were higher in aged rats than in young rats and higher in ovariectomized rats than in sham-operated rats. In contrast to male rats, plasma cholesterol concentrations were lower in female rats fed with a cholesterol-free taurine-supplemented diet than in those fed a cholesterol-free diet. Plasma cholesterol concentrations were increased in aged ovariectomized rats, but decreased by feeding with the taurine-supplemented diet. Faecal bile acid excretion was higher in rats fed with the taurine-supplemented diet than in those fed the cholesterol-free diet. The hypocholesterolemic effect of taurine was found to be greater in aged rats than in young rats. [Kishida T, Akazawa T, Ebihara K; Influence of age and ovariectomy on the hypocholesterolemic effects of dietary taurine in rats fed a cholesterol-free diet, *Nutr Res* **21**(7), 1025-33 (2001)].

Hypocholesterolemic effect of taurine has been studied on dietary hypercholesterolemia. [Yokogoshi H, Nishimura N, Oda H; Hypocholesterolemic effect of taurine on dietary hypercholesterolemia, *Nippon Nogeikagaku Kaishi* **75**(9), 958-60 (2001) Article in Japanese].

The effect of taurine on the plasma cholesterol concentration in genetic type 2 diabetic rats was studied. Diabetic rats (GK male rats) and normal rats (Wistar male rats) were fed with either a cholesterol-free or cholesterol-enriched (1% cholesterol + 0.25% sodium cholate) diet supplemented with or without 3% taurine for 21 or 14 days. At the start of the experiment, the plasma cholesterol concentration was significantly higher in the diabetic rats than in the normal rats. Taurine did not affect the plasma cholesterol level in rats fed with the cholesterol-free diet. However, taurine feeding significantly increased the plasma HDL-cholesterol concentration in the diabetic rats fed the cholesterol-free diet. In both the diabetic and normal rats fed with the cholesterol diet, the plasma cholesterol concentration was significantly lower in rats fed with the diet supplemented with taurine than in the rats fed the control diet. It was concluded that taurine has a hypocholesterolemic effect in both diabetic and normal rats fed with diets containing cholesterol. Further, taurine seemed to affect the HDL-cholesterol metabolism in diabetic rats fed with a cholesterol-free diet. [Nishimura N, Umeda C, Oda H, Yokogoshi H; The effect of taurine on plasma cholesterol concentration in genetic type 2 diabetic GK rats, *J Nutr Sci Vitaminol* **48**(6), 483-90 (2002)].

The effect of taurine on hypercholesterolemia, induced by feeding a highcholesterol diet (10 g/kg) to rats, was examined. When taurine was supplemented to high-cholesterol diet for 2 weeks, serum total cholesterol significantly decreased and serum HDL-cholesterol increased compared with the high-cholesterol diet group. In the diet-induced hypercholesterolemic rats, the excretion of faecal bile acids and hepatic cholesterol 7α-hydroxylase activity and its mRNA level increased significantly, and the supplementation of taurine further enhanced these indices, indicating an increase in cholesterol degradation. The serum level of VLDL increased significantly in high cholesterol diet-fed rats but taurine repressed this increase and normalised this pattern. The results suggest that the hypocholesterolemic effects of taurine observed in the high cholesterol diet-fed hypercholesterolemic rats were mainly due to the enhancement of cholesterol degradation and the excretion of bile acid. [Yokogoshi H, Oda H; Dietary taurine enhances cholesterol degradation and reduces serum and liver cholesterol concentrations in rats fed a high-cholesterol diet, *Amino Acids* (Vienna), **23**(4), 433- 39 (2002)].

The role of taurine on atherogenesis, induced by high fat diet, was studied on rats, a species which depends entirely on taurine for conjugation of bile acids. Taurine significantly increased faecal bile acids, which resulted in significant decrease of serum cholesterol. Aortic lesion index was significantly decreased in the taurine administered group suggesting the antiatherogenic effect of taurine. It was concluded that taurine attenuated the atherogenesis possibly by its hypocholesterolemic and antioxidant property. [Sethupathy S, Elanchezhiyan C, Vasudevan K, Rajagopal G; Antiatherogenic effect of taurine in high fat diet-fed rats, *Indian J Exp Biol* **40**(10), 1169-72 (2002)].

The effect of taurine on atherosclerotic lesions in Watanabe heritable hyperlipidemic (WHHL) rabbits was studied. Taurine had no apparent effect on blood pressure and serum cholesterol levels but the contents of thiobarbituric acid reactive substances (TBARS), a marker of lipid peroxidation, were reduced in serum and aorta by 29 and 50%, respectively, when taurine was ingested. In addition, LDL from taurine-treated rabbits was resistant to copper-induced oxidative modification. These results revealed that taurine prevents development of atherosclerosis and that the antiatherosclerotic effects of taurine are independent of serum cholesterol levels. The anti-oxidant action of taurine may be involved in inhibiting atherosclerosis in these rabbits. [Murakami S, Kondo Y, Sakurai T, Kitajima H, Nagate T; Taurine suppresses development of atherosclerosis in Watanabe heritable hyperlipidemic (WHHL) rabbits, *Atherosclerosis*. **163**(1), 79-87 (2002)].

The hypocholesterolemic effect of taurine was examined in mice fed with a high cholesterol diet containing 1% cholesterol and 0.25% sodium cholate. It transpired from the results of the investigation that taurine does not up-regulate LDL receptor protein level, and the decrease in cholesterol in the circulation is mainly due to its suppressive effect on triglycerides secretion from the liver. [Chen W, Matuda K, Nishimura N, Yokogoshi H; The effect of taurine on cholesterol degradation in mice fed a high-cholesterol diet, *Life Sci* **74**(15),: 1889-98 (2004)].

DIETARY CARBOHYDRATES: Monosaccharides, disaccharides and various kinds of starch can have varying effect on the cholesterol level in human and animal blood. The effect of the same carbohydrate may vary depending on the animal, e.g. glucose can be hypercholesterolemic in rabbits but not in rats. Disaccharides, sucrose and lactose have a weak effect on cholesterol metabolism. Various kinds of starch have different influence on cholesterol level in blood. It is usually found that wheat starch is hyper-and potato starch is hypo-cholesterolemic. The way starches exert their cholesterolemic effect is not known precisely. [Hanczakowski P; The effect of dietary carbohydrates on cholesterol level in blood, *Biuletyn Informacyjny Instytut Zootechniki* **36**(4), 29-34 (1998) Article in Polish].

DIETARY FATS: Whole body sterol balance, hepatic HMG-Co A reductase activity, hepatic low density lipoprotein (LDL) receptor levels and net tissue cholesterol concentrations were determined in guinea pigs fed with either a corn oil or lardbased purified diet for 6-7 weeks. In comparison to the saturated lard diet, the polyunsaturated corn oil diet resulted in a 34% reduction in plasma total cholesterol levels and a 40% lower triacylglycerol level. Feeding the corn oil diet altered very low density lipoprotein (VLDL) and LDL composition; the percent cholesterol ester in both particles was decreased and the relative percentages of VLDL triacylglycerol and LDL phospholipid increased. The results of the detailed investigation indicate that the hypocholesterolemic effects of dietary polyunsaturated fat in the guinea pig are not attributable to changes in endogenous cholesterol synthesis or catabolism but rather may result from a redistribution of plasma cholesterol to body tissue due to an increase in tissue LDL receptors. [Ibrahim JBT, McNamara DJ; Cholesterol homeostasis in guinea pigs-fed saturated and polyunsaturated fat diets, *Biochim Biophys Acta* **963**(1), 109-18 (1988)].

Effects of dietary soybean, egg yolk and krill-phospholipids, and soybean and sardine oil on serum and liver cholesterol concentrations were investigated using weanling rats fed with a hypercholesterolemic diet for 2 weeks. Serum total cholesterol concentrations were significantly lower and the ratio of HDL-cholesterol to total cholesterol was higher in all the experimental groups than those of the control group (olive oil). Liver cholesterol and triglyceride concentrations decreased in all the experimental groups, especially in the phospholipid groups. The excretory ratio of faecal to dietary cholesterol of the soybean and egg yolk phospholipid groups were higher than that of other groups. These results indicate that the different mecahnism in hypocholesterolemic effect exists between phospholipids and polyunsaturated fatty acids, and that the phospholipids containing a large amount of higher polyunsaturated fatty acids such as eicosapentaenoic acid probably prevent the hypercholesterolemic effect. [Kuroda K, Kobatake Y, Nishide E, Yamaguchi M; Comparison of hypocholesterolemic effect among three phospholipid containing different fatty acids and the related oils, *Japanese J Nutr* **48**(5), 213-20 (1990) Article in Japanese].

The effects of several dietary oils, rich in monounsaturated fatty acids and polyunsaturated fatty acids [(n-6) or (n-3)] on concentrations of cholesterol, triglycerides and phospholipids in serum and lipoproteins were investigated in rats. Oils rich in (n-3) polyunsaturated fatty acids had a more pronounced lowering effect on serum lipids than oils rich in (n-6) polyunsaturated fatty acids or monounsaturated fatty acids. The most striking effects of the dietary oils were observed on cholesterol and phospholipid concentrations in VLDL and HDL as well as VLDL-triglycerides. The hypocholesterolemic effect of salmon oil, rich in long-chain (n-3) polyunsaturated fatty, acids was more intensive than that of linseed oil rich in α-linolenic acid. Olive oil containing monounsaturated fatty acids had no effect on lipids in serum and lipoproteins. Safflower oil and evening primrose oils rich in (n-6) PUFA had only slight effects on serum lipids compared to cocoanut oil. [Stangl GI, Kirchgessner M, Reichlmayr Lais AM, Eder K; Serum lipids and lipoproteins from rats fed with different dietary oils, *J Animal Physiol Animal Nutr* **71**(2), 87-97 (1994)].

See *Echium plantagineum*: [Surette *et al.*; *J Nutr* **134**(6), 1406-11 (2004)].

DIETARY PROTEINS: The hypocholesterolemic effect of dietary proteins (whey, soybean, sunflower proteins and casein) was studied in rats. In comparison to casein, whey, soybean and sunflower proteins decreased the level of serum high density lipoprotein-cholesterol and these low cholesterol levels were accompanied by an increase in the daily faecal excretion of neutral sterols and bile acids in the case of soybean protein, and by a decrease in the liver cholesterol content, in the case of whey protein. Considering the amino acid composition of the four purified proteins, serum total and HDL-cholesterol levels had a significant positive correlation with tyrosine and glutamic acid and a negative correlation with cystine and alanine. The hypocholesterolemic effect of dietary proteins was not related to their animal or vegetable origin. [Sautier C, Dieng K, Flament C, Doucet C, Suquet JP, Lemonnier D; Effects of whey protein, casein, soybean and sunflower proteins on the serum tissue and faecal steroids in rats, *Brit J Nutr* **49**(3), 313-20 (1983)].

Effects of dietary protein (casein or soy protein) and fat (tallow or soybean oil) on cholesterol deposition and body composition of pigs were studied. Dietary protein was found to have no effect on plasma cholesterol concentration, body composition, bone weight or bone calcium. The type of dietary fat, however, affected the amount of whole body fat but did not affect whole body protein, bone weight or bone calcium. The hypocholesterolemic effect of polyunsaturated fats may function, in part, by stimulating deposition of cholesterol in adipose tissue.[Richard MJ, Julius AD, Wiggers KD; Effects of dietary protein and fat on cholesterol deposition and body composition of pigs, *Nutr Reports International* **28**(5), 973-82 (1983)].

Several reports suggest that plant protein sources are hypocholesterolemic relative to animal proteins. Weanling male rats were fed with complete diets, which contained 10% protein either as casein, heat-treated casein, egg albumin, wheat gluten, soy protein isolate, or a mixture (50:50) of wheat gluten and soy protein isolate. Plasma cholesterol and HDL-c were found to be inversely correlated with protein quality as indicated by protein efficiency ratio and final body weight. The study shows that in the rapid growing weanling rats, poorer quality proteins result in hypercholesterolemia perhaps due to less efficient plasma lipid clearance. [Lefevre M, Schneeman BO; Relationship between plasma cholesterol and protein quality in weanling rats, *Nutr Reports International* **28**(6), 1369-74 (1983)].

The relationship between the amino acid composition of various protein sources and serum and hepatic cholesterol levels was studied in rats. Eight groups of rats were fed for 45 days on one of eight semi-purified diets, containing 246 to 279g/kg of the following isolated proteins: Casein, lactoglobulin, ovalbumin, alfalfa, gluten, pea-, fava bean- or soya-protein with no added cholesterol. The final serum cholesterol level in comparison to the initial value decreased significantly with the ovalbumin diet and very significantly with the pea, fava and soya diets. Serum total and HDL-cholesterol levels were compared between the different groups and levels were high in the rats fed the casein and alfalfa diets and low in those fed the pea, fava and soya diets. The hypocholesterolemic effect of the dietary proteins was not related to their animal or vegetable origin. Higher faecal steroid excretion was observed with alfalfa, pea, gluten and soya diets than with casein and ovalbumin diets. Comparison of the amino acid proportions of the eight dietary proteins to the serum total cholesterol levels showed a positive correlation for proline and methionine and a negative one for arginine concentrations. [Sautier C, Flament C, Doucet C, Suquet JP; Effects of eight dietary proteins and their amino acid content on serum, hepatic and faecal steroids in the rat, *Nutr Reports International* **34**(6), 1051-62 (1986)].

Total serum cholesterol was measured in male Sprague Dawley rats fed with cholesterol-free or cholesterol-enriched (1% cholesterol, 0.5% cholic acid) semipurified diets containing protein from one of the nine different sources (casein, beef, fish, soy, pea, peanut meal, rapeseed, oatmeal, wheat gluten). Total serum cholesterol ranged from 70 mg/dl with the pea diet to 98 mg/dl with the peanut meal diet in rats fed with cholesterol-free diets and from 163 mg/dl with the wheat gluten diet to 313 mg/dl with the casein diet in rats fed the cholesteral-enriched diets. In rats fed with cholesterol-enriched diets, significant correlations were observed between total serum cholesterol and tyrosine content or leucine/isoleucine ratio of *in vitro* digestion products of the protein. [Jacques H, Deshaies Y, Savoie L; Relationship between dietary proteins, their *in vitro* digestion products and serum cholesterol in rats, *Atherosclerosis* **61**(2), 89-98 (1986)].

Young, growing pigs were fed with diets containing either soy protein isolate or ground beef as the main protein source and soybean oil or beef tallow as the main fat source for 8 weeks to examine effects of types of dietary protein and fat on cholesterol distribution between blood plasma, plasma lipoproteins and body organs. It was observed that type of dietary protein did not influence concentrations of cholesterol in plasma, low density lipoprotein (LDL)-cholesterol, high density lipoprotein (HDL)-cholesterol or cholesterol in several organs of pigs. Pigs fed tallow had greater concentrations of plasma cholesterol and LDL and HDL-cholesterol than did pigs fed soybean oil. Ratios of HDL to LDL were not altered by dietary fat.

Cholesterol concentrations were greater in heart, skeletal muscle and viscera of pigs fed soybean oil than in those fed tallow. Thus, dietary beef and soy protein isolate had similar effects on cholesterol concentrations in plasma, LDL, HDL and organs, whether pigs consumed soybean oil or beef tallow as a major fat source. Soybean oil, however, exerted a hypocholesterolemic effect, irrespective of major source of dietary protein. [Baldner Shank GL, Richard MJ, Beitz DC, Jacobson NL; Effect of animal and vegetable fats and proteins on distribution of cholesterol in plasma and organs of young growing pigs, *J Nutr* **117**(10), 1727-33 (1987)].

The effects of some dietary proteins on the level of serum cholesterol and triacylglycerol were studied in rats in a diphasic experiment. Dietary proteins were found to influence the serum level of cholesterol significantly. Rats fed with broilers were found to have lower serum cholesterol levels than those fed old layers in the first phase of the experiment but the difference was not significant in the second phase. Similarly, the rats fed with fatty fish had significantly higher values than those fed lean fish in the first phase while the difference in the second phase was not significant. Rats fed with animal proteins had significantly higher levels serum cholesterol than those fed cowpea. Cowpea (*Vigna unguiculata*) showed hypocholesterolemic effect. Methionine supplementation of cowpea resulted in a non-significant increase in the serum cholesterol and a decrease in the serum triacylglycerol level. [Adeyeye SO, Oyenuga VA, Fetuga BL; Serum cholesterol and triacylglycerol in rats fed different dietary protein sources, *Nutr Reports International* **40**(2), 323-34 (1989)].

The relationship between the amino acid composition of dietary proteins and the plasma cholesterol concentration was investigated. From these results, it is suggested that the plasma cholesterol concentration might be influenced by the methionine content of dietary proteins at least in part through an alteration of hepatic phospholipid metabolism. [Sugiyama K, Kanamori H, Akachi T, Yamakawa A; Amino acid composition of dietary proteins affects plasma cholesterol concentration through alteration of hepatic phospholipid metabolism in rats fed with a cholesterol-free diet, *J Nutr Biochem* **7**(1), 40-48 (1996)].

The relations between dietary protein and cardiovascular risk were first considered through their impact on blood cholesterol. Half a century after the first reports of hypocholesterolemic effect of plant proteins, this subject is still a mater of debate, notably because of the difficulty in distinguishing between an independent effect of proteins and that of phytochemicals present in proteins preparations. The recent advances in new areas of research that have recently gained attention have been reviewed. [Mariotti F, Huneau JF, Tome D; Dietary protein and cardiovascular risk, *J Nutr Health Aging* **5**(3), 200-04 (2001)].

DITERPENOIDS: Various tricyclic diterpenoid derivatives showed serum cholesterol lowering action in rats. Derivatives of totarol from *Thujopsis dolabrata* and abietane and pimarene groups of diterpenoids from *Cryptomeria japonica* were particularly effective. Inhibition of intestinal cholesterol absorption was apparently involved in the main mechanism of hypocholesterolemic action of totarol and abietic acid. [Enomoto H, Yoshikuni Y, Yasutomi Y, Ohata K, Sempuku K, Kitaguchi K, Fujita Y, Mori T; Hypocholesterolemic action of tricyclic diterpenoids in rats, *Chem Pharm Bull* (Tokyo) **25**(3), 507-10 (1977)].

FATTY ACIDS: The changes of plasma and liver cholesterol contents and fatty acid compositions in hypercholesterolemic rats in response to 4-day feeding of either (n-6) fatty acid-rich safflower oil or (n-3) fatty acid-rich fish oil were examined. Both dietary fats were found to be equally effective in lowering plasma and liver cholesterol. In plasma and liver phospholipids, the two fatty acids were metabolised in a similar pattern. The (n-3)- and (n-6)-polyunsaturated fatty acids in plasma cholesteryl esters were metabolised differently. In animals fed with safflower oil, the proportions of 18:2 (n-6) were elevated rapidly after one day on the diet, and remained constant thereafter, while the levels of 20:4 (n-6) increased after the second day. In animals fed with fish oil, the levels of 20:5 (n-3) increased steadily throughout the feeding, while those of 22:6 (n-3) increased only marginally. The implications of these results for the mechanism of the hypocholesterolemic effects of (n-3) and (n-6) fatty acids were discussed. [Huang YS, Mcadoo KR, Horrobin DF; Response of plasma and liver cholesterol and fatty acids in hypercholesterolemic rats to short-term feeding of vegetable and fish oils, *Nutr Reports International* **36**(6), 1171-84 (1987)].

Despite a recent conclusion by an ad hoc FDA panel that there need be little concern about the effects of *trans* fatty acids in the American diet on health, it is nevertheless proposed that on the basis of available evidence, unnatural dietary *trans* and *cis* unsaturated fatty acid isomers should be regarded as a definite risk factor in the etiology of coronary artery disease. [Booyens J, Louwrens CC, Katzeff IE; The role of unnatural dietary trans and cis unsaturated fatty acids in the epidemiology of coronary artery disease, *Med Hypotheses* **25**(3), 175-82 (1988)].

The effect of the degree of fatty acid saturation on cholesterol metabolism was studied in rats. The results of chronic feeding experiments in rats indicate that (a) high dietary cholesterol intake results in hypercholesterolemia, (b) the hypercholesterolemia is accentuated by high dietary saturated fat but is unaffected by polyunsaturated fat, (c) addition of polyunsaturated fat to high cholesterol diet leads to massive cholesterol accumulation in the liver which can partly account for the apparent hypocholesterolemic effect of polyunsaturated fat relative to saturated fat; and (d) differences in serum and tissue cholesterol levels between saturated and polyunsaturated fat supplemented groups are unlikely to be due to their effects on faecal sterol excretion. [Vaziri ND, Hollander D, Dearden L, Mallott K, Martin RA, Rosario L; Effects of dietary fatty acid saturation on serum and tissue cholesterol concentrations and faecal sterol excretion: A chronic metabolic study in the rat, *Res Comm Chem Pathol Pharmacol* **61**(2), 245-56 (1988)].

The plasma cholesterol-reducing effects of dietary omega-3 and omega-6 PUFA [(n-3) and (n-6)-poly unsaturated fatty acids] were compared in male Sprague Dawley rats, which were fed either sardine oil (omega-3 PUFA) or corn oil (omega-6 PUFA) as 5% added diet for 3 weeks. Liver microsome was separated by ultracentrifuge and HMG-CoA reductase activity was determined. HMG-CoA reductase activity from liver microsome was significantly lower in omega-3 PUFA diet when compared to omega-6 PUFA and saturated fatty acid diet. Omega-3 PUFA significantly increased the amount of cholesterol and bile acid excretion from faeces, omega-6 PUFA and saturated fatty acid diet were relatively less effective. Coprostanol and coprostanone contents from faeces excreted appeared to be highest for omega-6 PUFA diet. Levels of triglyceride, total cholesterol, LDL-c and VLDL-c in plasma or muscle were reduced by omega-PUFA diet but liver cholesterol contents were raised by omega-PUFA diet when compared to that of saturated fatty acid diet. The hypocholesterolemic effects of omega-PUFA could be due to the reduced HMGCoA reductase activity in liver microsome, resulting in the raised faecal steroid excretion., this effect being higher for omega-3 PUFA. [Park BS, Seong KS, Yoon CS, Hwangbo J, Lee HW, Lee NH, Rhee YC; Effect of dietary omega-PUFA on cholesterol synthesis and steroid excretion in rats, *Korean J Animal Nutr Foodstuffs* **16**(5), 283-90 (1992) Article in Korean].

The effect of dietary oleic acid on lipid metabolism was investigated using SD rats and different types of oleic acid (ethyl oleate, triolein, olive oil, and high-oleic sunflower oil) and compared with ethyl linoleate. Plasma cholesterol concentrations were significantly higher in rats fed ethyl oleate and olive oil than in those fed with triolein, high-oleic sunflower oil, ethyl linoleate, or the fat-free diet. The lowest plasma cholesterol concentration was observed in rats fed ethyl linoleate. Chylomicron plus VLDL and LDL-cholesterol concentrations were more markedly increased in rats fed the oleic acid-rich diets, especially ethyl oleate and olive oil, than in those fed with the ethyl linoleate diet. HDL-cholesterol concentrations were not different among the experimental groups. LCAT activity in rats fed with the ethyl linoleate was twice as high as that in any other group. The data suggest that oleic acid-rich oil does not induce a hypocholesterolemic response in rats fed with hypercholesterolemic diets. [Budijanto S, Ito M, Furukawa Y, Kimura S; Comparison of different types of dietary oleic acid on the reduction of plasma cholesterol levels in rats *J Clin Biochem Nutr* **13**(3), 161-67 (1992)].

Propionic acid moderated the increase of plasma cholesterol caused by the feeding of the casein diet but sodium propionate did not. [Ebihara K, Miyada T, Nakajima A; Comparison of propionic acid and sodium propionate infused to the cecum and stomach on hypocholesterolemic effect in rat fed with a cholesterol-free casein protein diet, *Nutr Res* **13**(11), 1305-11 (1993)].

The effect of a diet enriched in polyunsaturated fatty acids and antioxidants (α-tocopherol and carnosine at a dose of 2.5 mg/kg and 50 mg/kg, respectively, daily during 30 days) was studied in rabbits with experimental atherosclerosis. The diet exhibited a hypocholesterolemic effect accompanied by approximately a 10-fold decrease of the impaired aortic area, as well as lowered content of 2-thiobarbituric acid-positive lipid peroxidation products occurring in blood and, especially, in apoB lipoproteins. The diet may be recommended for the prophylaxis and treatment of atherosclerosis. [Sdvigova AG, Panasenko OM, Luk'yashchenko IV, Sergienko VI, Lopukhin YM; Correction of lipoprotein peroxidation in experimental atherosclerosis using a diet containing polyunsaturated fatty acids and antioxidants, *Vopr Med Khim* **39**(2), 30-33 (1993) [Article in Russian].

The effects of diets high in stearic acid and lauric + myristic acid on plasma lipids and lipoproteins of healthy young men were studied. The results of the investigation proved stearic acid to be a unique long-chain saturated fatty acid with an independent cholesterol-lowering effect. [Kris Etherton PM; Effects of chain length of saturated fatty acids on plasma total, LDL- and HDL-cholesterol levels, *Fett Wissenschaft Technol* **95**(12),: 448-51 (1993)].

The effects of whole food diets rich in different fatty acid were evaluated in normocholesterolemic young men using a randomised, crossover, double-blind experimental design. The study showed that whereas myristic and lauric acid rich dairy butter was hypercholesterolemic, linoleic acid rich soybean oil was hypocholesterolemic. Diets containing soybean oil and oleic acid rich olive oil were hypocholesterolemic compared with the diet containing stearic acid rich cocoa butter. Soybean oil significantly decreased apolipoprotein (apo B) levels compared with the other diets. Plasma very low density lipoprotein-cholesterol, high density lipoproteincholesterol (HDL-c), and apo A-I levels were unaffected by the experimental diets. Cocoa butter is hypocholesterolemic compared with butter because of its high proportion of stearic acid. Thus, stearic acid has unique effects on plasma total cholesterol levels compared with other long-chain saturated fatty acids; the mechanism by which stearic acid exerts this effect is not clear. It has also been shown that linoleic acid has a more potent hypocholesterolemic effect than oleic acid and does affect HDL cholesterol levels or HDL composition. [Kris Etherton PM, Derr J, Mitchell DC, Mustad VA, Russell ME, McDonnell ET, Salabsky D, Pearson TA; The role of fatty acid saturation on plasma lipids, lipoproteins, and apolipoproteins: I. Effects of whole food diets high in cocoa butter, olive oil, soybean oil, dairy butter, and milk chocolate on the plasma lipids of young men, *Metab Clin Exp* **42**(1), 121-29 (1993)].

The influence of dietary propionic acid and bile acid excretion on the hypocholesterolemic effect of fibres was studied. It was observed that absorption and further hepatic metabolism of large amounts of propionic acid are not sufficient to counteract the induction of HMG-CoA reductase resulting from bile acid faecal losses. The rise of these losses plays a major role in the hypocholesterolemic effect of β-cyclodextrin. [Levrat MA, Favier ML, Moundras C, Remesy C, Demigne C, Morand C; Role of dietary propionic acid and bile acid excretion in the hypocholesterolemic effects of oligosaccharides in rats, *J Nutr* **124**(4), 531-38 (1994)].

The effects of simultaneously lowering palmitic acid and increasing oleic acid levels in the diets on serum lipid responses in the absence and in the presence of dietary cholesterol were assessed in hamsters. Both the acids exhibited nonhypercholesterolemic effect in the absence and presence of low level of dietary cholesterol in hamsters but while palmitic acid exhibited hypercholesterolemic effect, oleic acid showed hypocholesterolemic effect in the presence of high level of dietary cholesterol. [Khor HT, Tan DTS; Serum lipid responses to simultaneous alterations in dietary palmitic and oleic acids in the absence and presence of dietary cholesterol in the hamster, *Nutr Res* **14**(8), 1191-99 (1994)].

Forty healthy volunteers were allocated in a double blind, randomised study to receive either 20 g of (n-3) polyunsaturated fatty acids (PUFA) or 20 g of (n-6) PUFA at their evening meal. The effect on plasma lipids and lipoproteins of this single dose of fish oil vs. corn oil was studied the next morning, Plasma triglycerides and very low density lipoprotein-cholesterol significantly decreased in case of fish oil having (n-3) PUFA but the total cholesterol decreased after both supplements. Experiments have shown that a single very high dose of (n-3)-PUFA has a pronounced hypotriglyceridemic effect, which is directly related to the initial plasma level. [Svaneborg N, Moller JM, Schmidt EB, Varming K, Lervang HH, Dyerberg J; The acute effects of a single very high dose of n-3 fatty acids on plasma lipids and lipoproteins in healthy subjects, *Lipids* **29**(2), 145-47 (1994)].

Addition of 5% linoleic acid or oleic acid to a 0.1% cholesterol-supplemented diet diminished the increases in plasma total and low density lipoprotein (LDL)-cholesterol, induced by cholesterol alone. Linoleic acid decreased high density lipoprotein cholesterol in comparison with cholesterol alone, whereas oleic acid did not. Linoleic acid and oleic acid each prevented hepatic LDL receptor suppression, although linoleic acid was more effective. Oleic acid prevented the increase in plasma cholesteryl ester transfer protein (CETP) activity induced by dietary cholesterol, whereas linoleic acid did not. Neither of the acids altered hepatic 3-hydroxy-3-methylglutaryl coenzyme A reductase activity but oleic acid increased hepatic cholesterol 7α-hydroxylase activity. These results suggest that dietary linoleic and oleic acids diminish the cholesterol-induced increases in plasma total and LDL-cholesterol by preventing hepatic LDL receptor suppression, and in the case of oleic acid by also preventing the increase in the plasma CETP activity. These effects on cholesterol 7α-hydroxylase activity may influence bile lipid metabolism. [Kurushima H, Hayashi K, Toyota Y, Kambe M, Kajiyama G; Comparison of hypocholesterolemic effects induced by dietary linoleic acid and oleic acid in hamsters, *Atherosclerosis* **114**(2), 213-21 (1995)].

The effects of stearic acid on total cholesterol, low density lipoprotein cholesterol (LDL-c), and high density lipoprotein-cholesterol (HDL-c) concentrations (mmol/L) were evaluated using regression analyses. The analyses revealed that unlike other long-chain saturated fatty acids, stearic acid had no effect on total cholesterol and lipoprotein cholesterol concentrations in men and women. Monounsaturated fatty acids elicited an independent hypocholesterolemic effect. [Yu S; Derr J; Etherton TD; Kris Etherton PM; Plasma cholesterol-predictive equations demonstrate that stearic acid is neutral and monounsaturated fatty acids are hypocholesterolemic, *Am J Clin Nutr* **61**(5), 1129-39 (1995)].

Saturated, monounsaturated and linoleic acids in diets accumulated relatively efficiently in the whole body but omega-3 fatty acids were catabolized preferentially in aged mice. The results of the investigation do not support the concept that an increased intake of high linoleate vegetable oils is useful for the prevention of hypercholesterolemia-associated diseases. However, dietary oils rich in omega-3 fatty acids may be useful. [Ishihara A, Ito A, Sakai K, Watanabe S, Kobayashi T, Okuyama H; Dietary high linoleate safflower oil is not hypocholesterolemic in aged mice after a long-term feeding-comparison with lard, perilla oil and fish oil, *Biol Pharma Bull* **18**(4), 485-90 (1995)].

Unlike other saturated fatty acids, stearic acid (18:0) exhibits mild hypocholesterolemic activity and this is generally believed to be due to desaturation of stearate into oleate in the system. Desaturation of stearate and palmitate and its effect on cellular accumulation of oleate were determined in primary culture of rat hepatocytes. The rate of oleate synthesis as measured by the formation of monounsaturated fatty acids from stearate was significantly higher than that from palmitate. The rate of (1-14C) stearate incorporation into oleate was 80% higher than that of (1-14C) palmitate. Despite the different rates of desaturation, the cellular oleate concentrations did not differ in the cells treated with stearate and palmitate. There was a dose-dependent increase in cellular stearate concentration by increasing stearate concentrations in culture medium. The results do not support the hypothesis that the hypocholesterolemic effect of stearate may be mediated by its conversion to oleate. [Pai T, Yeh YY; Desaturation of stearate is insufficient to increase the concentrations of oleate in cultured rat hepatocytes, *J Nutr* **127**(5), 753-57 (1997)].

Although there is a general agreement that saturated fatty acids elevate plasma cholesterol concentrations, the relative effects of individual fatty acids on cholesterol and bile acid metabolism are not very clear and, therefore, cholesterol and bile acid responses to diets enriched in different saturated fatty acids (C12-C18 fatty acids) were investigated in hamsters. Total plasma cholesterol concentration was significantly greater in hamsters fed myristic acid (14:0)-enriched diet relative to those fed the stearic acid (18:0)-enriched diet. Both plasma and liver cholesterol concentrations of hamsters fed stearic acid did not differ from those of the group fed no dietary cholesterol. There was greater deoxycholic acid excretion from hamsters fed myristic and palmitic acid (16:0) diets compared with those fed the stearic acid enriched diet. The observed relative hypocholesterolemic effect of stearic acid was not mediated by increased bile acid excretion. [Hassel CA, Mensing EA, Gallaher DD; Dietary stearic acid reduces plasma and hepatic cholesterol concentrations without increasing bile excretion in cholesterol-fed hamsters, *J Nutr* **127**(6), 1148-55 (1997)].

Current understanding of the cholesterolemic effects of individual fatty acids has been reviewed. In general, saturated fatty acids are hypercholesterolemic and that unsaturated fatty acids elicit a hypocholesterolemic effect compared with saturated fatty acids. On the basis of a limited number of well-controlled studies, it appears that myristic acid is the most potent saturated fatty acid. Of the saturated fatty acids, stearic acid is uniquely different in that it appears to be a neutral fatty acid. Monounsaturated fatty acids appear to exert a neutral effect or to be mildly hypocholesterolemic. *Trans* fatty acids elicit effects that are intermediate to those of the hypercholesterolemic saturated fatty acids and the *cis*-monounsaturated and *cis*-polyunsaturated fatty acids. Polyunsaturated fatty acids elicit the most potent hypocholesterolemic effects. [Kris Etherton PM, Yu S; Individual fatty acid effects on plasma lipids and lipoproteins: Human studies, *Am J Clin Nutr* **65**(5 Suppl.): 1628S-1644S (1997)].

Effect of unsaturated and saturated fats on cholesterol metabolism was studied in ascorbate sufficient and deficient guinea pigs. This study indicates that polyunsaturated fat intake with ascorbic acid deficiency may produce hypercholesterolemia. [Sen S; Mukherjee S; Interrelationship of dietary lipids and ascorbic acid with hepatic enzymes of cholesterol metabolic pathway, *Indian J Exp Biol* **35**(1), 42-45 (1997)].

From an investigation, undertaken to study the effect of the composition of monounsaturated and saturated fatty acids in a test meal on postprandial lipid metabolism, it was concluded that varying the levels of monounsaturated fatty acids and saturated fatty acids in test meals has little or no effect on postprandial lipid metabolism. [Roche HM, Zampelas A, Jackson KG, Williams CM, Gibney MJ; The effect of test meal monounsaturated fatty acid:Saturated fatty acid ratio on postprandial lipid metabolism, *Brit J Nutr* **79**(5), 419-24 (1998)].

The effects of diets containing equal amounts of α - or γ-linolenic acid on lipid metabolism were compared in rats. The results indicate that α-linolenic acid exhibits a larger hypocholesterolemic effect than γ-linolenic acid, and it may be displayed mainly through the repression of the activity and mRNA expression of HMG-CoA reductase. [Ihara Watanabe M, Umekawa H, Takahashi T, Furuichi Y; Effects of dietary *α*- or *gamma*-linolenic acid on levels and fatty acid compositions of serum and hepatic lipids, and activity and mRNA abundance of 3-hydroxy-3-methylglutaryl CoA reductase in rats, *Comparative Biochem Physiol* A. **122**(2), 213-20 (1999)].

Effects of dietary fat amount and saturation on the regulation of hepatic mRNA and plasma apolipoprotein A-I were studied in rats. From the results of the investigation it was concluded that different fatty acid containing diets regulate apolipoprotein A-I through different mechanisms, and these mechanisms could be modulated by the fat intake. [Calleja L, Trallero MC, Carrizosa C, Mendez MT, Palacios Alaiz E, Osada J; Effects of dietary fat amount and saturation on the regulation of hepatic mRNA and plasma apolipoprotein A-I in rats, *Atherosclerosis* **152**(1), 69-78 (2000)].

From an investigation, it has been concluded that unlike saturated fatty acids with chain length less than 18 carbon atoms, monounsaturated fatty acids, especially oleic acid, have hypocholesterolemic properties. [Hanczakowski P; The effect of saturated and monounsaturated fatty acids on cholesterol content in the body, *Biuletyn Informacyjny Instytut Zootechniki* **39**(4), 45-52 (2001)].

Epidemiological studies indicate that dietary n-3 PUFAs (polyunsaturated fatty acids like linolenic acid) reduce mortality due to coronary heart disease. At high doses, dietary n-3 PUFAs have several beneficial properties. First, they act favourably on blood characteristics; they are hypocholesterolemic and hypotriglyceridemic and reduce platelet aggregation and exhibit antithrombotic and fibrinolytic activities. Second, they reduce ischemia/reperfusion-induced cellular damage, apparently due to the incorporation of eicosapentaenoic acid in membrane phospholipids. Third, they reduce ischemia and reperfusion arrhythmias. Numerous experimental studies have indicated that low concentrations of exogenous n-3 PUFAs reduce the severity of cardiac arrhythmias. This effect is probably responsible for the protective action of n- 3 PUFA on mortality due to coronary heart disease. Further studies are necessary to confirm this assumption in animals. [Demaison L, Moreau D; Dietary n-3 polyunsaturated fatty acids and coronary heart disease-related mortality: A possible mechanism of action, *Cell Mol Life Sci* **59**(3), 463-77 (2002)].

The effects of positional and geometric isomers of conjugated linoleic acid (*cis*-9 *trans*-11 and *trans* 10, *cis*-12, known to exist in dairy products and meat) on body fat accumulation and serum lipids were studied in hamsters, fed an atherogenic diet. The addition of *trans* 10, *cis*-12-linoleic acid reduced fat accumulation and led to lower serum cholesterol, as compared with linoleic acid group. The reduction in serum cholesterol was limited to LDL-c. This isomer also reduced triacylglycerol content in liver but did not modify serum triacylglycerol level. However, *cis*-9, *trans*-11 isomer showed no effect on lipid metabolism in hamsters. [Navarro V, Zabala A, Macarulla MT, Fernandez Quintela A, Rodriguez VM, Simon E, Portillo MP; Effects of conjugated linoleic acid on body fat accumulation and serum lipids in hamsters fed an atherogenic diet, *J Physiol Biochem* **59**(3), 193-200 (2003)].

Though short-term feedings of dietary polyunsaturated fatty acids are known to exhibit hypocholesterolemic activity, long-term feedings are suspected to accelerate ageing through tissue accumulation of lipid peroxides and age pigments (lipofuscin). The long-term effects of fats and oils were studied on female mice, which were fed a conventional basal diet supplemented with lard, high-linoleic safflower oil, rapeseed oil, high- α-linolenic perilla oil, or a mixture of ethyl docosahexaenoate and soybean oil from 17 weeks to 71 weeks. The docosahexaenoate and soybean oil and perilla oil groups had decreased serum cholesterol levels compared with the lard and safflower oil groups, but the difference between the lard and safflower oil groups was not significant. The HMG-CoA reductase activity in the liver was also significantly lower in the perilla oil and docosahexaenoate groups. However, no significant difference in lipofuscin contents in the brain and liver was observed among the 5 dietary groups, despite significant differences in peroxidizability indices of the dietary and/or tissue lipids. These results indicate that oils rich in high- α-linolenic acids exhibit hypocholesterolemic activity by suppressing hepatic HMG-CoA reductase activity compared with animal fats and oils rich in linoleic acid, but tissue lipofuscin contents are not affected by a long-term feeding of fats and oils with different degree of unsaturation in mice. [Du C, Sato A, Watanabe S, Wu CZ, Ikemoto A, Ando K, Kikugawa K, Fujii Y, Okuyama H; Cholesterol synthesis in mice is suppressed but lipofuscin formation is not affected by long-term feeding of n-3 fatty acid-enriched oils compared with lard and n-6 fatty acid-enriched oils, *Biol Pharm Bull* **26**(6), 766-70 (2003)].

FLAVONOIDS: Among isoflavones, biochanin A and formononetin showed hypolipidemic activity but diadzein did not. p-Coumaric acid also produced a significant reduction in serum cholesterol levels. [Sharma RD; Isoflavones and hypercholesterolemia in rats, *Lipids* **14**(6), 535-9 (1979)].

Hypolipidemic activity of the natural isoflavones prunitrin, genistrin, daidzin and their aglycones was studied and a correlationship between chemical structure and activity was established. [Kazakov A; Study of hypolipidemic activity of natural isoflavones, *Khim Farma Zh* **13**(1), 58-60 (1979)].

The effect of oral administration of quercetin, a vitamin P-like compound, on serum and liver lipid parameters was studied in rats, fed stock and 1% cholesterol diet for a period of 6 and 12 weeks. Quercetin exhibited hypolipidemic activity in cholesterol fed rats but had no such effect in rats, fed stock diet both at the end of 6 and 12 weeks. The significance of these findings with respect to development of atherosclerosis is discussed. [Basarkar PW, Nath N; Hypocholesterolemic and hypolipidemic activity of quercetin, a vitamin P-like compound in rats, *Indian J Med Res* **77**(Jan.), 122-26 (1983)].

The hypolipidemic activity of isoflavones, flavonols, flavones, and flavanones, isolated from *Allium cepa, Ammothamnus* sp, *Cicer moglotavicum, Ferula varia, Glycyrrhiza glabra, Haplophyllum perforatum, Lagonychium faretum, Raphanus radicula, Rhapanticum carthamoides, Saussurea elegans, Sophora japonica, Thermopsis alterniflora, Thermopsis dolichocarpa* and *Vexibia alopecuroides* were investigated. The compounds in question were found to largely prevent rat serum cholesterol and triglyceride accumulation in triton (WR-1339) -treated animals. They substantially diminished the manifestations of an atherosclerotic process in rabbits. The correlationship between -chemical structure and hypolipidemic activity was discussed. [Khushbaktova ZA, Syrov VN, Batirov EKH; Experimental study of the effect of flavonoids on the course of hyperlipidemia and atherosclerosis, *Khim Farma Zh* **25**(4), 53-57 (1991)].

Quercetin and related bioflavonoids have shown hypocholesterolemic activity and other important clinically relevant functions. [Bravo JM, Bravo F; Hygienic, therapeutic value of quercetin and other wine bioflavonoids, *Alimentaria* **35**(281), 131-33 (1997) Article in Spanish].

Hesperetin is a naturally occurring flavonoid that has hypolipidemic properties. The supplementation of hesperetin and its metabolites (mhydroxycinnamic acid, 3,4-dihydroxyphenylpropionic acid and ferulic acid) significantly lowered the plasma total cholesterol and triglyceride concentrations compared to the control group. The hepatic HMG-CoA reductase and acyl- CoA:cholesterol acyltransferase (ACAT) activities were significantly lower in the hesperetin and its metabolite supplemented groups than in the control group. The excretion of acidic sterol was significantly higher in the hesperetin and its metabolite supplemented groups than in the control group. These results demonstrated that the metabolites of hesperetin played a role as potent as hesperetin in plasma lipidlowering activities *in vivo* and further suggested that hesperetin and its metabolites reduced cholesterol biosynthesis and esterification, as indicated by the decreased HMG-CoA reductase and ACAT activities. [Kim HK, Jeong T, Lee MK, Park YB, Choi MS, Sank YD, Puk Ku T; Lipid-lowering efficacy of hesperetin metabolites in high-cholesterol fed rats, *Clin Chim Acta* **327**(1-2), 129-37 (2003)].

The antiatheroscleroic activity of two classes of naringenin derivatives was investigated. In high cholesterol-fed rabbits, administration of naringenin-7-O-oleate and naringenin 7-O-acetate inhibited the aortic atherosclerotic plaque formation. [Lee S, Lee CH, Moon SS, Kim CT, Kim BH, Bok SH, Jeong TS; Naringenin derivatives as antiatherogenic agents, *Biorg Med Chem Lett* **13**(22), 3901-903 (2003)].

Antioxidative effect of rutin, a flavonoid, *gamma*-terpinene and ascorbic acid on the LDL oxidation was studied. Rutin alone inhibited the LDL oxidation. It was shown that redox active copper rutin complex initiated the LDL oxidation but prevented copper from reacting at the binding sites of Apo B-100. Ascorbic acid exerted synergistic effect with rutin in preventing LDL oxidation by trapping of copper in a complex. Similarly, γ-terpinene also exhibited synergism with rutin in inhibiting LDL oxidation. [Milde J, Elstner EF, Rassmann J; Synergistic inhibition of low density lipoprotein oxidation by rutin, *gamma* terpinene and ascorbic acid, *Phytomedicine* **11**(2-3), 105-13 (2004)].

FLOWER POLLEN: Hepatoprotective, hypolipidemic and hypocholesterolemic effects of lipid extract of flower pollen in subchronically testosterone-androgenised rats were shown. [Polanski M, Czarnecki R, Woron J; The hepatoprotective and hyoplipidemic effect of flower pollen lipid extract in androgenized rats, *Folia Med Cracov* **37**(1-2), 89-95 (1996) [Article in Polish].

GUM ARABIC True gum arabic is the product of *Acacia senegal*, abundant in dry tropical west Africa from Senegal to northern Nigeria. *Acacia arabica* (babool) is the gum Arabic tree of India, but it yields a gum inferior to the true gum Arabic. Exudations of various other *Acacia* species are commonly known gum arabic or gum *Acacia*:

Administration of gum Arabic to human volunteers for three weeks reduced the serum cholesterol levels without any significant increase in faecal bile acids and neutral sterols excretion. Gum Arabic showed little effect on glucose tolerance. [Ross

AHM, Eastwood MA, Brydon WG, Anderson JR, Anderson DMW; A study of the effect of dietary gum Arabic in humans, *Am J Clin Nutr* **37**(3), 368-75 (1983)].

Fifteen grams of gum acacia, administered twice daily to seven subjects for 30 days, reduced their serum cholesterol by approximately 10.4% but had little effect on HDL-cholesterol and triglycerides. LDL + VLDL-cholesterol also decreased significantly. [Sharma RD; Hypocholesterolemic effect of gum acacia in men, *Nutr Res* **5**(12), 1321-26 (1985)].

Serum cholesterol level was signifivcntly reduced in rats fed, diet containing 7.5% gum Arabic and 1 % cholesterol as compared to rats maintained on a diet supplemented with 7.5 % cellulose and cholesterol. On the other hand, liver cholesterol was increased in animals fed with diet containing gum Arabic than those given cellulose in diet. [Al-Othanman AA, Al-Shagrawi RA, Hewedy FM, Hamdi MM; Plasma total lipoprotein cholesterol and organs cholesterol and growth performance in rats fed with dietary gum Arabic, *Food Chem* **62**(1), 67-72 (1998)].

A study on 110 hypercholesterolemic men and women was made to determine whether a soluble dietary fibre supplement containing gum Arabic and pectin in apple juice would lower serum lipids. The results of the study failed to support the hypothesised hypocholesterolemic effect of the gum arabic/pectin (4:1) mixture, but underlined the importance of selecting appropriate vehicles for delivery of dietary fibre mixtures. [Davidson MH, Dugan LD, Stocki J, Dicklin MR, Maki KC, Coletta F, Cotter R, McLeod M, Hoersten K; A low-viscosity soluble-fibre fruit juice supplement fails to lower cholesterol in hypercholesterolemic men and women, *J Nutr* **128**(11), 1927-32 (1998)].

INOSITOL HEXAPHOSPHATE: Inositol hexaphosphate, ubiquitous in plants and eukaryotic cells, is believed to be an active compound of high fibre diet, responsible for many of the beneficial effects of fibre. Hypocholesterolemic and antiplatelet effects of inositol hexaphosphate may be important in preventing and controlling cardiovascular disorders. It may bring about its beneficial action by acting as an anti-oxidant and/or by entering into intracellular inositol phosphates pool, and affecting signal transduction, thereby controlling cellular proliferation, differentiation and other biological processes. Being a natural and a non-toxic compound, inositol hexaphosphate has great potential in controlling cancer and preventing cardiovascular diseases. [Vucenik Vvana, Abulkalam MS; Inositol hexaphosphate (IP-6) reduces risk for cancer and cardiovascular diseases, *Periodicum Biologorum* **99**(1), 25-30 (1997)].

LECITHIN: An investigation was taken up to find out whether the consumption of lecithin has a more beneficial effect on serum cholesterol than does the consumption of equivalent amounts of polyunsaturated oils. No clear evidence for a specific effect of lecithin on serum cholesterol independent of its linoleic acid content or secondary changes in food intake was observed. The observed lecithin-induced hypocholesterolemic effects found in various studies were artifacts caused by the design and the manner of data analysis or were due to the linoleic acid present in lecithin. [Knuiman JT, Beynen AC, Katan MB; Lecithin intake and serum cholesterol, *Am J Clin Nutr* **49**(2), 266-68 (1989)].

MISCELLANEOUS PLANT CONSTITUENTS: Serum and liver cholesterol depressing activity of **Cu-Na-chlorophyllin**, a water-soluble derivative of chlorophyll, was markedly confirmed in the hypercholesterolemic rats placed on the diet containing 1% cholesterol and 0.25% bile salts. The hypocholesterolemic activities of β-carotene, rutin, quercetin and xanthophyll were not recognised. [Tsuji K, Tsuji E, Suzuki S; Effects of plant pigments on serum and liver cholesterol levels in rats, *Annual Report National Inst Nutr* (24), 100-06 (1975)].

In male cynomologus monkeys, oral administration of **gossypol acetate** (10mg/kg/d) significantly decreased total plasma cholesterol, LDL cholesterol and VLDL cholesterol levels without affecting HDL-cholesterol. No noticeable change in total cholesterol and LDL + VLDL-cholesterol was observed in animals treated with gossypol (5mg/kg) as compared to controls. It was suggested that gossypol acetate acted in a dose dependant manner. [Shandilya LN, Clarkson TB; Hypolipidemic effect of Gossypol in cyanomologus monkeys (*Macaca fasicularis*), *Lipids* **17**(4), 285-90 (1982)].

Administration of some natural compounds of plant origin (**alizole, berberine, pheonol and pheoniphlorine**) in doses of 30-100 μg/ml in the culture of the atherosclerotic human aortic intimal cells decreased the content of intracellular cholesterol by 35-41% and reduced the proliferative activity of the cells. [Ren LH, Vasil'ev AV, Orkehov AN, Tertov VV, Tutel'ian VA; Evaluation of the antiatherosclerotic properties of natural compounds of plant origin on cell cultures of the human aortic intima, *Farmakol Toksikol* **52**(5), 44-6 (1989) [Article in Russian].

Solasodin, a Solanaceae alkaloid and a nitrogen analogue of diosgenin, markedly decreased serum cholesterol and LDL-cholesterol levels in cholesterol-fed rabbits and prevented atherogenesis. Solasodin prevented accumulation of cholesterol in liver and aorta and reduced the plaque size in aorta. Faecal excretion of cholesterol and phospolipid was also significantly enhanced in treated animals. [Dixit VP, Verma M, Mathur NT, Mathur R, Sharma S; Hypocholesterolemic and antiatherosclerotic effects of Solasodin (C27H42O2N) in cholesterol fed rabbits, *Phytother Res* **6**(5), 270- 73 (1992)].

Oxidative modification of low density lipoproteins are now believed to play a major part in the initiation and progression of arterial lesions. Nutrients with antioxidant properties such as **vitamins C and E, β-carotene, and monounsaturated fatty acids** can reduce the susceptibility of LDL to oxidation. Antioxidant therapy, if proven useful, should be considered an adjunct to lipid-lowering therapy in order to have the greatest impact on coronary heart disease. [Harris WS; The prevention of atherosclerosis with antioxidants, *Clin Cardiol* **15**(9), 636-40 (1992)].

Indole-3-carbinol, a plant product, lowered serum LDL / VLDL-cholesterol levels in mice, and this effect was considered to be mediated by the inhibition of the enzyme, acyl-CoA: cholesterol acyltransferase (ACAT), effected by some of the acid condensation products of the indole-3-carbinol. These results provide a possible mechanism, by which indole-3-carbinol -rich vegetables lower serum cholesterol levels. [Dunn SE, LeBlanc GA; Hypocholesterolemic properties of plant indoles. Inhibition of acyl-CoA:cholesterol acyltransferase activity and reduction of serum LDL/VLDL cholesterol levels by glucobrassicin derivatives, *Biochem Pharmacol* **47**(2), 359-64 (1994)].

The effect of catechin on lipid metabolism was investigated in rats. **Catechin** at doses ranging from 0.1 to 100 mg/kg body weight was administered daily by gastric intubation to rats fed with a normal laboratory diet. Maximum hypocholesterolemic activity was detected at a dose of 10 mg/kg bw/d. The hypocholesterolemic activity of the drug was found not to be due to a decreased cholesterogenesis, but to a higher rate of degradation and excretion of cholesterol. As hydrolysis (breakdown) of glucobrassicin, a compound found in cruciferous vegetables, is known to give Indole-3-carbinol, vegetables rich in glucobrassicin derivatives also exhibit similar activity. [Valsa AK, Ushakumari B, Vijayalakshmi NP; Effect of catechin on lipid metabolism, *J Clin Biochem Nutr* **19**(3), 175-82 (1995)].

A mixture of (-)-epicatechin and three of its congeners **[(-) epigallocatechin gallate** (51.2%) **epigallocatechin** (18.7%), **(-) epicatechin** (12.3%), and **(-) epicatechin gallate** (11.8%)], present in jasmine green tea polyphenol, demonstrated strong antioxidant activity in Cu^{2+}-mediated oxidation of human LDL. The inhibitory effect of these epicatechins on LDL oxidation was dose-dependent at the concentrations ranging from 5 to 40 μM. (-)-Epicatechin and (-)-epigallocatechin were less protective against LDL oxidation than their gallate derivatives, which seemed to have similar antioxidant activity. The inhibitory effect of jasmine green tea epicatechins on Cu^{2+}-mediated oxidation was also characterized by their protective activity against oxidative degradation of docosahexaenoic, arachidonic, α-linolenic, and linoleic acid in LDL. Oxidative modification of low density lipoproteins (LDL) is thought to play an important role in the development of atherosclerosis and jasmine tea may serve as a source of natural antioxidative agents in human diet. [Zhang A, Chan PT, Luk YS, Ho WKK, Chen ZY; Inhibitory effect of jasmine green tea epicatechin isomers on LDL-oxidation, *J Nutr Biochem* **8**(6), 334-40 (1997)].

Lycopene and **β-carotene** augmented the activity of the macrophage LDL receptor, similar to the effect of fluvastatin. In agreement with these *in vitro* observations, dietary supplementation of tomato's lycopene (60 mg/day) to 6 males for 3 months resulted in a significant reduction in their plasma LDL-cholesterol concentrations. From these observations, it was concluded that dietary supplementation of carotenoids might act as moderate hypocholesterolemic agents, secondary to their inhibitory effect on macrophage 3-hydroxy-3-methyl glutaryl coenzyme A (HMG-CoA) reductase, the rate limiting enzyme in cholesterol synthesis. [Fuhrman B, Elis A, Aviram M;

Hypocholesterolemic effect of lycopene and β- carotene is related to suppression of cholesterol synthesis and augmentation of LDL receptor activity in macrophages, *Biochem Biophys Res Commun* **233**(3), 658-62 (1997)].

Resveratrol, a natural phytoalexin showed hypolipidemic, antiaggregatory and anti-inflammatory activities. In small doses, resveratrol decreased two adhesion molecules expressed in atherogenesis, metastasis and inflammatory process. [Bertelli AAE; Modulatory effect of Resveratrol, a natural phytoalexin on endothelial adhesion molecules and intracellular signal transduction, *Pharm Biol* **36**(Suppl.), 44- 52 (1998)].

Natural products that are known to exhibit hypocholesterolemic activity include **β-carotene, lycopene, cycloartenol, β-sitosterol, sitostanol, saponin**, soybean protein, **indoles**, dietary fibre, **propionate, mevinolin** (β-hydroxy- β- methylglutaryl coenzyme A reductase inhibitor) and polysaccharides. Garlic compounds are known to possess antiatherosclerotic activity. [Wang HX, Ng TB; Minireview: Natural products with hypoglycemic, hypotensive, hypocholesterolemic, antiatherosclerotic and antithrombotic activities, *Life Sci* **65**(25), 2663-77 (1999)].

Reports of plants added to milk and meat-based soups by the Maasai and Batemi tribes in East Africa support a role for **phenolic antioxidants** and hypocholesterolemic agents in the diet, and provide explanation of the low incidence of cardiovascular disease in populations that traditionally consume high levels of dietary fat and cholesterol. A total of 81% of the Batemi additives and 82% of additives known to be used by the Maasai tribes, contain potentially hypocholesterolemic saponins and/or phenolics. [Johns T, Mahunnah RL, Sanaya P, Chapman L, Ticktin T; Saponins and phenolic content in plant dietary additives of a traditional subsistence community, the Batemi of Ngorongoro District, Tanzania, *J Ethnopharmacol.* **66**(1), 1-10 (1999)].

Hypocholesterolemic potentials of different plant products have been reviewed. [Mukherjee PK; Plant products with hypocholesterolemic potentials. *Adv Food Nutr Res* **47**, 277-338 (2003)].

In hypercholesterolemic rats, administration of α-**asarone** (80mg/kg) for 8 days decreased serum cholesterol by 38%. It mainly lowered LDL-cholesterol without affecting HDL-cholesterol levels. Consequently LDL/HDL-cholesterol ratio was decreased (74%) following treatment with α-asarone. It also stimulated bile flow (60%) in hypercholesterolemic rats. α-Asarone decreased the gall bladder bile cholesterol contents, which led to the lowering of cholesterol saturation index. It was suggested that a decrease in cholesterol saturation index and enhancement of bile flow may account for cholelitholytic activity of α-asarone. [Rodriguez Paez L, Jurarez Sanchez M, Antunez Solis J, Baeza I, Wong C; α-Asarone inhibits HMG CoA reductase, lowers serum LDL cholesterol levels and reduces biliary CSI in hypercholesterolemic rats, *Phytomedicine* **10**(5), 397-404 (2003)].

OLIGOSACCHARIDES: The hypo cholesterolemic effects of β-glucans in barley diets, fed to broiler chicks were evaluated by measuring blood lipids, feed to gain ratios, excreta dry matter and exreta fats. For the chicks fed diets based on Washonupana variety of barley, inclusion of β-glucanase resulted in a significant increase in blood cholesterol to a level higher than that observed for Franubet variety of barley or control (corn) diet. However, blood triglycerides and high density lipoprotein cholesterol (HDL-c) levels were similar for chicks fed with either of two barley varieties. LDL levels for chicks fed the Washonupana diet without the enzyme were significantly lower than all other diets but increased on inclusion of β-glucanase. The LDL to HDL ratios were lowest for chicks fed the Washonupana diet without the enzyme but not significantly different when compared to the other barley diets. In general, excreta fats were higher, excreta dry matter lower and feed to gain ratios were significantly higher for the chicks fed with the Washonupana diet without the enzyme. The results show that some barley diets have hypocholesterolemic effects on broiler chicks and this effect is apparently due to the β-glucans in barley. [Fadel JG, Newman RK, Newman CW, Barnes AE; Hypocholesterolemic effects of β-glucans in different barley diets fed to broiler chicks, *Nutr Reports International* **35**(5), 1049-58 (1987)].

The effect of increasing amounts of a cyclic oligosaccharide, β-cyclodextrin, included in the diet on plasma cholesterol and triglycerides, was investigated in male genetically hypercholesterolemic Rico rats and in male Syrian hamsters. The results of the investigation suggest that β-cyclodextrin does not alter the microbial degradation of bile acids, but rather stimulates their synthesis and increases their pool size. β-Cyclodextrin prevents the intestinal absorption of lithocholic acid and washes this cytotoxic bile acid from the colon. The hypocholesterolemic effect of β- cyclodextrin appears to be due to stimulation of bile acid synthesis. [Riottot M, Olivier P, Huet A, Caboche JJ, Parquet M, Khallou J, Lutton C; Hypolipidemic effects of β-cyclodextrin in the hamster and in the genetically hypercholesterolemic Rico rat, *Lipids* **28**(3), 181-88 (1993)].

The cholesterol lowering effect of steroid sequestering compounds, such as cholestyramine or β-cyclodextrin, was examined to assess the respective importance of bile acids excretion and the fermentation process. In contrast to cholestyramine, β- cyclodextrin is metabolised by the large intestine microflora to yield short chain fatty acids, especially propionic acid, which is absorbed in the portal vein and metabolised by the liver. β-Cyclodextrin was found to be less potent than cholestyramine at elevating the faecal excretion of bile acids and depressing soluble bile acids in the large intestine. Changes in circulating lipoproteins (depressed HDL1 and apoE abundance) were observed only in the β-cyclodextrin-fed group. Cholestyramine was more potent than β-cyclodextrin to induce the activity of hepatic HMG-CoA reductase or cholesterol-7α-hydroxylase, whereas that of fatty acid synthetase was depressed only in the β-cyclodextrin. It appears that fermentable bile acid sequestrants are the most effective at depressing plasma cholesterol, probably in relation to the capacity of fermentation end-products to counteract the up- regulation of bile acids and cholesterol biosynthesis. [Moundras C, Demigne C, Mazur A, Remesy C; The cholesterol lowering effect of steroid sequestrants is modulated by large intestine fermentations, *J Nutr Biochem* **6**(3), 158-62 (1995)].

The effects of β-cyclodextrin on lipid metabolism were examined in growing pigs that were fed a 0.3% cholesterol-enriched diet for 4 weeks or this diet containing 5% or 10% β-cyclodextrin. Addition of β-cyclodextrin to the cholesterol-rich diet prevented the elevation of plasma cholesterol due to dietary cholesterol excess and produced a dose-dependent effect in reducing liver cholesterol storage, stimulating hepatic cholesterogenesis, increasing the proportion of primary bile acids in bile and in faeces, and the faecal loss of neutral sterols and bile acids. Pigs receiving 10% β- cyclodextrinon differed markedly from controls, especially for HMG-CoA reductase and cholesterol-7α-hydroxylase hepatic activities and faecal output of total bile acids. β-cyclodextrin possesses the ability to bind cholesterol and bile acids *in vitro*, and in view of this property, the results suggest that this non-absorbable carbohydrate accelerates body cholesterol turnover by reducing cholesterol absorption, increasing cholesterol and bile acid synthesis, and altering the action of the intestinal microflora. [Ferezou J, Riottot M, Serougne C, Cohen Solal C, Catala I, Alquier C, Parquet M, Juste C, Lafont H, Mathe D, Corring T, Lutton C; Hypocholesterolemic action of β-cyclodextrin and its effects on cholesterol metabolism in pigs fed a cholesterolenriched diet, *J Lipid Res* **38**(1), 86-100 (1997)].

The effect of feeding a cyclic oligosaccharide, β-cyclodextrin, on plasma cholesterol and triglyceride concentrations were investigated in rats fed a diet, either rich in cholesterol or in saturated fat. The β-cyclodextrin diet caused a marked decrease in plasma total lipid, triglyceride, total cholesterol and low density lipoprotein-cholesterol (LDL-c) concentrations. The plasma total bile acid contents of β-cyclodextrin group was significantly increased in all the groups as compared to control group. The hepatic HMG-CoA reductase activity was significantly lowered and faecal steroid excretion was significantly increased in the β-cyclodextrin-fed group compared to normal diet-fed rats. The bleeding time was significantly prolonged and the whole blood clotting time was significantly increased in β- cyclodextrin fed group. These results suggest that the β-cyclodextrin possesses antithrombotic activity and is a hypolipidemic, hypotriglyceridemic and hypocholesterolemic agent. [Park BS; The biological effects of β-cyclodextrin on antithrombotic activity and plasma lipid metabolism in rats, *J Animal Sci Technol* **45**(2), 199-210 (2003)].

PECTINS: Pectins are polymers of galacturonic acid and are widely spread in ripe fruits of terrestrial plants.

See Polysaccharides: [Tsuji *et al.*; *Annual Report National Inst Nutr.* (24), 83- 91 (1975)].

Pectin, gum arabic, cellulose, wheat bran and two polymers of galactose or its derivatives (agar and carragheenan) were each fed to rats at a level of 5 to 7% to examine their effect on serum, liver and tissue cholesterol levels. Among the fibres tested, pectin displayed the most hypocholesterolemic effect. In some experiments, pectin lowered the level of cholesterol in the serum, liver and aorta. Carragheenan was inconsistent in lowering serum cholesterol levels and tended to increase liver cholesterol levels. Gum Arabic and agar did not lower serum cholesterol levels and in some experiments they elevated liver cholesterol levels. Wheat bran or cellulose had no significant effect on either serum or liver cholesterol levels. From the results of the investigation, it appeared that the effect of dietary fiber is dependent on the composition of the diet. [Tsai AC, Elias J, Kelley JJ, Lin RS, Robson JR; Influence of certain dietary fibres on serum and tissue cholesterol levels in rats, *J Nutr* **106**(1), 118-23 (1976)].

Incorporation of 5% citrus pectins and 0.5% ascorbic acid in the high fat diet-fed to guineapigs inhibited accumulation of cholesterol in liver and blood. Administration of 15 g pectins and 450mg ascorbic acid for 6 weeks to 21 healthy mild hypercholesterolemic and 11 hyperlipidemic patients lowered the cholesterol levels without affecting HDL-cholesterol. The changes in triglycerides were not very consistent. [Ginter E, Kubec FJ, Vozar J, Bobek P; Natural hypocholesterolemic agent: Pectin plus ascorbic acid, *Int J Vitam Nutr Res* **49**(4), 406-12 (1979).

See *Cyamopsis tetragonoloba* (Guar): [Jenkins *et al.*; *Am J Clin Nutr* **32**(12), 2430-5 (1979)].

Feeding of *C. tetragonoloba* (1g/kg bw), pectin (0.5g/kg bw), *Plantago ovata* (1g/kg bw), and wheat bran (2g/kg bw), with the standard diet to different groups of mongrel dogs for one week did not affect the serum cholesterol levels. However, at the end of 15 days, pectin significantly lowered the cholesterol levels. [Sharma S, Kishore N, Sharma RK, Sharma BB; Hypocholesterolemic effcets of dietary fibre, *Indian J Physiol Pharmacol* **24**(2), 136-38 (1980)].

The mechanism responsible for the hypolipidemic action of pectin was investigated. The intestinal binding of dietary and biliary lipids by pectin was considered to be a major mechanism of action of this hypolipidemic polysaccharide. [Falk JD, Nagyvary JJ, Exploratory studies of lipid-pectin interactions, *J Nutr* **112**(1), 182-88 (1982)].

Pectins are non-digestible polysaccharides, which are known to be hypocholesterolemic. The mechanism of this effect was studied by measuring rates of absorption of the bile salt sodium cholate (and also of glucose) from perfused loops of small intestine, *in vivo*, in the rat. The results of the investigation suggest that the hypocholesterolemic activity of pectins cannot be due to binding of bile salts or to inhibition of the various processes of cholate absorption by the high viscosity of pectin solutions. [Oakenfull DG, Sidhu GS; Effects of pectins on intestinal absorption of glucose and cholate in the rat, *Nutr Reports International* **30**(6), 1269-78 (1984)].

The hypocholesterolemic activity of different pectins was studied in Sprague Dawley rats. Plasma cholesterol levels were lower in all pectin-fed groups compared with rats given the control diets containing 100 g Solkafloc (Food grade fiber and silicon dioxide as a low-calorie additive) and 100 g oil/kg. Liver lipid and cholesterol levels increased with increasing fat content of the diet, but were still significantly lower in all pectin-fed groups compared with the control group. The effects of molecular weight and degree of methoxylation of pectins were studied in 5 groups of rats given either a control diet containing 100 g Solkafloc/kg or pectins of high or low molecular weights with high or low degree of methoxylation. All diets in this experiments contained 100 g fat and 10 g cholesterol/kg. Plasma cholesterol levels were significantly lower than control values only in the high molecular weight high methoxyl pectin group. Compared with controls, animals given high molecular weight pectins had lower levels of liver lipid and liver cholesterol; but only liver cholesterol but not the liver lipid was lower in low molecular weight high methoxyl pectin. The results of the detailed investigation suggest that the hypocholesterolemic effects of pectins are at least partly due to their viscosity. Gut length and weight was increased in pectin-fed animals compared with controls despite their lower body-weight. [Judd PA, Truswell AS; The hypocholesterolemic effects of pectins in rats, *Brit J Nutr* **53**(3), 409-26 (1985)].

A significant decrease in the level of total cholesterol was observed in rats fed with high cholesterol diet supplemented with either cholestyramine or pectin, and this was due exclusively to the lowering of low density lipoprotein. Statistical evaluation of data revealed no significant difference between the cholesterol levels of rats fed either cholestyramine or pectin. Both cholestyramine and pectin are comparable and effective hypocholesterolemic agents and the observed hypocholesterolemic effect of these agents is mediated through lowering of cholesterol associated with the low density lipoprotein. [Baig MM, Burgin CW, Cerda JJ; Hypocholesterolemic agents: A comparison of the relative effectiveness of cholestyramine and pectin in rats, *Drug Nutrient Interactions* **3**(2), 109-14 (1985)].

Pectin is a type of water-soluble fibre that might exert distinct hypocholesterolemic effects. Fifteen adult male mice were divided into three groups and fed three levels of dietary pectin (2%, 5%, and 10%), respectively, for four weeks. Higher pectin intake was associated with lower mean total serum cholesterol levels. [Chen Y, Yuhas JA; Effects of pectin on food intake and total serum cholesterol in adult mice, *Bull Inst Zoology Academia Sinica* (Taipei) **25**(1), 7-12 (1986)].

In six male adult hypercholesterolemic minipigs, the effects of oral and intracecal pectin administration for 4 weeks on blood lipids were examined. Total serum cholesterol concentration was about 50% lower after feeding 75 g pectin per day than during the control period, during which water was infused into the cecum. The intracecal infusion of the same amount of pectin had no effect on total serum cholesterol concentration compared to the control period. The cholesterol level in the low density lipoproteins (LDL), in the very low density lipoproteins (VLDL) and in the high density lipoproteins (HDL) was lower after feeding pectin than in the control period. The HDL-cholesterol, but not LDL or VLDL-cholesterol, was at a lower level after intraceal infusion of pectin than during the control period. The study clearly demonstrates that the passage of pectin through the small intestine is necessary for its hypocholesterolemic action. [Ahrens F, Hagemeister H, Pfeuffer M, Barth CA; Effects on oral and intracecal pectin administration on blood lipids in minipigs, *J Nutr* **116**(1), 70-76 (1986)].

Supplementation of diet to rats with low methoxyl pectin (100 g/kg) displayed the most hypocholesterolmic effect and decreased the cholesterol content of the very low density lipoprotein (VLDL) and low density lipoproteins (LDL), when the low-fat diet (50 g/kg) was given. When rats were fed on the high fat diet (250 g/kg), pectin no longer had a hypocholesterolaemic effect but still decreased the VLDL-cholesterol content. Pectin lowered serum triglyceride and VLDL-triglyceride levels only when the low fat diet was given. Supplementation of diet with wheat bran (100 g/kg) exerted no hypocholesterolemic effect in rats fed on the low and high fat diets, but decreased the cholesterol content of VLDL and lowered serum triglycerides and VLDL-tryglycerides when the high fat diet was given. Purified cellulose had no significant effect on plasma lipids. Low-methoxyl pectin and wheat bran both beneficially modified the serum triglyceride and cholesterol variables except VLDL-triglycerides. [Vigne JL, Lairon D, Borel P, Portugal H, Pauli AM, Hauton JC, Lafont H; Effect of pectin , wheat bran and cellulose on serum lipids and lipoproteins in rats fed on a low or high fat diet, *Brit J Nutr* **58**(3), 405-14 (1987)].

Cholesterol absorption was not significantly different between the two groups of pigs fed a high cholesterol (1%) diet and a high cholesterol (1%) pectin (1%) diet. There was on the average less faecal fat, less faecal sterol and less bile acid per gram of dry faeces in the pectin-fed group compared to the other group. There was less protein absorption in both groups compared to the control. The results of this study lend support to the hypothesis that the hypocholesterolemic effect of pectin may not be related to intestinal absorption. [Shireman RB, Campbell D, Muth J, Corbett K, Combs GE Jr; The short-term effect of dietary pectin on fat absorption from the small intestine of swine, *Nutr Reports International* **35**(6), 1313-20 (1987)].

The hepatic and serum triglyceride as well as hepatic carnitine concentrations were analysed in rats, fed the purified diet free from fibre source or the diet containing varying amounts of citrus pectin. Both hepatic and serum triglyceride concentration decreased as the dietary levels of pectin increased. Cholesterol concentrations in the serum but not in the liver also decreased in rats fed with pectin but to a much lesser extent. In the situation where dietary pectin exerted a potent triglyceride lowering effect, hepatic carnitine concentrations were noi affected by the dietary fibre. [Ide T; Horii M; Hepatic carnitine and triglyceride lowering effect of dietary pectin in the rat, *Nutr Reports International* **39**(4), 861-66 (1989)].

See *Glycine max* (Soya bean, soybean): [Lanksy PS, *Acta Horticulturae* (332), 131-36 (1993)].

See *Amorphophallus konjac:* [Wu and Peng; *Acta Nutr Sin* **15**(2), 130-36 (1993) [Article in Chinese].

Various sources of food fibres were compared for efficacy in correction of carbohydrate and lipid metabolism disorders, induced by diabetes mellitus type II. The results showed a hypocholesterolemic effect of citrus pectin and hypoglycemic effect of wheat bran. [Sharafetdinov KK, Plotnikova OA, Tsagikyan TA; Carbohydrate and lipid metabolism correction in patients with diabetes mellitus type II: Comparative efficacy of food fibres, *Vopr Pitan* (3), 9-13 (1993) [Article in Russian].

See *Plantago psyllium:* [Matheson *et al.*; *J Nutr* **125**(3), 454-8 (1995)].

See Plant fibres: [Fernandez *et al.*; *J Lipid Res* **36**(10), 2191-202 (1995)].

The low molecular weight pectin (Mr = 66,000), obtained by decomposition of original pectin (Mr = 750,000), had the properties of low viscosity and high solubility but it lost hypocholesterolemic activities in rats. On the other hand, the medium molecular weight pectin (Mr = 185,000) had characteristics of both low viscosity and hypocholesterolemic activities. [Yamaguchi F, Uchida S, Watabe S, Kojima H, Shimizu N, Hatanaka C; Relationship between molecular weights of pectin and hypocholesterolemic effects in rats, *Biosci Biotech Biochem* **59**(11), 2130-31 (1995)].

An examination of hypocholesterolemic action of dietary pectin indicates that this effect is due to a shift of cholesterol from plasma to the hepatic pools. [Basu TK, Ooraikul B; Lipid-lowering effects of dietary fibre, *J Clinical Biochem Nutr* **18**(1), 1-9 (1995)].

Pectin-rich fruits and vegetables are known to exert antihyperlipidemic activity. However, all pectins are not equally effective in dyslipidemia. Of 11 pectins investigated, the pectins from *Carica papaya, Coccinia indica, Lycopersicon esculentum* and *Cucumis sativus* exhibited highly significant hypolpidemic activity. These pectins appear to lower lipid levels by increasing their rate of degradation and elemination along with a decrease in the absorption of lipid. Higher activity of lecithin cholesterol acyl tranferase (LCAT) in pectin-fed rats may also be responsible for hypolpidemic effect. Lowering of serum triglyceride following feeding of pectins may be attributed to higher activity of lipoprotein lipase in the adipose tissue of heart of these animals [Prasanna Kumar G, Sudheesh S, Usha Kumari B, Valsa AK, Vijaya Kumar S, Sandhya C, Vijaya Lakshmi NR; A comparative study on the hypolipidemic activity of 11 different pectins, *J Food Sci Technol* **34**(2), 103-07 (1997)].

The effects of the dietary fibres (Pectin vs cellulose) on plasma apolipoproteins and lipoproteins and liver cholesterol were studied in rats. Pectin lowered plasma cholesterol, but not triglyceride levels. Liver cholesterol was significantly lower in the rats fed with pectin compared with cellulose. Apolipoprotein A-IV and E levels were lower in the pectin group but apo B levels were lower in the rats fed the cellulose diets. The study confirmed the hypocholesterolemic effect of pectin and further showed its effects on plasma apolipoproteins which were even more pronounced than those on plasma lipids. [Suprijana O, Terpstra AHM, Van Lith HA,

Van Tol A, Lemmens AG, Geelhoed Mieras MM, Beynen AC; Plasma lipids and apolipoproteins in rats fed with diets with type of fat (fish oil versus corn oil) and fibre (pectin versus cellulose) as variables, *Nutr Res* **17**(7), 1187-97 (1997)].

See gum Arabic: [Davidson *et al.*; *J Nutr* **128**(11), 1927-32 (1998)].

See *Allium sativum* (Garlic): [Ismail *et al.*; *Pharmacol Res* **39**(2), 157-66 (1999)].

Hybrid F1B hamsters were fed with cholesterol-enriched (0.1% w/w) semipurified diets containing 3% of lemon pectin or 3% of the polygalacturonic acid regions fraction (smooth regions fraction) of the lemon pectin for a period of 8 weeks. A control group was fed cellulose and a positive control group was fed psyllium. The hamsters fed the psyllium, pectin, or the polygalacturonic acid regions fraction had significantly lower plasma cholesterol levels than the cellulose fed group throughout the experimental period. Liver cholesterol concentrations were also lower in the hamsters fed with the psyllium, pectin or the polygalacturonic acid regions fraction than in the hamsters fed the cellulose, but this effect reached statistical significance only in the hamsters fed the polygalacturonic acid regions fraction. The results of these studies suggest that the polygalacturonic acid region of the pectin molecule is responsible for the cholesterol-lowering properties of pectin. [Terpstra AHM, Lapre JA, De Vries HT, Beynen AC; Intact pectin and its polygalacturonic acid regions have similar hypocholesterolemic properties in hybrid F1B hamsters, *Nahrung* **46**(2), 83-86 (2002)].

PEPTIDES: Experiments were designed to verify the validity of the hypothesis that small quantity of intraluminal peptides enters into circulatory system and affects on lipid metabolism and this was confirmed. [Asato L; Kina T; Sugiyama M; Shimabukuro T; Yamamoto S; Effect of dietary peptides on plasma lipids and its mechanism studied in rats and mice, *Nutr Res* **14**(11), 1661-69 (1994)].

PHYTOSTEROLS: Evidence in support of a nonabsorptive antihypercholesterolemic action of phytosterols in the chicken was produced. [Konlande JE, Fisher H; Evidence for a nonabsorptive antihypercholesterolemic action of phytosterols in the chicken, *J Nutr* 98(4), 435-42 (1969)].

The efficacy of plant sterol preparations from two different sources (soy oil and tall oil from pine trees) and in two different physical forms (suspension and powder) in lowering the plasma cholesterol of patients with type II hyperlipoproteinemia was evaluated. Sterol balance data showed that plant sterols inhibit cholesterol absorption with maximal negative cholesterol balance in adults at a dose of 3 g/day of a tall oil sterol suspension. Maximal plasma cholesterol reduction in the adult outpatients on this preparation was seen at the same dose level. Since the tall oil sterol suspension is relatively palatable and is poorly absorbed, it has a potential value as an adjunct to dietary therapy in patients with mild hypercholesterolemia. [Lees AM, Mok HYI, Lees RS, McCluskey MA, Grundy SM; Plant sterols as cholesterol –lowering agents: Clinical trials in patients with hypercholesterolemia and studies of sterol balance,

Atherosclerosis **28**(3), 325-38 (1977)].

The hypocholesterolemic activity of β-sitosterol was compared with that of its hydrogenated product, β-sitostanol, in young male rats. When cholesterol was included in the diet, sitostanol exhibited significantly greater hypocholesterolemic activity than sitosterol. There was no apparent difference in the effects of the sterol and the stanol on the concentration of liver cholesterol and triglyceride. Increases in plasma triglyceride due to feeding sitosterol were not observed with sitostanol. Incorporation of dietary sitostanol into plasma, liver and other tissues was always negligible, and thus sitostanol was almost completely recovered in faeces, while there was considerable deposition of sitosterol. The increase in faecal output of dietary cholesterol was significantly greater with the stanol than with the sterol. The hydrogenation of phytosterols is a novel approach to enhance their hypocholesterolemic activities without influencing the relative safety of the initial sterols. [Sugano M, Morioka H, Ikeda I; A comparison of hypocholesterolemic activity of β-sitosterol and β-sitostanol in rats, *J Nutr* **107**(11), 2011-19 (1977)].

A comparison of absorption and metabolism of β-sitosterol and β-sitostanol was made by oral or i.v. administration of labeled sterols in rats. Excretion into faeces of oral β-sitostanol was significantly higher than that of β-sitosterol. More than 97% of sitostanol and 88% of sitosterol were recovered in the faeces within 7 days. Deposition of β-sitostanol was negligible in the tissues that were examined. The rate of excretion of labeled cholesterol was slightly greater when β-sitostanol was administered simultaneously. The liver contained significantly less radioactivity after labeled β-sitostanol than after β-sitosterol administration. The ratio of sterol in very low density lipoprotein to that in high density lipoprotein was less for sitostanol or sitosterol than for endogenous cholesterol; this was particularly marked with β- sitostanol, which may be a more effective hypocholesterolemic agent than β- sitosterol. [Ikeda I, Sugano M; Comparison of absorption and metabolism of β- sitosterol and β-sitostanol in rats, *Atherosclerosis* **30**(3), 227-38 (1978)].

Intravenous adminstration of phytosterol to rats fed on high fat diet containing 3 % cholesterol for 5 days, significantly decreased plasma and liver cholesterol levels. Bile acid excretion (without alterations in its composition) was enhanced following phytosterol treatment. The phytosterol was mainly accumulated in liver in treated rats and it decreased hepatic cholesterol by enhancement of conversion of cholesterol to bile acids. [Tabata T, Tanaka M, Yoden K, Iio T; Hypocholesterolemic activity of phytosterol I. *Yakugaku Zasshi* **99**(3), 315-18 (1979)].

In a long-term feeding experiment with diets free of cholesterol to rats, β- sitostanol exhibited significantly greater hypocholesterolemic activity than β- sitosterol did. Inhibitory effect on the absorption of endogenous and exogenous cholesterol was apparently much greater in β-sitostanol than in β-sitosterol. [Ikeda I, Morioka H, Sugano M; The effect of dietary β-sitosterol and β-sitostanol on the metabolism of cholesterol in rats, *Agric Biol Chem* **43**(9), 1927-34 (1979)].

Administration of different phytosterols to rats receiving 3% cholesterol containinmg diet caused lowering of hepatic cholesterol. The hepatic cholesterol lowering effect of the phytosterols were in the following decreasing order: Stigmasterol > β-sitosterol > stigmastanol >ergosterol >7-keto –cholesterol. Palmitate and stearate esters of stigmasterol exhibited much less activity than free sterol. These observations indicated that the presence of a free –OH group at C-3 position, a double bond at C-5 position and a side chain at C-17 position are essential for hypocholesterolemic activity. [Tabata T, Tanaka M, Iio T; Hypocholesteolemic activity of phytosterols, *Yakugaku Zasshi* **100**(5), 546-52 (1980)].

Male rats were fed on semipurified cholesterol-free diets containing butter fat with or without supplementary β-sitosterol. The plant sterol effectively lowered the liver cholesterol level in rats as well as in mice. The distribution of cholesterol in serum lipoproteins remained unchanged among different dietary regimens. A trend toward higher serum apoA-I with supplementation of β-sitosterol in a butter-fat diet was noticed. The effect of the plant sterol on serum apoB was rather variable. Satisfactory estimation of the changes in cholesterol metabolism in these rodents was not possible by the serum cholesterol parameter alone and the concentrations of hepatic cholesterol and serum apolipoproteins are considered to be more appropriate measure for this purpose. [Sugano M, Ikeda I, Imaizumi K, Watanabe M, Andoh M; Effects of β-sitosterol on the concentrations of serum and liver cholesterol and lipoproteins in rats fed butter fat, *J Nutr Sci Vitaminol* **28**(2), 117-26 (1982)].

The possible synergistic effect of cycloartenol in the hypocholesterolemic effect of β.sitosterol was studied in two strains of rats fed on cholesterol-enriched (0.5%) diets. In the experiment using Wistar rats, the decrease in serum apo A-I due to feeding cholesterol was ameliorated more effectively when a combination of cycloartenol and β-sitosterol was used than when β-sitosterol was used alone. The hepatic deposition of cholesterol was mitigated by dietary β-sitosterol, and further, although slightly, by a combination of β-sitosterol and cycloartenol except in the experiment with diets containing sodium cholate. Cycloartenol itself was not as effective as β-sitosterol in mitigating lipid disorders due to dietary cholesterol but it was absorbed at a rate approximately 4-fold higher than that of β-sitosterol. A preference for cycloartenol in cholesterol dynamics was thus suggested. [Ikeda I, Nakashima Yoshida K, Sugano M; Effects of cycloartenol on absorption and serum levels of cholesterol in rats, *J Nutr Sci Vitaminol* (Tokyo) 31(3), 375-84 (1985)].

See *Glycine max* (Soya bean, soybean): [Lanksy PS *Acta Horticulturae* (332), 131-36 (1993)].

Small amounts of dietary plant sterols (<1g/d), especially sitostanol esters dissolved in dietary fats, decrease serum total and LDL-cholesterol by a proportional decrease in cholesterol absorption which, in turn, is associated with a compensatory increase in cholesterol synthesis. The effects are most consistent in subjects with epsilon 4 allele, but for effective hypocholesterolemic treatment dietary amount of sitostanol ester should exceed 1g/day. [Miettinen TA, Vanhanen H; Dietary sitostanol related to absorption, synthesis and serum level of cholesterol in different apolipoprotein E phenotypes, *Atherosclerosis* **105**(2), 217-26 (1994)].

Partial replacement of normal dietary fat consumption by sitostanol ester (3g/d) dissolved in rapeseed oil margarine appears to be an effective and safe hypocholesterolemic treatment in children with familial hypercholesterolemia. [Gylling H, Siimes MA, Miettinen TA; Sitostanol ester margarine in dietary treatment of children with familial hypercholesterolemia, *J Lipid Res* **36**(8), 1807-12 (1995)].

Plant sterols and stanols lower serum cholesterol by inhibiting intestinal absorption of cholesterol. The use of fatty acid esters of stanols is particularly helpful because stanols readily mix with dietary fats in this form and their hypocholesterolemic efficacy is greater than in the free form. [Ikeda I, Sugano M; Inhibition of cholesterol absorption by plant sterols for mass intervention *Curr Opin Lipidol* **9**(6), 527-31 (1998)].

Plant sterols and stanols derived from wood pulp and vegetable oils lower total and LDL-cholesterol by inhibiting cholesterol absorption from the intestine in humans. Plant stanols are virtually unabsorbable, which makes them more ideal hypocholesterolemic agents than plant sterols. Plant stanol esters at a level of 2-3 g/day have been shown to reduce LDL-cholesterol by 10-15% without side effects. [Nguyen TT; The cholesterol-lowering action of plant stanol esters, *J Nutr.* **129**(12), 2109-12 (1999)].

An intake of 2-3 grams of plant sterols/day is associated with a 10% reduction of total cholesterol and a 13-15% reduction of LDL-cholesterol, whereas HDL-cholesterol remains largely unchanged. This amount of plant sterols may be incorporated into approximately 20 grams of margarine. Subjects that are poor responders to treatment with statins may benefit from such margarine, and also children with familial hypercholesterolaemia. [Almendingen K, Lia A; Presence of plant sterols in the diet and the hypocholesterolemic effects of plant sterols, *Tidsskr Nor Laegeforen* **120**(22), 2661-65 (2000) [Article in Norwegian].

From appropriate experiments, it has been shown that vegetable oil and wood based stanol ester mixtures, with a different sitostanol/campestanol ratio, have similar LDL-cholesterol lowering effects in a non-hypercholesterolemic population. [Plat J, Mensink RP; Vegetable oil-based versus wood based stanol ester mixtures: Effects on serum lipids and hemostatic factors in non-hypercholesterolemic subjects, *Atherosclerosis* **148**(1), 101-12 (2000)].

See *Quillaja saponaria:* [Ueda & Tanoue; *Animal Sci J* **71**(4), 393-99 (2000)].

Feeding of plant stanol esters, independent of their sources, dramatically reduced the extent and severity of atherosclerotic lesions, by decreasing VLDL, IDL and to a lesser extent LDL-cholesterol in apoE*3-Leiden transgenic mice. [Volger OL, Mensink RP, Plat J, Hornstra G, Havekes LM, Princen HM; Dietary vegetable oil and wood derived plant stanol esters reduce atherosclerotic lesion size and severity in apoE*3-

Leiden transgenic mice, *Atherosclerosis* **157**(2), 375-81 (2001)].

The mechanisms involved in the plasma cholesterol-lowering of sitostanol were evaluated using male Hartley guinea pigs. The results suggest that sitostanol might have its hypocholesterolaemic effect by reducing cholesterol absorption, which results in lower concentration of cholesterol in liver. This reduction in hepatic cholesterol might possibly alter hepatic cholesterol metabolism and affect lipoprotein concentration and composition. [Ramjiganesh T, Roy S, McIntyre JC, Fernandez ML; The hypocholesterolaemic effects of sitostanol in the guinea pig are in part related to changes in hepatic lipids and lipoprotein composition, *Brit J Nutr* **85**(2), 165-72 (2001)].

A decreased intestinal cholesterol absorption due to a competition between plant stanols and cholesterol for incorporation into mixed micelles is considered to be the reason for the hypocholesterolemic effect of plant stanols. It is now hypothesised that plant stanols—and possibly plant sterols—increase ATP binding cassette transporters (ABCA1)-mediated cholesterol efflux back into the intestinal lumen and that intracellular levels of plant stanols are monitored by the same sensors as those that monitor cholesterol. Consequently, increased plant stanol levels within the enterocyte activate cholesterol efflux. [Plat J, Mensink RP; Increased intestinal ABCA1 expression contributes to the decrease in cholesterol absorption after plant stanol consumption, *FASEB J* **16**(10), 1248-53 (2002)].

It has been demonstrated that daily consumption of 2-3 g of plant sterols or stanols reduces LDL-cholesterol concentrations by 9-14%. Functional foods enriched with plant sterols and stanols have been shown to be effective in various population groups. [Kerckhoffs DA, Brouns F, Hornstra G, Mensink RP; Effects on the human serum lipoprotein profile of β-glucan, soy protein and isoflavones, plant sterols and stanols, garlic and tocotrienols, *J Nutr* **132**(9), 2494-505 (2002)].

The cholesterol-lowering activity of dietary phytosterols is known to be due to their interference with the intestinal absorption of cholesterol. The effects of phytosterols on cholesterol biosynthesis in human cells, particularly in the sterolconversion pathway were studied. For this, both Caco-2 (intestinal mucosa) and HL- 60 (promyelocytic) human cell lines were incubated with 14C-acetate, and the incorporation of radioactivity into sterols was determined using standard procedure. Sterols containing a double bond at C-22 in the side chain (stigmasterol, brassicasterol and ergosterol) dramatically inhibited the activity of sterol *DELTA*-24-reductase but phytosterols with saturated side chain (β-sitosterol and campesterol) were inactive in this regard. The phytosterols with a double bond at C-22 position acted as competitive inhibitors of sterol *DELTA*-24-reductase. The sterol 5,22-cholestedien-3β-ol that lacks the alkyl groups characteristic of phytosterols, acted as a much stronger inhibitor of *DELTA*-24-reductase. Inhibition of sterol *DELTA* - 24-reductase may represent an additional mechanism for the cholesterol-lowering action of phytosterols. [Fernandez C, Suarez Y, Ferruelo AJ, Gomez Coronado D, Lasuncion MA; Inhibition of cholesterol biosynthesis by *DELTA*-22-unsaturated phytosterols via competitive inhibition of sterol *DELTA*-24-reductase in mammalian cells, *Biochem J* **366**(1), 109- 19 (2002)].

The effects of consuming bakery products enriched with sterol esters, α- tocopherol and β-carotene on plasma lipid and fat-soluble antioxidant concentrations in normocholesterolemic, habitual consumers of bakery products following their usual diet and lifestyle were investigated using a randomised, double-blind, placebocontrolled design. The investigation showed that bakery products are excellent carriers for phytosterols and their consumption is associated with a decrease in total and LDL-c concentrations, with no changes in α-tocopherol and β-carotene. The ability of bakery products to include sufficient quantities of β-carotene to compensate for a potential deficiency and the fact that their efficacy was not associated with the time of day at which they were consumed, are interesting findings. [Quilez J, Rafecas M, Brufau G, Garcia Lorda P, Megias I, Bullo M, Ruiz JA, Salas Salvado J; Bakery products enriched with phytosterol esters, α-tocopherol and β-carotene decrease plasma LDL-cholesterol and maintain plasma β-carotene concentrations in normocholesterolemic men and women, *J Nutr* **133**(10), 3103-09 (2003)].

Dietary phytosterols are known to reduce plasma cholesterol concentrations when consumed in different food matrices, but their effectiveness in nonfat or low fat beverages has not been established. An investigation was, therefore, made on moderately hypercholesterolemic men and women to examine whether phytosterols alter plasma lipid levels when incorporated into nonfat or low fat beverages. The results show that intake of phytosterols in a low fat beverage format is not efficacious for lipid level modification. [Jones PJH, Vanstone CA, Raeini Sarjaz M, St Onge MP; Phytosterols in low and nonfat beverages as part of a controlled diet fail to lower plasma lipid levels, *J Lipid Res* **44**(9), 1713-19 (2003)].

The effect of a phytosterol-enriched spread (margarines) in subjects with type-2 diabetes mellitus on serum lipids, glycosylated haemoglobin (HbA1c), and blood glucose under free-living conditions was investigated. The clinical study shows that a phytosterol-enriched spread is effective in lowering total and LDL-cholesterol in subjects with type-2 diabetes. Although this effect is modest, it may contribute to decreasing the elevated risk of cardiovascular disease in type-2 diabetes. [Lee YM, Haastert B, Scherbaum W, Hauner H; A phytosterol-enriched spread improves the lipid profile of subjects with type 2 diabetes mellitus: A randomized controlled trial under free-living conditions, *European J Nutr* **42**(2), 111-17 (2003)].

The cholesterol-lowering efficacy and anti-atherogenic properties of hydrogenated versus non-hydrogenated tall oil-derived phytosterols were compared in Apo E-deficient mice. The elevated plasma cholesterol levels observed in controls, were significantly reduced by the addition of either 0.5%, 1% or 2% nonhydrogenated or hydrogenated phytosterols at week 4. Cholesterol-lowering effect of the hydrogenated phytosterols was lower at all doses in comparison to non-hydrogenated phytosterols. By contrast, both hydrogenated and non-hydrogenated phytosterols showed comparable non-significant anti-atherogenic properties in treated animals after 14-week treatment. In conclusion, this study did not show statistically significant differences between hydrogenated and non-hydrogenated plant sterols with regard to their cholesterol-lowering and anti-atherosclerotic properties in Apo E-deficient mice. [Pritchard PH, Li M, Zamfir C, Lukic T, Novak E, Moghadasian MH; Comparison of cholesterol-lowering efficacy and anti-atherogenic properties of hydrogenated versus non-hydrogenated (PhytrolTM) tall oil-derived phytosterols in Apo E-deficient mice, *Cardiovasc Drugs Ther* **17**(5-6), 443-49 (2003)].

The antioxidant effects of phytosterols (β-sitosterol, stigmasterol, and campesterol) against lipid peroxidation were examined and compared with that of 2,2,5,7,8-pentamethyl-6-chromanol (PMC). The phytosterols exerted antioxidant effects on the oxidation of methyl linoleate in solution and PMC was most active and stigmasterol was the least active one. The study showed that phytosterols act chemically as an antioxidant, a modest radical scavenger, and physically as a stabiliser in the membranes. [Yoshida Y, Niki E; Antioxidant effects of phytosterol and its components, *J Nutr Sci Vitaminol* **49**(4), 277-80 (2003)].

While the hypocholesterolemic effect of plant sterols is well known, it is not clear whether plant sterols regulate lipoprotein production and secretion from the liver and intestines, thereby decreasing the levels of circulating atherogenic lipoproteins. The effect of the three main phytosterols (stigmasterol, campesterol and β-sitosterol) on lipoprotein production in HepG2 human liver cells and Caco2 human intestinal cells were studied. Secretion levels of apoB100 were significantly decreased after incubation with all plant sterols compared to control. Cholesterol ester concentrations were significantly decreased when HepG2 cells were incubated with these plant sterols. Secretion of apoB48 from intestinal cells was significantly decreased by these sterols. From the results of the investigation it was concluded that plant sterols limit lipid (cholesterol ester) availability in cells leading to increased degradation of apoB100 in HepG2 liver cells and apoB48 in Caco2 intestinal cells, which, in turn, results in a decreased production of VLDL from the liver and chylomicrons from the intestine. Plant sterols were thus found to decrease the numbers of the atherogenic lipoproteins LDL and thus reduce the risk of developing cardiovascular disease. [Ho SS, Pal S; Phytosterols decrease the secretion of atherogenic lipoproteins from HepG2 liver and Caco2 intestinal cells, *Asia Pac J Clin Nutr* **13**(Suppl), S68 (2004)].

The recent findings concerning the effect of phytosterols on the blood cholesterol have been reviewed emphasizing the results from experimental and human studies. The hypocholesterolemic effect is observed with the intake of 2.5g/day of phytosterols or phytostanols. Daily intake, usually of stanols, for 4 weeks has shown to to be effective in lowering blood total as well as LDL-cholesterol by about 10%. The mechanism of action in lowering blood cholesterol comes from their structural similarity to cholesterol, hence they act by competing with cholesterol at the luminal absorption site. The adverse effects of a high intake of phytosterols and phytostanols are the lower absorption of some fat-soluble vitamins and antioxidants. [Martins SL, Silva HF, Novaes MR, Ito MK; Therapeutic effects of phytosterols and phytostanols in cholesterolemia, *Arch Latinoam Nutr* **54**(3), 257-63 (2004). Article in Portuguese].

The cholesterol-lowering properties of plant sterols have been known for some time and many clinical studies have confirmed the efficacy of sitosterol in lowering plasma LDL-cholesterol concentrations. Plant sterols are known to compete with cholesterol for space within bile salt micelles in the intestinal lumen and thereby reduce cholesterol absorption. The discovery of the adenosine binding cassette transporters has clarified the function of plant sterols in impeding cholesterol absorption. Compared to cholesterol and other sterols, sitosterol is preferentially pumped out to the intestinal lumen by the adenosine binding cassette transporters. This selective binding of sitosterol to the transporters ultimately results in significant lowering of plasma cholesterol. From the review of these studies, it is apparent that sitosterol is a useful dietary supplement for the lowering of plasma cholesterol. Nevertheless, this plant sterol should be used with caution in certain individuals who have a higher absorption rate of sitosterol. [Fernandez ML, Vega-Lopez S; Efficacy and safety of sitosterol in the management of blood cholesterol levels, *Cardiovasc Drug Rev* **23**(1), 57-70 (2005)].

The molecular effects of phytosterols were studied in small intestines and livers of apolipoprotein E-deficient (apoE(-/-)) mice. From the results of the investigation, it was concluded that inhibition of intestinal cholesterol absorption by phytosterols is not mediated *via* transcriptional changes in ABCA1, ABCG5, ABCG8 or NPC1L1. Changes suggestive of immunomodulation are associated with the hypocholesterolemic effect of phytosterols and with apoE deficiency. [Calpe Berdiel L, Escola-Gil JC, Ribas V, Navarro-Sastre A, Garces-Garces J, Blanco-Vaca F; Changes in intestinal and liver global gene expression in response to a phytosterol enriched diet, *Atherosclerosis* **181**(1), :75-85. (2005)].

PLANT FIBRES: It has been postulated that dietary fibre's protective effect against the development of colon cancer, diverticular disease and atherosclerosis may be due to the adsorption and/or dilution of intestinal sterols such as bile acids and neutral sterols and their bacterial metabolites by components of fibre. Of the plant fibres, hemicellulose and pectin may induce an increase in faecal bile acid excretion in man, which may be accompanied by a decrease in serum cholesterol. Natural fibres, such as rolled oats, alfalfa, guar gum and Bengal gram have hypocholesterolemic properties and some of these fibres were found to bind considerable amounts of bile acids *in vitro*. The fibre theory linking fibre deficiency with the development of colon cancer and other diseases is simple, attractive and appears firmly based in common sense but the research data are often contradictory and confusing, probably due to lack of adequate documentation on fibre intake and/or the absence of detailed information on the chemistry of the fibre itself. [Huang CTL, Gopalakrishna GS, Nichols BL; Fibre, intestinal sterols and colon cancer, *Am J Clin Nutr* **31**(3), 516-26 (1978)].

Certain soluble plant fibres are known to have hypocholesterolemic effects. In view of the fact that information about soluble fibres of most foods is not available, a modification of Southgate's method was used to separate plant fibre into soluble and insoluble fractions. Both fractions were hydrolysed with dilute sulphuric acid or trifluoracetic acid and the hydrolysed sugars were measured by gas-liquid chromatography. Fibre content of selected cereals and vegetables were examined. Oat, corn, and cooked beans have greater proportions of soluble fibre than wheat and green vegetables. Acid hydrolysis products of soluble fibres of cereals and beans were mainly glucose whereas in green vegetables uronic acids were the major components. The differing fibre composition of various plant food sources is probably important in determining their physiological effects. [Chen WJ, Anderson JW; Soluble and insoluble plant fibre in selected cereals and vegetables, *Am J Clin Nutr* **34**(6), 1077-82 (1981)].

The effects of dietary cellulose, pectin and guar gum on the concentrations of serum cholesterol in the major serum lipoprotein fractions were compared in rats in 2 separate experiments of 6 and 15 wk duration. Dietary pectin, when fed for 6 weeks, produced a significant decrease in the percent of serum cholesterol associated with high-density lipoprotein and elevation in that associated with low-density lipoproteins, compared with the group fed cellulose or guar gum. The long-term (15 weeks) feeding resulted in a further decline in HDL-cholesterol in all three groups but most markedly in the rats fed guar gum. No differences in the concentration of serum triglycerides were noticed among the groups in either the 6 or 15 weeks experiment. In the light of the current evidence for the inverse relationship between HDL-cholesterol and coronary heart disease, the lowering of HDL concentration by dietary pectin and guar gum may not be regarded as favourable, despite their distinct hypocholesterolemic effects, compared with dietary cellulose. [Koo S, Stanton P; Effects of cellulose, pectin and guar gum on the distribution of serum cholesterol among lipoprotein fractions, *Nutr Reports International* **24**(2), 395-402 (1981)].

The effects of propionate, a metabolic product of fibre fermentation, on serum and liver lipid concentrations were studied in cholesterol-fed rats. Both serum and liver cholesterol levels were significantly lower in rats fed with cholesterol-sodium propionate diet than in rats fed cholesterol diet without propionate. Liver triglyceride levels were also significantly lower in the propionate-treated group. Serum triglyceride concentrations were not influenced by propionate feeding. Thus propionate may mediate some of the hypocholesterolemic effects of certain soluble plant fibres. [Chen WJL, Anderson JW, Jennings D; Propionate may mediate the hypocholesterolemic effects of certain soluble plant fibres in cholesterol fed rats, *Proc Soc Exp Biol Med* **175**(2), 215-18 (1984)].

The effects of various whole vegetables on blood and liver lipids and excretion of faecal steroids in chickens fed with cholesterol-containing diets were studied. The levels of vegetable powders and cholesterol in the experimental diets were 10.0%

and 1.0% (w/w), respectively. Vegetable supplemented diets resulted in a marked decrease in serum cholesterol, phospholipids and VLDL + LDL-cholesterol compared to the fibre free diet. In contrast, levels of faecal cholesterol and bile acid excretion were increased in the vegetable supplemented diets. Vegetable supplementation of diets did not affect the serum triglycerides and HDL-cholesterol levels. Lower concentrations of liver cholesterol were obtained in vegetable supplemented groups than the fibre-free group. There were no differences in liver triglycerides and phospholipids between vegetable supplemented and fibre-free groups. Among the vegetable supplemented diets, the diets containing bellflower (*Campanula lactiflora*) roots and wild aster (*Aster* species) leaves, whose crude fibre contents were higher than the others, resulted in the lowest serum cholesterol. The study suggests that dietary vegetables exert hypocholesterolemic effects by increasing faecal cholesterol and bile acid excretion. Further studies are needed to elucidate the exact mechanisms by which fibres in vegetables decrease serum cholesterol. [Kim KN, Han IK; Effects of different dietary sources of cholesterol, protein and fibre on lipid metabolism in chicks. Effects of various dietary vegetables on blood and liver lipids and the excretion of faecal steroids in cholesterol-fed chicks, *Korean J Animal Sci* **27**(6), 374- 80 (1985)].

Binding of bile acids and phospholipids to a number of dietary fibres and cholestyramine within the small intestine was determined. Of the fibres used, guar gum and lignin bound significant quantities of bile acids. However, only cholestyramine reduced the bile acid concentration within the aqueous phase of the intestinal contents. The failure of guar gum and lignin to significantly decrease the amount of solubilised lipid suggests that the hypocholesterolemic effect of these fibres is due more to their bile acid binding capacity than to an effect on lipid solubilisation. [Gallaher D, Schneeman BO; Intestinal interaction of bile acids, phospholipids, dietary fibres and cholestyramine, *Am J Physiol* **250**(4 Part 1), G420- G426 (1986)].

Certain cultivars of hulless barley, rich in water-soluble fibre, have a hypocholesterolemic effect in the chick. The type of dietary fibre, soluble versus insoluble, and level of serum cholesterol are considerations in predicting the degree of hypocholesterolemic effect in cereal grains. [Newman RK, Lewis SE, Newman CW, Boik RJ, Ramage RT; Hypocholesterolemic effect of barley foods on healthy men, *Nutr Reports International* **39**(4), 749-60 (1989)].

Dietary fibres from blackgram, barley, ragi and rice bran were isolated as neutral detergent fibre and their effect on cholesterol metabolism studied in rats, fed high fat-cholesterol diet. It was seen that the hemicellulose content of different fibres correlated with their effect on cholesterol metabolism. Neutral detergent fibre from barley with its maximum hemicellulose content produced lowest concentration of serum and tissue cholesterol, highest concentration of hepatic and faecal bile acids and faecal sterols. [Thomas M, Leelamma S, Kurup PA; Neutral detergent fibre from various foods and its hypocholesterolemic action in rats, *J Food Sci Technol* **27**(5), 290-93 (1990)].

The hypocholesterolemic effects of psyllium were compared with those of methylcellulose, calcium polycarbophil, and placebo as dietary adjuncts in treating mild to moderate hypercholesterolemia. In managing mild to moderate hypercholesterolemia, methylcellulose and calcium polycarbophil proved little or of no additional benefit, while psyllium significantly enhanced the American Heart Association diet effects. [Anderson JW, Floore TL, Geil PB, O'neal DS, Balm TK; Hypocholesterolemic effects of different bulk-forming hydrophilic fibres as adjuncts to dietary therapy in mild to moderate hypercholesterolemia, *Arch Internal Med* **151**(8), 1597-602 (1991)].

Dietary fibres from seed coat of wheat, maize, green seeded gram and soybean lowered the levels of plasma as well as tissue total lipids, cholesterol and glycerides, the effect being prominent with soybean and green seeded gram, which also appeared to be potent anti-atherogenic agents. The hypocholesterolemic action of fibre could be directly correlated with their bile acid binding capacity and inverse relationship to water holding capacity. In general, higher the lignin content of fibre, better was its hypocholesterolemic effect. [Uberoi SK, Vadhera S, Soni GL; Role of dietary fibre from pulses and cereals as hypocholesterolemic and hypolipidemic agent, *J Food Sci Technol* **29**(5), 281-83 (1992)].

The cholesterol-lowering effects of a fibre supplement were evaluated in patients with mild to moderate hypercholesterolemia. After a nine-week diet stabilisation period, patients were randomly assigned to treatment with 10 or 20 g/d of the fibre supplement or with a matching placebo. Among patients who completed the 15-weeks treatment period, total cholesterol, LDL-cholesterol, and the ratio of LDL to HDL were significantly reduced for the 10 and 20 g/d groups compared with the placebo group The fibre supplement had no significant effects on HDL cholesterol or triglycerides. [Hunninghake DB, Miller VT, Larosa JC, Kinosian B, Brown V, Howard WJ, Diserio FJ, O'Connor RR; Hypocholesterolemic effects of a dietary fibre supplement, *Am J Clin Nutr* **59**(5), 1050-54 (1994)].

The hypocholesterolemic effects of long-term treatment (36 to 51 weeks, 20 g/d, twice a day) with a mixture of dietary fibres (guar gum, pectin, soy, pea, corn bran) were evaluated. There were no significant effects on the levels of either triglycerides or high-density lipoprotein cholesterol (HDL-c). Levels of total cholesterol and low density lipoprotein cholesterol (LDL-c) and the LDL/HDL ratio were significantly reduced during treatment. [Hunninghake DB; Miller VT; Larosa JC; Kinosian B; Jacobson T; Brown V; Howard WJ; Edelman DA; O'Connor RR; Long-term treatment of hypercholesterolemia with dietary fibre, *Am J Med* **97**(6),:504-08 (1994)].

Soluble dietary fibres have been shown to reduce total plasma cholesterol and LDL-cholesterol, the two important risk factors for coronary heart disease. The mechanisms, which have been suggested, include binding of bile acids and interference with their enterohepatic circulation, interference with micelle formation, and reduced hepatic cholesterol synthesis. [Basu TK, Ooraikul B; Lipid-lowering effects of dietary fibre, *J Clin Biochem Nutr* **18**(1), 1-9 (1995)].

The results of investigation suggest that the degree of intestinal fermentation and bile acid excretion, which are considered to be associated with the hypocholesterolemic action of dietary fibre, varies with each kind of dietary fibre. [Kishimoto Y, Wakabayashi S, Takeda H; Hypocholesterolemic effect of dietary fibre: Relation to intestinal fermentation and bile acid excretion, *J Nutr Sci Vitaminol* **41**(1), 151-61 (1995)].

Significant lowering of plasma low density lipoprotein (LDL) cholesterol concentrations in humans and animals by dietary soluble fibres is well documented. While such activity has been reported in male guinea pigs, it was important to know whether dietary fibres elicited similar hypocholesterolemic responses in both genders. To test whether dietary fibre elicited similar hypocholesterolemic responses in both genders, female guinea pigs were fed with diets containing 12.5% pectin, 12.5% guar gum, 7.5% psyllium or 12.5% cellulose (control diet). In addition, low (0.04%) or high (0.25%) amounts of cholesterol were tested with the fibres to determine whether dietary cholesterol altered the plasma cholesterol response. Significant reductions in plasma cholesterol were observed in females fed with low cholesterol diets with pectin, guar gum or psyllium while the responses to fibre with high cholesterol intake were more moderate. The study demonstrated that female, compared to male guinea pigs are more responsive to a dietary cholesterol challenge and that with high cholesterol intake effects of fibres are moderate compared to males. In contrast, with low cholesterol intakes, the cholesterol lowering effects of fibre are similar in both genders. [Fernandez ML, Vergara Jimenez M, Romero AL, Erickson SK, McNamara DJ; Gender differences in response to dietary soluble fibre in guinea pigs: Effects of pectin, guar gum, and psyllium, *J Lipid Res* **36**(10), 2191-202 (1995)].

Semipurified diets containing 5% cellulose, psyllium hydrocolloid, pectin or oat bran as dietary fibre sources or 2% cholestyramine were fed to groups of 10 male Wistar rats for 4 weeks and the activity of the rate-limiting step in bile acid synthesis, cholesterol-7α-hydroxylase, was measured. The activity of cholesterol-7α- hydroxylase was highest in the cholestyramine-treated group, followed by groups fed psyllium or pectin, which exhibited more than twice the enzyme activity of groups fed with cellulose or oat bran. Feeding cholesterol resulted in significantly higher enzyme activity when cellulose, oat bran and rice bran were fed but no difference in activity was observed when cholesterol was added to the psyllium-containing diet. The data support the hypothesis that the hypocholesterolemic effect of soluble fibres is modulated through increased synthesis and therefore pool size of bile acids. [Matheson HB, Colon IS, Story JA; Cholesterol 7α-hydroxylase activity is increased by dietary modification with psyllium hydrocolloid, pectin, cholesterol and cholestyramine in rats, *J Nutr* **125**(3), 454-58 (1995)].

In order to examine possible mechanisms for the hypocholesterolemic effects of dietary fibres, both biochemical changes and morphometric parameters of the intestine following fibre intake were evaluated. Thirty male Sprague Dawley rats were divided into 3 groups and fed either a fibre-free, 15% high methoxy pectin fibre, or 15% cellulose diet for a 4 - week period. Plasma cholesterol levels, hepatic enzyme activity and faecal bile acid excretion were determined and changes in the intestinal structure were evaluated. Daily faecal bile acid excretion was significantly higher in rats fed with the pectin diet accompanied by elevated HMG-CoA reductase activity. Pectin feeding also led to significant elongation of both the small and large intestine whereas cellulose only affected colon length. Computerized image analysis of intestinal crosssections showed enlarged muscle area in the ileum and midcolon of pectin-fed rats and greater mucosal area in the colon. Circular muscle cell hypertrophy was also observed in the colon. In contrast, the effects of cellulose feeding were limited to elongation of the colon accompanied by muscle cell hypertrophy. These data indicate that the hypocholestrolemic effects of pectin may be due to increased bile acid secretion accompanied by significant morphological changes in the ileum and colon. [Stark A, Nyska-A, Madar-Z; Metabolic and morphometric changes in small and large intestine in rats fed with high-fibre diets, *Toxicologic Pathol* **24**(2), 166-71 (1996)].

Sites and mechanisms for the hypocholesterolemic actions of soluble dietary fibres have been studied. [Marlett JA; Sites and mechanisms for the hypocholesterolemic actions of soluble dietary fibre sources, *Adv Exp Med Biol* **427**, 109-21 (1997)].

The effects of lignin on growth performance and blood metabolites, mostly those related to lipid metabolism, were studied on piglets of 21 days of age. The results of the study indicate that lignin supplementation has a hypolipemic but no hypocholesterolemic property when fed to the piglets. [Valencia Z, Chavez ER; Lignin as a purified dietary fibre supplement for piglets, *Nutr Res* **17**(10), 1517-27 (1997)].

In order to make a comparative evaluation of different dietary fibres, ten diets containing 10% dietary fibre as cellulose (control), psyllium, barley bran, sugarbeet or oat bran, with or without 0.5% added cholesterol and 0.1% cholic acid, were fed to Sprague Dawley rats for 6 weeks. Among rats fed hyperlipidemic diets, the psyllium diet not only lowered total serum cholesterol, serum LDL-cholesterol, total liver lipids and liver cholesterol, but also significantly increased HDL-c/LDL-c ratio, compared to the cellulose-fed controls. The group fed barley bran had significantly lower total serum cholesterol, serum LDL cholesterol, total liver lipids and liver cholesterol but no effect was seen on HDL-c/LDL-c ratio when compared to cellulose fed controls. The rats fed with oat bran had lower serum total and LDL-cholesterol concentrations relative to the controls. However, the total liver lipid and liver cholesterol were higher in the oat bran diet. The group fed with sugarbeet fibre showed only a lowering in total serum cholesterol concentrations. Thus, of the different dietary fibres, psyllium showed the strongest therapeutic effect. [Ismail S, Smolyar I, Navder KP; Four different dietary fibres have different effects on serum and liver lipids, in rats, *Biochem Arch* **13**(3), 161-70 (1997)].

The effects of refined konjac (*Amorphophallus konjac*) meal (RKM) in comparison to pectin, algin and agar on lipid levels in serum and liver and on liver histopathology in rats were studied. All four kinds of dietary fibre were given at a level of 5% of diet to young male rats of Wistar strain fed on a lipid-rich diet containing 5% lard, 1% cholesterol and 0.25% cholate. All the dietary fibres prevented increases in total cholesterol in fasting serum but the level of triglyceride was unchanged. The concentrations of total cholesterol and triglyceride in the liver were lower in the RKM group than in the control group and the other three groups. Hepatic histopathological examination also showed the most significant lipotropic effect in the RKM group. The daily output of faecal bile acids was significantly increased in all the four experimental groups than in the normal group and the control group. [Wu Jie; Comparison of hypolipidemic effect of refined konjac meal with several common dietary fibres and their mechanisms of action, *Biomed Environ Sci* **10**(1), 27-37 (1997)].

The effects of indigestible dextrin and polydextrose—soluble dietary fibres with low molecular weight— on lipid metabolism and disaccharidase activities of intestinal mucosa in rats fed with a high sucrose diet were investigated. Their effects were compared with those of well known soluble fibres, pectin, and guar gum, and also with an insoluble fibre, cellulose. Body weight gain was the lowest in rats fed guar gum, the highest in rats fed cellulose and in between these two extremes were the rats fed with other diets. Like guar gum and pectin, feeding of indigestible dextrin showed lower plasma lipid values than cellulose feeding. Liver triglyceride level of rats fed with polydextrose, indigestible dextrin, and pectin were lower than that of cellulose. Liver cholesterol and phospholipid concentrations were similar among groups. Daily faecal excretion of total lipid, cholesterol, and bile acids were highest in rats fed with guar gum, followed by pectin-fed and cellulose-fed rats, and the lowest in rats fed with indigestible dextrin and polydextrose. Jejunal sucrase activity was low in the order of guar-gum, polydextrose, indigestible dextrin, pectin, and cellulose. The results indicate that the hypolipidemic effect of soluble dietary fibres would be lessened with reduction in molecular weight. [Choi YS, Cho SH, Kim HJ, Lee HJ; Effects of soluble dietary fibres on lipid metabolism and activities of intestinal disaccharidases in rats, *J Nutr Sci Vitaminol* **44**(5), 591-600 (1998)].

The effects of various cereal fibres and various amounts of β-glucan on cholesterol and bile acid metabolism were examined. Hamsters were fed with semisynthetic diets containing 0.12% cholesterol, 20% fat and either 16% total dietary fibre from wheat bran (control) or dietary fibres from oat bran, oat bran concentrate, barley grains, oat fibre concentrate, barley flakes, or rye bran. After five weeks, plasma total cholesterol and liver cholesterol concentrations were significantly lower only in hamsters, fed rye bran. Diets containing oat ingredients or barley had no effect on total cholesterol. Changes in the pattern of biliary bile acids occurred in hamsters-fed total dietary fibres from barley flakes (16%) or from oat bran (10%). Hamsters fed with rye bran had a significantly higher faecal bile acid excretion when compared with controls fed wheat bran. Because rye bran caused the most pronounced lowering effect of total cholesterol despite the lowest content of β-glucan and soluble fibres, components other than β-glucan and soluble fibres seem to be involved in its hypocholesterolemic action. [Rieckhoff D, Trautwein EA, Maelkki Y; Erbersdobler HF; Effects of different cereal fibres on cholesterol and bile acid metabolism in the Syrian golden hamster, *Cereal Chem* **76**(5), 788-95 (1999)].

POLYSACCHARIDES: The hypocholesterolemic effects of various polysaccharides, gums, carrageenan (same as carragheenan and carrageenin), xylan, pectin, inulin, derivatives of alginic acid, cellulose, starches, bacterial gums and konjac flour on rats fed with a hypercholesterolemic diet containing 1% cholesterol and 0.25% bile salts were examined. Serum and liver cholesterol depressing activities of pectin, konjac flour and guar gum were reconfirmed in rats with fed a hypercholesterolemic diet. Locust bean gum, alginic acid and Na-alginate also decreased elevation of the liver cholesterol level. [Tsuji E, Tsuji K, Suzuki S; Effects of polysaccharides on cholesterol metabolism. Part 6: Effects of various polysaccharides on serum and liver cholesterol levels in cholesterol fed rats, *Annual Report National Inst Nutr* (24), 83-91 (1975)].

The hypolipidemic and antisclerotic properties of polysaccharides, isolated from *Peganum harmala, Ungernia sewerzowii, Eremurus regelii, Gossypium hirsutum, Allium cepa, U. ferganica, A. suworowii,* and *Polygonatum sewezowii,* were studied. Experiments were carried out in male rats and rabbits. The administration of the polysaccharides reduced blood cholesterol and triglyceride levels. A direct correlation was established between the molecular weight of the polysaccharides and their hypocholesterolemic and hypotriglyceridemic activity. [Zhushbaktova ZA; Syrov VN; Dzhukharova MKH; Rakhimov DA; Study of the hypolipidemic properties of polysaccharides isolated from Central Asian flora, *Khim Farma Zh* **21**(11), 1348-52 (1987) Article in Russian].

PROANTHOCYANIDIN POLYMER: Hypolipidemic and antiatherosclerotic activities of proanthocyanidin polymers, derived from *Hypericum perforatum, Rheum palmatum, Ephedra equisetina, Punica* sp, *Polygonum* sp. and other plants were examined. The compounds in question were found to prevent an increase in rat serum cholesterol and triglycerides. On addition of Tween-80 and Triton, these compounds diminished the manifestation of the atherosclerotic process in rabbits. In addition to the hypolipidemic activity, these compounds are believed to enhance resistance of the vascular wall providing its protection from cholesterol penetration into the composition of atherogenic lipoproteins. [Khushbaktova ZA, Syrov VN, Kuliev Z; Study of the hypolipidemic properties of polymer proanthocyanidines from plants used in folk medicine, *Khim Farma Zh* **23**(9), 1111- 15 (1989)].

RETROGRADED STARCH: Retrograded or resistant starch is a type of starch that is resistant to (not easily broken down by) digestive enzymes, so it is absorbed much more slowly into the bloodstream than other starches.

Diets enriched in retrograded amylose have been shown to lower serum cholesterol concentrations in rats. The possibility, that this hypocholesterolaemic effect of retrograded starch is caused by an increased influx of neutral steroids and bile acids into the caecum and increased faecal excretion of bile acids, was considered appropriate from the results of the investigation. [Verbeek MJF, De Deckere EAM, Tijburg LBM, Van Amelsvoort JMM, Beynen AC; Influence of dietary retrograded starch on the metabolism of neutral steroids and bile acids in rats, *Brit J Nutr* **74**(6), 807-20 (1995)].

The influence of retrograded high amylose corn starch on cholesterol metabolism in normocholesterolemic as well as in hypercholesterolemic rats was studied. No effect on cholesterol metabolism was observed in normocholesterolemic rats but in hypercholesterolemic animals plasma free and total cholesterol concentrations were significantly lower, when enzyme resistant starch was fed. Liver cholesterol concentrations were significantly decreased in rats given the hypercholesterolemic diet supplemented with retrograded high amylose corn starch. Enzyme resistant starch consumption, however, did not change total faecal bile acid excretion. Plasma total cholesterol concentrations showed a significantly negative correlation with faecal coprostanol excretion in hypercholesterolemic rats. However, no evidence that coprostanol is the only factor responsible for the observed hypocholesterolemic effect of enzyme resistant starch in cholesterol-fed rats could be secured. [Vanhoof K, De-Schrijver R; Consumption of enzyme resistant starch and cholesterol metabolism in normo- and hyper-cholesterolemic rats, *Nutr Res* **17**(8), 1331-40 (1997)].

The effects of resistant starch and cholestyramine on cholesterol metabolism were tested in guinea pigs. The data from this study suggest that although both resistant starch and cholestyramine lower plasma LDL-cholesterol concentrations, the order of magnitude is different, and the distinct effects of these two treatments on hepatic cholesterol homeostasis suggest that different mechanisms are involved in the plasma cholesterol lowering. [Fernandez ML, Roy S, Vergara Jimenez M; Resistant starch and cholestyramine have distinct effects on hepatic cholesterol metabolism in guinea pigs fed with a hypercholesterolemic diet, *Nutr Res* **20**(6), 837-49 (2000)].

SAPONINS and SAPOGENINS: Saponins are steroid or triterpene glycosides, which occur in a number of important plants. The non-sugar part of saponins are sapogenins.

In albino rats the effect of tomatin, an almost non-absorbable saponin, on lipid metabolism was studied. Administration of tomatin (1%) with the diet decreased the uptake of dietry cholesterol by liver, enhanced hepatic and intestinal cholesterol synthesis and increased the sterol excretion without affecting bile acid excretion. Unlike cholestyramine, tomatin did not sequester cholic acid *in vitro*. Tomatin affected cholesterol absorption and other aspects of lipid metabolism similar to cholestyramine excepting that tomatin increased sterol excretion while cholestyramine enhanced bile acid excretion. [Cayen MN; Effect of dietary tomatin on cholesterol metabolism in the rat, *J Lipid Res* **12**(4), 482-90 (1971)].

Saponins occur in a variety of plants especially in legumes of *Glycine max, Cicer arietinium, Lens culinaris, Phaseolus mungo, Phaseolus aconitifolius, Cicia faba, Pisum sativum, Medicago sativa* and *Avena sativa*. Various experimental studies have demonstrated that these dietary saponins possess hypocholesterolemic activity and may thereby reduce the risk of cardiovascular disorders. [Khokhar S, Chauhan BM; Saponins in food: Their physiological and nutritional significance, *Sci Cult* **52**(9), 287-91 (1986)].

The reported hypocholesterolemic activity of some saponins might be due to their ability to form insoluble complexes with cholesterol and thereby preventing the absorption of cholesterol from the small intestine, while some others might cause an increase in the faecal excretion of bile acids, an indirect route for elimination of cholesterol. The effects of different saponins on absorption of the bile salt sodium cholate from perfused loops of small intestine were investigated, *in vivo*, in rats. Purified saponins from soapwort (*Saponaria officinalis*) and soybeans (*Glycine max*) substantially reduced the rate of absorption of the bile salt but quillaja (*Quillaja saponaria*) saponin reduced the absorption to a much lesser extent. These results were explained by the formation of large mixed micelles by bile acid and saponin molecules in aqueous solution, making the bile acid molecules unavailable for absorption. [Sidhu GS, Oakenfull DG; A mechanism for the hypocholesterolemic activity of saponins, *Brit J Nutr* **55**(3), 643-50 (1986)].

The occurrence of saponins in plants and their various effects including hypocholesterolemic effects when consumed by animals and man have been reviewed. [Price KR, Johnson IT, Fenwick GR; The chemistry and biological significance of saponins in foods and feeding stuffs, *Crit Rev Food Sci Nutr* **26**(1), 27-135 (1987)].

There is evidence that diosgenin, when given orally or parenterally decreases plasma cholesterol levels in rats, chicken and rabbits that have had a diet-induced hypercholesterolemia. [Juarez Oropeza MA, Diaz Zagoya JC, Rabinowitz JL; *In*-vivo and *in vitro* hypocholesterolemic effects of diosgenin in rats, *Int J Biochem* **19**(8), 679-84 (1987)].

Effects of *Gypsophila* saponins on performance and plasma cholesterol concentration in chicks fed with diets different in casein content were investigated. In chicks fed the cholesterol-free casein diet containing 18% protein, supplementation of 0.25% saponins depressed body weight gain to about half. Addition of 1% cholesterol was completely effective in alleviating the growth retardation even when 0.5% saponins was added. Saponin supplementation partially suppressed the elevated plasma total cholesterol caused by added cholesterol. However, hypocholesterolemic effect of saponins disappeared when 25% or more dietary casein was replaced on the protein basis with soybean protein isolate fortified with methionine. Increasing protein content itself was very effective in lowering plasma total cholesterol and feeding suboptimal protein markedly increased plasma total cholesterol level so that suppression by saponins was not observed. These results indicated that hypocholesterolemic effect of *Gypsophila* saponins was little as compared with that of protein source or protein content. [Ueda H; Effect of *Gypsophila* saponins on performance and plasma cholesterol concentration in chicks fed the diets different in casein content, *Animal Sci Technol* **63**(9), 905-11 (1992)].

See *Glycine max* (Soya bean, soybean): [Lanksy PS; *Acta Horticulturae* (332), 131-36 (1993)].

The majority of saponins form insoluble complexes with 3β-hydroxysteroids and are known to interact with and form large mixed micelles with bile acids and cholesterol. In rats, saponin intake has been correlated with a hypocholesterolemic effect by some authors, whilst others have disputed this claim. Saponins are also known to form insoluble saponin-mineral complexes, with iron, zinc and calcium. The beneficial effects on plasma cholesterol may be somewhat speculative in humans. Intakes up to 500 mg/day have not had particularly marked effects on plasma cholesterol although alteration in enterohepatic circulation of bile acids and neutral sterol excretion may be of benefit. The association between saponin intake and cholesterol metabolism has been reviewed in this article. [Milgate J, Roberts DCK; The nutritional and biological significance of saponins, *Nutr Res* **15**(8), 1223-49 (1995)].

The dietary proteins were found to modify the cholesterol-lowering effect of saponins in chicks. The effects of casein, casein hydrolysate and soybean protein isolate on the cholesterol-lowering action of *Quillaja* or tea saponin were investigated. Casein and casein hydrolysate diets suppressed the elevation of serum total cholesterol and liver cholesterol, but casein hydrolysate was less effective than casein in lowering LDL-cholesterol concentrations. Soybean protein isolate diet was more effective than casein hydrolysate in lowering serum total cholesterol and liver cholesterol concentrations. *Quillaja* or tea saponins also lowered serum total cholesterol and liver cholesterol concentrations in chicks fed with casein diet, but their concentrations were still higher than those of chicks given other protein diets. Thus, in addition to the interference between saponins and steroids in the intestine, it seems likely that dietary proteins affect the cholesterol-lowering action of saponins. [Ueda H, Yokoyama A; Dietary protein sources modify the cholesterol-lowering effect of saponins in chicks, *J Poultry Sci* **38**(3), 225-33 (2001)].

The different biological activities including hypocholesterolemic activity of saponins have been reviewed. [Francis G, Kerem Z, Makkar HPS, Becker K; The biological action of saponins in animal systems: A review, *Brit J Nutr* **88**(6), 587-605 (2002)].

TANNIC ACID: The RAIF and RICO rats, when fed on high fat diet with tannic acid, showed beneficial changes in serum lipids compared to the rats fed only high fat diet. [Yugarani T, Tan BKH, Das NP; The effects of tannic acid on serum and liver lipids of RAIF and RICO rats fed on high fat diet, *Comparative Biochem Physiol A-Comparative Physiol* **104**(2), 339-43 (1993)].

TANNINS: Tannin comprises a large group of natural polyphenolic compounds possessing antioxidant effects.

In search of a specific HMG-CoA reductase inhibitor like pravastatin, tannin derivatives, isolated from different traditional Chinese herbs, were tested by well established methods using Vero cells, a cell line obtained from kidneys of African green monkeys. More than 50 tannin derivatives were used for the study, but only two compounds - proanthrocyanidin A-2 and 1,2,3,6-tetra-O-galloyl-β-D-glucose showed significant growth inhibition of Vero cells. This study showed that some isolated tannin derivatives from traditional herbs were effective HMG-CoA reductase inhibitors which might be developed into new hypocholesterolemic agents. [Chang JJ, Chen TH, Chan P, Chen YJ, Hsu Feng Lin, Lo MY, Lin JY; The *in vitro* inhibitory effect of tannin derivatives on 3-hydroxy-3-methylglutaryl-coenzyme A reductase on Vero cells, *Pharmacology* (Basel) **62**(4), 224-28 (2001)].

TOCOPHEROLS and TOCOTRIENOLS: α-, β-, γ- and δ- Tocopherols and α-, β-, γ- and δ-tocotrienols are the eight members of vitamin E family.

Plasma cholesterol level in rabbits fed on a basal synthetic diet supplemented with stripped corn oil and varying amount of vitamin E was depressed as the supplementation of vitamin E was increased. This hypocholesterolemic effect was accompanied by an increase in hepatic cholesterol-7α-hydroxylase activity and cytochrome P-450 level and by a redistribution of plasma lipoprotein-cholesterol resulting in the elevation of high density to low density lipoprotein-cholesterol ratio. [Komaratat P, Chupukharoen N, Wilairat P; Effect of vitamin E on cholesterol, plasma lipoprotein distribution and metabolism in rabbits, *Int J Vitamin Nutr Res* **55**(2), 167-72 (1985)].

Tocotrienols (the farnesylated benzopyran natural products), present in large amounts in several cereals (barley, oats, rice, wheat and rye) and certain vegetable oils (palm oil and rice bran oil), were found to elicit hypocholesterolemic activity *in vitro* and *in vivo*. These compounds reduced lipids by post-transcriptional suppression of HMG-CoA reductase. γ-Tocotrienols have been found to be more potent than α-tocotrienols in inhibiting cholesterol biosynthisis *in vitro*. An improved method for isolation of tocotrienols from palm oil distillate has also been described. [Pearce BC, Parker RA, Deason ME, Queshi AA, Wright KJ; Hypocholesterolemic activity of synthetic and natural tocotrienols, *J Med Chem* **35**(2), 3595-606 (1992)].

An experiment was designed to determine whether incorporation of γ- tocotrienol or α -tocopherol in an atherogenic diet would reduce the concentration of plasma cholesterol, triglycerides and fatty acid peroxides, and attenuate platelet aggregability in rats. The results of the investigation suggested that the combination of γ-tocotrienol and α-tocopherol, as present in palm oil distillates, deserved further evaluation as a potential hypolipemic agent in hyperlipemic humans at atherogenic risk. [Watkins T, Lenz P, Gapor A, Struck M, Tomeo A, Bierenbaum M; *Gamma-* Tocotrienol as a hypocholesterolemic and antioxidant agent in rats fed atherogenic diets, *Lipids* **28**(12), 1113-18 (1993)].

The effects of dietary tocopherol and cholesterol on the levels of serum tocopherol, cholesterol and amino acid were determined using female rats, and the relationships among their levels were studied. There was no significant change in the levels of serum cholesterol with increases in serum tocopherol but supplementing the diet with cholesterol caused serum tocopherol to increase together with the level of serum cholesterol. The results of the investigation indicated that the ratio of tocopherol / cholesterol in serum, as an indicator of the status of vitamin E nutrition, increased with dietary tocopherol and decreased with dietary cholesterol. Dietary tocopherol and cholesterol may be involved in the metabolism of threonine, lysine and arginine and may affect the hypocholesterolemic action by changing the ratio of arginine / lysine. [Hirai K, Amagase S, Maeda A, Ishitani A; Effects of dietary tocopherol and cholesterol on the ratios of tocopherol to cholesterol and arginine to lysine in rats, *Nutr Res* **14**(11), 1701-10 (1994)].

The effect of α-tocopherol on the hypocholesterolemic action of sesamin (a lignan from *Sesamum indicum* and other plants) was examined in rats, given a cholesterol-enriched diet. When different levels (0.05 and 0.2%) of sesamin were fed, the supplementation of 1% α-tocopherol significantly accentuated the hypocholesterolemic action of sesamin, particularly with the higher sesamin level, although α-tocopherol alone did not affect the concentration of serum cholesterol. The dose-dependent promoting effect of α-tocopherol on the hypocholesterolemic action of sesamin was confirmed by supplementing different levels (0.2 and 1%) of α- tocopherol to a fixed level of sesamin (0.2%). The metabolism of sesamin in the liver S9 fraction appeared to be interfered with α-tocopherol *in vitro*, suggesting a possible role of α-tocopherol in maintenance of the availability of sesamin. [Nakabayashi A, Kitagawa Y, Suwa Y, Akimoto K, Asami S, Shimizu S, Hirose N, Sugano M, Yamada H; α-Tocopherol enhances the hypocholesterolemic action of sesamin in rats, *Int J Vitamin Nutr Res* **65**(3), 162-68 (1995)].

Supplementation of palm olein triglycerides (POTG), isolated from commercial palm olein, with 72 ppm of tocopherols raised the serum total cholesterol, LDL-and HDL-cholesterol levels and lowered the serum triglyceride level as compared to that of the POTG when tested on male Syrian Golden hamsters. Supplementation of POTG with 162 ppm of tocatrienols lowered the serum total cholesterol level significantly, but did not significantly lower the levels of LDL-and HDL-cholesterol and serum triglyceride as compared with the POTG group. Hypocholesterolemic effect of tocotrienols and mild hypercholesterolemic effect of tocopherols in hamsters were indicated by the experiment. Supplementation with high level of tocotrienols did not increase the hypocholesterolemic effect of the tocotrienols. [Khor HT, Chieng DY; Effect of dietary supplementation of tocotrienols and tocopherols on serum lipids in the hamster, *Nutr Res* **16**(8), 1393-401 (1996)].

γ-Tocotrienol, a naturally occurring analog of tocopherol, has been shown to have a hypocholesterolemic effect in animals and humans. Unlike tocopherol, it has also been shown to reduce plasma apoB levels in hypercholesterolemic subjects. The mechanism of action of γ-tocotrienol on hepatic modulation of apoB production was studied using cultured HepG2 cells as the model system. The results of the study suggest that γ-tocotrienol stimulates apoB degradation possibly as the result of decreased apoB translocation into the endoplasmic reticulum lumen. It is speculated that the lack of cholesterol availability reduces the number of secreted apoB-containing lipoprotein particles by limiting translocation of apoB into the endoplasmic reticulum lumen. [Theriault A, Wang Qi, Gapor A, Adeli K; Effects of *gamma*- Tocotrienol on apoB synthesis, degradation, and secretion in HepG2 cells, *Arterioscler Thromb Vasc Biol* **19**(3), 704-12 (1999)].

In the vitamin E group, α-tocopherol is considered to be the most active antioxidant but recent research has suggested tocotrienol to be a better antioxidant. Moreover, tocotrienol has been shown to possess novel hypocholesterolemic effects together with an ability to reduce the atherogenic apolipoprotein B. In addition, tocotrienol has been suggested to have an anti-thrombotic activity, which makes it an effective agent in the prevention and/or treatment of cardiovascular diseases. The physiological activities of tocotrienol suggest it to be superior to α-tocopherol in many situations. [Theriault A, Chao JT, Wang Qi, Gapor A, Adeli K; Tocotrienol: A review of its therapeutic potential, *Clin Biochem* **32**(5), 309-19 (1999)].

Effects of administration of α-tocopherol and tocotrienols on serum lipids and liver HMG CoA reductase activity have been studied. The results of the investigation indicate that the α-tocopherol is hypercholesterolemic in the hamster and its effect on liver HMG CoA reductase is dose-dependent. Tocotrienols exhibited inhibitory effect on liver HMG CoA reductase and α-tocopherol attenuated the inhibitory effect of tocotrienols on liver HMG CoA reductase. [Khor HT, Ng TT; Effects of administration of α-tocopherol and tocotrienols on serum lipids and liver HMG CoA reductase activity, *Int J Food Sci Nutr* **51**(supplement), S3-S11 (2000)].

Tocotrienols are known to exhibit hypocholesterolemic, antioxidant and other activities that might interfere with the formation of atherosclerotic placques. A comparison of the effects of α-tocopherol, the tocotrienol-rich fraction (TRF25) and didesmethyl tocotrienol (d-P25-T3) of rice bran was made on the pathogenesis of atherosclerotic lesions in C57BL/6 apolipoprotein (apo)E-deficient mice, which are excellent model because they become hyperlipidemic even when they consume a low fat diet and they develop complex atherosclerotic lesions similar to those of humans. A significant reduction in the size of atherosclerotic lesion was observed in all three genotypes of apoE mice fed a novel tocotrienol (d-P25-T3) of rice bran. Tocotrienols were superior in efficacy in compaison to α-tocopherol. Dietary tocotrienol supplements may provide a unique approach in promoting cardiovascular health. [Qureshi AA, Salser WA, Parmar R, Emeson EE; Novel tocotrienols of rice bran inhibit atherosclerotic lesions in C57BL/6 apoE-deficient mice, *J Nutr* **131**(10), 2606- 18 (2001)].

Both tocotrienols and lovastatin (a fungal product) exert hypocholesterolemic action in humans and animals by suppressing the activity of β-hydroxy- β- methylglutaryl coenzyme A reductase through different mechanisms, post- transcriptional vs competitive inhibition. A human study with 28 hypercholesterolemic subjects indicates the synergistic effect of these two agents without any side effect. [Qureshi AA, Sami SA, Salser WA, KhanFA; Synergistic effect of tocotrienol-rich fraction (TRF25) of rice bran and lovastatin on lipid parameters in hypercholesterolemic humans, *J Nutr Biochem* **12**(6), 318-29 (2001)].

Both lovastatin and α tocotrienol rich fraction {TRF25, a mixture of tocols isolated from stabilised and heated rice bran containing desmethyl (d-P21-T3) and didesmethyl (d-P25-T3) tocotrienols} are potent hypocholesterolemic agents, although they suppress cholesterol biosynthesis by different mechanisms. The additive and/or synergistic effects of both agents were determined on chickens. The mixture of TRF25 + lovastatin inhibited the activity of HMG CoA reductase compared to lovastatin alone reflecting possible additive pharmacological actions. Combinations of d-P25-T3 with lovastatin were found most effective in reducing serum total cholesterol and low density lipoprotein (LDL)-cholesterol compared to the control diet or individual supplements. However, the effects of d-P25- T3/lovastatin combination were no greater than that of d-P25-T3 alone, possibly indicating that d-P25-T3 produced a maximum cholesterol lowering effect at the concentration used. [Qureshi AA; Peterson DM; The combined effects of novel tocotrienols and lovastatin on lipid metabolism in chickens, *Atherosclerosis* **156**(1), 39-47 (2001)].

Tocotrienols, a lesser-known member of the vitamin E family, have increasingly received global attention. Structurally, the only difference between tocotrienols and tocopherols is that the former possess three double bonds in the isoprenoid side chain. Recent findings have found that tocotrienols possess superior pharmacological properties as compared with tocopherols including antioxidant, anticancer, hypocholesterolemic, antithrombotic and neuroprotective properties. Several theories on the mechanism of action of tocotrienols with respect to antioxidant, hypocholesterolemic and anti-cancer activities have been postulated. Tocotrienols are concluded to have great potential for the prevention and/or treatment of cardiovascular disease, cancer and neuro-degenerative disease. The pharmacological properties and potential mechanism(s) of action of palm tocotrienols have been reviewed. [Lean TNg, Leong WH, Ho D; The pharmacological properties of palm tocotrienols, *Chinese Pharm J* (Taipei) **54**(2), 63-75 (2002)].

TRITERPENOIDS: In experimentally induced hypercholesterolemic animals betulin glycoside (incorporated in lecithin liposomes) was found to potentiate the effect of liposomal drugs by decreaseing the blood cholesterol levels. [Ivanov AA, Zakharova TS, Odinokova LE, Uvarova NI; Hypolipidemic properties of Betulin glycosides, *Khim Farma Zh* **29**(9), 1091-94 (1987)].

In normal and experimentally induced hyperlipidemic animals, single administration of yuccagenin bisrhamnoside in the doses of 10, 25, 50 and 75 mg/kg significantly lowered the serum cholesterol and triglyceride levels. [Pal'yants N Sh, Khusbaktova ZA, Pshenichnov EA, Syrov VN, Karimov AK; Synthesis and biological activity of yuccagenin bisrhamnoside, *Khim Prir Soedin* No 3, 242-43 (2000); Translated in *Chem Nat Comp* **36**(3), 299-301 (2000)].

The antihyperlipidemic, antioxidant, antihypertensive and hypoglycemic activities of oleanolic acid and ursolic acid were studied in Dahl salt sensitive (DSS) insulin resistant rat model. Both triterpenoids significantly lowered LDL-cholesterol, triglyceride and blood sugar levels in these animals. The triterpene acids also enhanced the activity of antioxidant enzymes (superoxide dismutase and glutathione peroxidase) to varying degrees. Administration of these triterpenoids (60mg/kg ip) for six weeks also prevented the development of severe hypertension. [Somova LO, Nadar A, Rammanan P, Shode FO; Cardiovascular, antihyperlipidemic and antioxidant effects of oleanolic and ursolic acids in experimental hypertension, *Phytomedicine* **10**(2-3), 115-21 (2003)].

INDEX